A Primer of Drug Action

A Primer of Drug Action

A Concise, Nontechnical Guide
to the Actions, Uses, and Side Effects
of Psychoactive Drugs

Sixth Edition

Robert M. Julien, M.D.

St. Vincent Hospital and Medical Center
Portland, Oregon

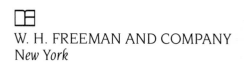
W. H. FREEMAN AND COMPANY
New York

Library Of Congress Cataloging-in-Publication Data

Julien, Robert M.
    A primer of drug action: a concise, nontechnical guide to the actions, uses, and side effects of psychoactive drugs / Robert M. Julien. — 6th ed.
      p.   cm.
    Includes bibliographical references and index.
    ISBN 0-7167-2260-7. — ISBN 0-7167-2261-5 (pbk.)
    1. Psychotropic drugs. 2. Psychopharmacology. I. Title.
    [DNLM: 1. Psychopharmacology. 2. Psychotropic drugs. QV 77 J94p]
    RM315.J75 1992
    615'.78—dc20
    DNLM/DLC
    for Library of Congress   91-16511
                                         CIP

Printed in the United States of America
2 3 4 5 6 7 8 9 0 VB 9 9 8 7 6 5 4 3 2

To my wife, Judi,
for her understanding and support

Contents

Preface

In this age of science and discovery, it seems strange that many of us know very little about our own bodies, especially about the responses of our bodies to drugs. Perhaps this is because we take drugs so casually, but perhaps it is also because those who are not trained in medical or biological science have neither sought nor received information about drugs that is scientifically correct yet comprehensive and relevant to their lives. The purpose of *A Primer of Drug Action* is to provide readers with concise, accurate, and timely information about psychoactive drugs, that is, those drugs that exert their primary effect on the brain, thus altering mood or behavior, or that are used in the treatment of mental disorders.

My overall premise is that psychoactive drugs all act in predictable fashions, understood by examining their mechanisms of action. Each drug has inherent benefits, uses, risks, side effects, toxicities, and societal consequences. My objective has been to describe this information about drugs in clear language, as free of technical jargon as possible, so that it can be easily understood by students and general readers with little background in the biological sciences.

Since 1975, when the first edition of *A Primer of Drug Action* was published, vast amounts of new information have become available about both the actions of these drugs and the brain processes underlying neuropsychological function. Accompanying this growth of knowledge have been frequent updates of this text, culminating now in this sixth edition. This latest edition reflects the most recent developments and describes in new detail the mechanisms of action of psychoactive drugs; their pharmacological effects, uses, limitations, and toxicities; and the current state of knowledge of the brain mechanisms involved in mental illness or dysfunction.

Public awareness of drug risks and toxicities has markedly increased during the last two decades. This awareness is evidenced by the proliferation of rehabilitation and treatment programs, the recognition of drug dependence as a medical problem, the willingness of insurance programs to pay for rehabilitation, the increased enforcement of drug laws, and the growing public intolerance of cigarette smoking, driving by alcohol-intoxicated persons, and other drug use.

Despite this increased awareness, there is much about drug use that is still distressing: every year, more than 450,000 people still fall victim to cigarette toxicities, alcohol burdens the lives of millions of people, cocaine use is seriously damaging an increasing number of users as well as their offspring, marijuana has become a part of our culture, experimentation with various psychedelic drugs continues, and drug use by minors continues to be a problem. Hence, the emphasis of *A Primer of Drug Action* remains focused on those drugs that primarily affect human thought and behavior as well as on the broader field of neuropsychopharmacology. This text can also be coupled with my companion text, *Drugs and the Body* (New York: W. H. Freeman and Company, 1988), to provide a comprehensive introduction to the wider science of pharmacology.

Features of the Sixth Edition

A Primer of Drug Action has become a classic text for courses in psychopharmacology and drug education. Now, in this sixth edition, I have completely revised and updated the entire book with the aim of making it the most current and understandable drug education text for the 1990s.

Two new chapters have been added to this edition (Chapter 5, "Benzodiazepines," and Chapter 7, "Caffeine and Nicotine"). These topics were included in earlier editions, but they are now given expanded discussion and emphasis. All other chapters have been revised to update and clarify the presentation of pharmacology, drug mechanisms, and the physiological basis of psychological disorders. In addition, I have reorganized the presentation to more clearly separate pharmacokinetics (how the body handles drugs) and pharmacodynamics (how drugs affect the body, including their mechanisms of action). References have been updated throughout; indeed, most are from the years 1989 and 1990. I have included discussions of both current and future directions in drug research (including new drugs that are, as of this date, on the horizon but not yet available), and I have added study questions at the end of each chapter. Much new material is included:

- The mechanisms of action of both psychoactive drugs and those drugs used in the treatment of neuropsychological illness

- The toxicities associated with the use and abuse of alcohol, cigarettes, caffeine, opioids, marijuana, oral contraceptives, and phencyclidine

- Psychoactive drugs as behavioral reinforcers and the role of such action in drug dependence

- The effects of psychoactive drugs on the fetus

- The neurochemical basis of anxiety and panic disorders, excessive alcohol ingestion, manic-depressive affective disorders, schizophrenia, dementia, attention-deficit hyperactivity disorder, parkinsonism, and both central and peripheral components of pain and analgesia

- New drugs, including
    serotonin-reuptake blocking antidepressants
    benzodiazepine antagonist
    atypical antidepressants
    selective MAO-A inhibitors
    newer opioid analgesics
    atypical antipsychotics
    new drugs for parkinsonism
    injectable analgesic–anti-inflammatory agents
    implantable female contraceptives
    injections for male contraception
    abortifacient

I hope that this expanded and rewritten text will continue to serve the needs of all those who desire a concise, clearly presented introduction to the field of neuropsychopharmacology.

Robert M. Julien
June 1991

Principles of Drug Action

HOW DRUGS ARE HANDLED BY THE BODY: PHARMACOKINETICS

A drug must be present in the body and in an adequate concentration (or amount) for it to act at its target site—the specific site in the body where it can exert its effect. Usually the time course of a particular drug's action simply reflects the amount of time required for the rise and fall of its concentration at the target site. Thus, most drugs that are ingested must somehow get from the external world into the bloodstream and, ultimately, to their target sites, where they can exert their effects. (A few drugs, which are classified as topical drugs, act on the skin, genitalia, or gastrointestinal tract; they do not actually enter the body. Topical drugs are not discussed in this text.)

Simple though this may sound, the process of transporting a drug from outside the body to its ultimate site of action is very complex. The action of any drug (that is taken by any means other than intravenous injection) depends on the *absorption* of that drug into the bloodstream, the *distribution* of the drug by the circulating blood to all regions of the

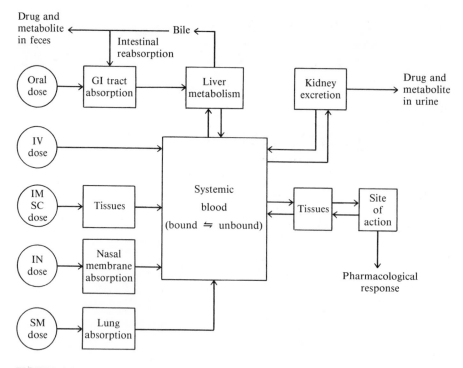

FIGURE 1.1

Schematic representation of the fate of a drug in the body. IV = intravenous; IN = intranasal; SM = smoked. [Adapted from C. N. Chiang and R. L. Hawks, "Implications of Drug Levels in Body Fluids: Basic Concepts," in R. L. Hawks and C. N. Chiang, eds., *Urine Testing for Drugs of Abuse*, NIDA Research Monograph No. 73 (Rockville, Md.: National Institute on Drug Abuse, 1986), p. 63.]

body, the tissue action of the drug itself, the eventual breakdown of the drug into an inactive compound, and, finally, the excretion of the drug (Figure 1.1). *Pharmacokinetics* is the term applied to that area of pharmacology in which the factors that influence the absorption, distribution, metabolism, and excretion of drugs are elucidated.[1,2] Thus, let us consider briefly the processes that are involved.

Drug Absorption

The term *drug absorption* refers to those mechanisms by which non-injected drugs pass from the point of entry into the bloodstream. When administering any drug, one must be able to select a *route* of administration, a *dose* of the drug, and a *dosage form* (liquid, tablet, capsule, or injection) that will place the drug at its site of action in a pharmacologically effective concentration and maintain that concentration for an adequate period of time.

Drugs are most commonly administered in one of five ways: *orally* (through the mouth), *rectally* (into the rectum), *parenterally* (by injection), by *inhalation* through the lungs, and by *absorption* through mucous membranes. Let us consider these methods of administration and absorption in more detail.

Oral Administration

Drugs are most commonly taken by mouth and swallowed. To be effective when administered orally, the drug must be soluble and stable in stomach fluid, be carried to the intestine, penetrate the lining of the intestine, and pass into the bloodstream. Indeed, the amount of drug that can be absorbed depends on its solubility (in stomach fluid) and permeability (through the lining of the intestine).

Because they are already in solution, drugs that are administered in liquid form tend to be absorbed more rapidly than those given in tablet or capsule form. Alcohol, for example, is taken in liquid form. As a result, about one-fourth to one-third of the alcohol that is ingested is absorbed directly from the stomach into the bloodstream. Thus, absorption is rapid and the effects of the alcohol may be felt very rapidly, especially if no food contents are present in the stomach. When a drug is taken in solid form, the rate at which it dissolves will limit its rate of absorption.

After a drug dissolves in the stomach, its subsequent absorption into the bloodstream begins with the passive transfer of that drug across the stomach or intestinal lining. This process occurs against a developing concentration gradient of drug at a rate that is determined by the ratio of water solubility to lipid solubility of the drug molecules. Indeed, once they are in in the body, drugs exist as a mixture of two interconvertible forms: one that is water-soluble (the ionized, or electrically charged, form) and one that is lipid soluble (the un-ionized, or uncharged, form). When the drug molecule is in the water-soluble form, it does not readily cross lipid membranes; in the lipid-soluble form, it can freely permeate the membrane.

The extent to which a drug is present in each form depends on the relative acidity (pH) of the fluid in which it is dissolved and on a characteristic of the drug molecule itself (its pK_a—the pH at which 50 percent of the drug is ionized).[*] Gastric juice is very acidic; intestinal contents are less acidic; and plasma (the noncellular component of blood) is slightly alkaline. As we have already stated, only lipid-soluble molecules diffuse readily across cell membranes—the level of lipid-soluble drug is the limiting factor that determines the passage of a drug across a lipid membrane.

If the pH is different on the two sides of a membrane (as, for example, between the stomach and the bloodstream), the ratio of water-soluble drug to lipid-soluble drug will also be different on the two sides of the membrane. At equilibrium, the concentration of the lipid-soluble drug will be equal on both sides of the membrane (because, as we have said, the lipid soluble form of the drug can freely permeate the membrane); but the *total* quantity of drug will be higher on the side where the ratio of water-soluble drug to lipid-soluble drug is greater (because the water-soluble drug molecules are unable to traverse the membrane). Thus, a drug is *absorbed* against its concentration gradient by passive transfer, without expenditure of the energy that would be necessary to maintain an active (energy-requiring) pump to move molecules against a concentration gradient.

Although oral administration of drugs is common, it does have disadvantages. First, it may lead to occasional vomiting and stomach distress. Second, although the amount of a drug that is put into a tablet or capsule can be calculated, how much of it will be absorbed into the bloodstream cannot always be predicted accurately because of unexplained differences between individuals and differences in the manufacturing of drugs. (Indeed, different brands of the same drug may be absorbed at widely differing rates.) Third, some drugs, such as the local anesthetics (Chapter 13) and insulin, when administered orally, are destroyed by the acid in the stomach before they are absorbed. To be effective, such drugs must be administered by injection.

Despite the disadvantages, in general, about 75 percent of an orally-administered drug will be absorbed by the body within about 1 to 3

---

[*]The ratio of lipid-soluble (un-ionized) drug to water-soluble (ionized) drug at each pH (and, therefore, in each body compartment) can be calculated from the Henderson-Hasselbalch equation:

$$pH = pK_a + \log\left(\frac{base}{acid}\right)$$

For drugs that are weak acids, the *acid* form of the drug is the un-ionized form; for drugs that are weak bases, the *base* form is un-ionized. The reader who is interested in a more in-depth discussion of this chemistry is referred to any of the several textbooks of pharmacology listed in the bibliography.

hours. Wide variance is allowed for multiple factors, including particle size, formulation, blood flow to the stomach, and so on.

Absorption through the Rectum

Although the primary route of drug administration is oral, some drugs are administered rectally (usually in suppository form) if the patient is vomiting, unconscious, or cannot swallow. However, absorption is often irregular, unpredictable, and incomplete; and many drugs irritate the membranes that line the rectum.

Absorption through the Lungs

Administration by inhalation is an increasingly used alternative to oral administration. Inhalation of drugs bypasses the problems and unpredictable factors that are associated with administration through the gastrointestinal tract. Drugs that are administered as gases or aerosols penetrate the cell linings of the respiratory tract easily and rapidly. Anesthetic gases (such as nitrous oxide or halothane) are composed of small molecules that are highly lipid-soluble. Therefore, those gases pass through the membranes of the lungs nearly as fast as they are inhaled. They are absorbed promptly because of the close contact between the blood and the membranes of the lung. With very volatile substances (such as anesthetic gases), inhalation produces effects almost as fast as intravenous administration.

Despite our knowledge about the rapid absorption of gases, very little is known about the pulmonary absorption of other, nongaseous drugs. Such drugs are administered as very small particles that are carried in a gas or smoke. Cigarette smoke and marijuana smoke are examples, because the active ingredients in each are not gases but, rather, particles that are carried in the smoke. Although many drugs *appear* to be absorbed readily when they are inhaled as sprays, aerosols, smoke, or dust, knowledge about the extent and rate of their absorption is incomplete. However, from hundreds of years of experience with nicotine, opium, and marijuana, it is clear that inhalation is an effective mode of administration.

It is also well known that inhalation of substances that are not volatile, such as tars, which are abundant in inhaled cigarette smoke, can injure the sensitive tissues of the lung. Lung cancer, which can be induced by long-term inhalation of cigarette smoke, is thought to be fatal in more than 90 percent of cases and is estimated to result in more than 75,000 deaths a year in the United States. It is not yet clear what undesirable effects will be produced by long-term inhalation of smoke obtained from marijuana.

Absorption through the Mucous Membranes

Occasionally, drugs are administered through the *mucous membranes of the mouth or nose.* Examples of those drugs include nasal decongestants, nitroglycerin, cocaine, and nicotine-containing snuff or gum. A heart patient taking nitroglycerin, for instance, places the tablet under the tongue and the drug is absorbed into the bloodstream directly from the mouth. Cocaine powder, when sniffed, is absorbed through the nose, because the powdered drug adheres to the membranes on the inside of the nose and is absorbed directly into the bloodstream. Nasal decongestants are sprayed directly onto mucous membranes. Nicotine that is contained in snuff or gum (for example, Nicorette) is applied to the buccal membranes and is absorbed directly into the bloodstream.

Absorption by Injection

Administration of drugs by injection can be *intravenous* (directly into a vein), *intramuscular* (directly into a muscle), or *subcutaneous* (just under the skin). Each of these routes of administration has its advantages and disadvantages (Table 1.1), but some features are shared by all. In general, administration by injection produces a more prompt response than is obtainable by oral administration, because absorption is more rapid after injection. Also, a more accurate dose is attained by injection, because the unpredictable processes of absorption are bypassed.

Administration of drugs by injection, however, has several drawbacks. First, because of the rapid rate of absorption (the absorption processes through the stomach and intestine are bypassed), there is often little time to respond to an unexpected drug reaction or accidental overdose. Second, administration by injection requires the use of sterile techniques. The ongoing AIDS crisis is a vivid example of the drastic consequences that can occur as a result of unsterile injection techniques. Third, once a drug is administered, it cannot be recalled.

INTRAVENOUS ADMINISTRATION   In an intravenous injection, a drug is introduced directly into the bloodstream. This technique avoids all the variables related to oral absorption, so the drug arrives in the circula-

TABLE 1.1

Some characteristics of drug adminsitration by injection.

Route	Absorption pattern	Special utility	Limitations and precautions
Intravenous	Absorption circumvented Potentially immediate effects	Valuable for emergency use Permits titration of dosage Suitable for large volumes and for irritating substances when diluted	Increased risk of adverse effects Must inject solutions *slowly* as a rule Not suitable for oily solutions or insoluble substances
Subcutaneous	Prompt, from aqueous solution Slow and sustained from repository preparations	Suitable for some insoluble suspensions and for implantation of solid pellets	Not suitable for large volumes Possible pain or necrosis from irritating substances
Intramuscular	Prompt, from aqueous solution Slow and sustained from repository preparations	Suitable for moderate volumes, oily vehicles, and some irritating substances	Precluded during anticoagulant medicine May interfere with interpretation of certain diagnostic tests (e.g., creatine phosphokinase)

Modified from L. Z. Benet, J. R. Mitchell, and L. B. Sheiner,[1] p. 6.

tion with minimum delay. In addition, the dose of the drug can be controlled. The injection can be made slowly and it can be stopped instantaneously if untoward effects develop. Finally, the intravenous route permits great accuracy in dosage, and it enables the practitioner to dilute and administer in large volumes drugs that would at higher concentration be irritants to the muscles or blood vessels.

The intravenous route has several important drawbacks, however. First, it is the most dangerous of all routes of administration, because it has the fastest speed of onset of pharmacological action. Second, a normally safe dose may be given too rapidly, causing catastrophic, life-threatening effects (such as collapse of respiration or of heart function). Third, allergic reactions to a drug may be mild when it is administered orally, but they may be extremely severe when the same drug is administered intravenously. Fourth, drugs that are not soluble in the blood or drugs that are dissolved in oily liquids may not be given intravenously because of the danger of blood clots forming. Finally, infection by bacterial contaminants is a continual danger, and infectious diseases or abscesses may be induced when sterile techniques are not employed.

INTRAMUSCULAR ADMINISTRATION   Drugs that are injected into skeletal muscle (usually in the arm, thigh, or buttock) are generally absorbed fairly rapidly. Absorption of a drug from muscle is more rapid than absorption of the same drug from the stomach, but it is slower than when the drug is administered intravenously. The absolute rate of absorption of a drug from muscle is variable, depending on the rate of the blood flow to that muscle, the solubility of the drug, and the volume of the injection.

In general, most of the precautions that apply to intravenous administration also apply to intramuscular injection. However, drugs that are intended for intramuscular administration should not be given intravenously as a rule, and one must be careful to avoid hitting a blood vessel when inserting a needle into muscle. Such an accident would result in an inadvertent intravenous injection.

SUBCUTANEOUS ADMINISTRATION   Absorption of drugs that have been injected under the skin (subcutaneously) is quite rapid. The exact rate depends mainly on the ease of blood-vessel penetration and the rate of blood flow through the skin. Irritating drugs should not be injected subcutaneously because they may cause severe pain and local tissue damage. The usual precautions to maintain sterility apply.

Self-administration of any drug by injection is to be discouraged except in certain circumstances (such as the injection of insulin by a diabetic) when oral administration is not effective or when the drug is being taken therapeutically under the direction of a physician. The risks associated with injection of a drug (infection, overdose, allergic responses, AIDS, and so forth) are far greater than those associated with the oral administration of the same drug.

Distribution of Drugs throughout the Body

Once it is absorbed into the bloodstream, a drug is distributed throughout the body by the circulating blood. However, even after the drug reaches the bloodstream, it must still pass across various barriers to reach its site of action. At any given time, only a very small portion of the total amount of a drug that is in the body reaches the specific target sites (*receptors*) that produce its pharmacological action. Most of the total amount of administered drug is found in areas of the body that are remote from the drug's site of action. In the case of psychoactive drugs (drugs that alter mood or behavior as a result of their effect on the central nervous system [CNS]), most of the drug is circulating outside of the brain and, therefore, does not contribute directly to its pharmacological effect. Indeed, this wide distribution often accounts for many of the side effects of a drug. *Side effects* are those actions that are different from the primary, or therapeutic, effect for which a drug is taken.

Most discussions about psychoactive drugs are focused solely on the amount of a drug that actively produces a pharmacological and a psychological action in the brain. Yet it is the total amount of a drug in the body that (1) governs the movements of that drug through the tissues and its ultimate elimination, (2) determines both the duration and the intensity of the drug's effect, and (3) underlies many of the drug's side effects.

Distribution of Drugs by Blood

Each minute the heart pumps approximately 5 liters (1 liter = 2.1 pints) of blood. Because the total amount of blood in the circulatory system equals about 6 liters, the entire blood volume circulates in the body about once every minute. Once a drug is absorbed into the bloodstream, it is quite rapidly (usually within this one-minute circulation time) distributed throughout the circulatory system.

A schematic diagram of the circulatory system is presented in Figure 1.2. Blood returning to the heart through the veins is first pumped into the pulmonary (lung) circulation system, where carbon dioxide is removed and replaced by oxygen. The oxygenated blood then returns to the heart and is pumped into the great artery (the aorta). From there, blood flows into the smaller arteries and finally into the capillaries, where nutrients (and drugs) are exchanged between the blood and the cells of the body.

To perform this exchange, the body has an estimated 10 billion capillaries, which have a total surface area of more than 200 square meters. Probably no single functioning cell of the body is more than 20 to 30 micrometers away from a capillary (1 micrometer = 0.0004 inch). (A discussion of the structure and function of capillaries follows.) After the blood passes through the capillaries, it is collected by the veins and returned to the heart to circulate again.

Thus, drugs are fairly evenly distributed throughout the bloodstream. A normal, lean, 150-pound man contains approximately 41 liters of water (60 percent of the total body weight). Therefore, 41 liters represents the total amount of water in his body; 6 liters represents the

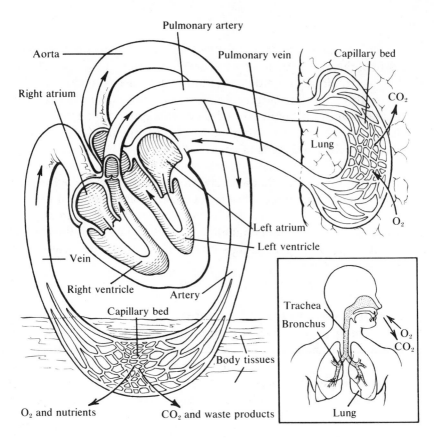

FIGURE 1.2

The heart and circulatory system. Blood returning from the body tissues to the heart via the veins passes through the right atrium into the right ventricle and, with the contraction of the heart, is pumped into the arteries leading to the lungs. In the lungs, carbon dioxide (CO_2) is lost and replaced by oxygen (O_2). This oxygenated blood returns to the heart through the left atrium, is pumped out of the left ventricle into the aorta, and is carried to the body tissues, where oxygen and nutrients are exchanged in the capillary beds. Oxygen and nutrients are supplied to the body tissues through the walls of the capillaries; CO_2 and other waste products are returned to the blood. The CO_2 is eliminated through the lungs, and the other waste products are excreted through the kidneys.

volume of the water in his circulating blood; and 35 liters represents the amount of water in his body tissues. However, that 35 liters of water is not isolated from his blood, because fluids (and most drugs) are freely exchanged, or equilibrated, between the blood, other body fluids, and most cells of the body. Thus, drugs are diluted not only by the blood but also by the total amount of water that is contained in the body.

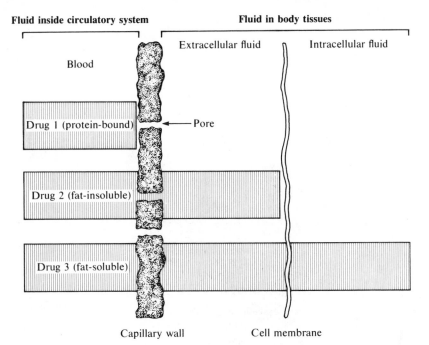

Fluid inside circulatory system

Fluid in body tissues

Extracellular fluid

Intracellular fluid

Blood

Drug 1 (protein-bound)

←— Pore

Drug 2 (fat-insoluble)

Drug 3 (fat-soluble)

Capillary wall

Cell membrane

FIGURE 1.3

Distribution of three hypothetical drugs into different body compartments. Drug 1 is bound to blood proteins; *drug* 2 is unbound, soluble in water but insoluble in fat; *drug* 3 is unbound and soluble in both water and fat. Note that *drug* 1 is largely restricted to the bloodstream; *drug* 2 is distributed in the blood and in the fluid outside the body cells; and *drug* 3 is distributed through all the body compartments and readily passes into the brain, easily crossing the blood-brain barrier.

In addition to solubility, there is another factor that often limits the distribution of a drug in the body. Large amounts of many drugs may actually bind reversibly to proteins that are contained in the blood plasma. Protein-bound drug exists in equilibrium with free (unbound) drug, as shown in Figure 1.1. Because plasma proteins (albumin, for example) are quite large and thus unable to leave the bloodstream, the proportion of drug that is bound to plasma proteins remains confined within the blood vessels. This obviously limits drug distribution.

The unequal distribution of three drugs in the different body compartments is illustrated in Figure 1.3. After absorption from the stomach into the bloodstream, drug 1 becomes almost completely protein-bound and is largely confined to the bloodstream. Drug 2 does not bind to blood proteins and passes easily out of the bloodstream into tissue

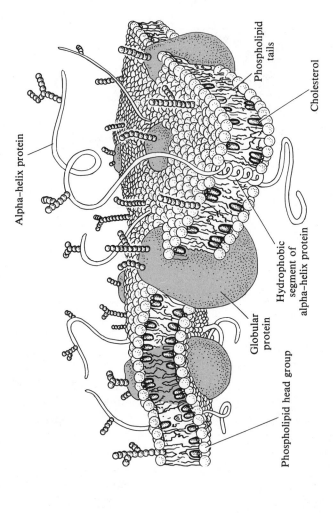

Alpha-helix protein

Phospholipid tails

Cholesterol

Hydrophobic segment of alpha-helix protein

Globular protein

Phospholipid head group

FIGURE 1.4

A diagrammatic representation of the cell membrane: a phospholipid bilayer in which cholesterol and protein molecules are embedded. Both globular and helical kinds of protein traverse the bilayer. Cholesterol molecules tend to keep the tails of the phospholipids relatively fixed and orderly in the regions closest to the hydrophilic phospholipid heads; the parts of the tails closer to the core of the membrane move about freely. [From M. S. Bretscher, "The Molecules of the Cell Membrane," *Scientific American* 253 (1985): 104.]

fluid, but it is unable to pass into cells and, therefore, does not have access to the fluid inside them. Drug 3 is a compound that passes easily from the bloodstream and readily penetrates cell membranes into the fluid inside the cell. An example of this last drug is thiopental (Pentothal), a commonly used anesthetic that induces anesthesia within a matter of seconds after i.v. injection. Thiopental is extremely soluble in the fat of cell membranes, so it can leave the bloodstream rapidly and pass into brain cells, where it quickly depresses the brain and abolishes consciousness.

Body Membranes That Affect Drug Distribution

The absorption and distribution of drugs are affected by various types of membranes in the body. The four types of membranes most pertinent to this discussion are those of (1) the cell, (2) the walls of the capillary vessels in the circulatory system, (3) the blood-brain barrier, and (4) the placental barrier. Let us consider each of these.

CELL MEMBRANES   To be absorbed from the intestine or to gain access to the interior of a cell, a drug must penetrate the cell membranes. What, then, is known of the structure and properties of such membranes that determine their permeability to drugs? The generalized picture that has emerged from chemical, physiological, and electron micrograph studies is represented in Figure 1.4. In this figure, the two layers of circles represent the water-soluble head groups of complex lipid molecules called *phospholipids*. These phospholipid heads form a rather continuous layer on both the inside and the outside of the cell membrane. The wavy lines that extend from the heads into the central core of the membrane are the lipid chains of the phospholipid molecules. Therefore, for our present purposes, the interior of the cell membrane can be considered to consist of a sea of liquid lipid in which large proteins are suspended. This structure has been named the *fluid mosaic model*.

Notice in Figure 1.4 that several large globules and spiral strands appear to be situated on the outer layer of the membrane and extend either into or, in some cases, through the three layers of the membrane. These globules and spirals represent protein structures. The total thickness of this membrane is about 80 angstroms. (The angstrom, which is abbreviated Å, is equal to 0.0001 micrometer, or 0.00000004 inch.) This membrane, consisting of protein and fat, provides a barrier that is permeable to many drug molecules but impermeable to others. Using this model, it is not surprising to find that the penetration of a drug molecule through the membrane, and thus into a cell, is determined by the solubility of that drug in oil (since oil is a fat, and the core of this membrane consists of fat molecules). In addition to this layered structure of protein and fat, the membrane also appears to contain small pores (about 8 Å in diameter) that permit the passage of small water-soluble molecules, such as alcohol and water.

These cellular membranes (as barriers to the absorption and distribution of drugs) are important for the passage of drugs (1) from the stomach and intestine into the bloodstream, (2) from the fluid that closely surrounds tissue cells into the interior of cells, (3) from the interior of cells back into the body water, and (4) from the kidneys back into the bloodstream. Because most drugs are too large to penetrate the small pores, most water-soluble, fat-insoluble drugs cannot pass through the cellular barriers.

BLOOD CAPILLARIES   As we have already discussed, drug molecules are distributed throughout the body by means of the circulating blood. Within a minute or so after a drug enters the bloodstream, it is distributed fairly evenly throughout the entire blood volume. However, most drugs are not confined to the bloodstream, because they are exchanged back and forth between blood capillaries and tissues.

Figure 1.5 is a cross-sectional diagram of a capillary. Capillaries are tiny cylindrical blood vessels that have walls formed by a thin, unicellular layer of cells packed tightly together. Between the cells are small passageways (pores) that connect the interior of the vessel (the capillary) with the exterior (the body tissues). These pores have a diameter that is between 90 and 150 Å, and they are larger than most drug molecules. Because it is only in the capillaries that drugs are exchanged between the blood and the body cells, the capillaries must be small (to bring water and essential body nutrients into close contact with the surrounding cells) and numerous (10 billion, it has been estimated).

Because most drug molecules are smaller than the pores, drugs are able to pass out of the capillaries and into the surrounding tissue with little difficulty. As a result, most drugs reach the cells of most body tissues within a fairly short period of time, limited, primarily, by the rate of blood flow to the tissue. Therefore, in the transport of drug molecules out of blood capillaries and into tissues (and, conversely, from tissues back into the blood through the capillaries), it does not matter whether a drug is soluble in fat, because the membrane pores are large enough for even fat-insoluble drug molecules to

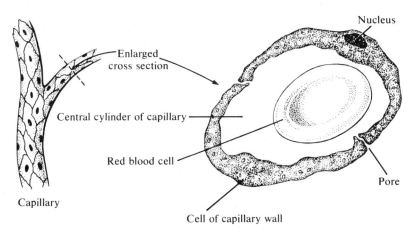

Nucleus

Enlarged
cross section

Central cylinder of capillary

Red blood cell

Pore

Capillary

Cell of capillary wall

FIGURE 1.5

Cross section of a blood capillary. Within the capillary are the fluids, proteins, and cells of the blood, including the red blood cells. The capillary itself is made up of cells that completely surround and define the central cylinder (or lumen) of the capillary. Water-filled pores form channels, allowing communication between the lumen and the fluid outside the capillaries.

penetrate. These drug molecules traverse the capillary pores at a rate that is roughly proportional to the difference in concentration of the drug on either side of the capillary membrane; that is, the higher the concentration of the drug in the blood and the lower the concentration in the tissues, the faster the drug will diffuse out of the capillaries and into the tissues.

The pores in the capillary membrane are not large enough to permit the red blood cells and the plasma proteins to leave the bloodstream. Thus, the only drugs that do not readily penetrate capillary pores are those rare drugs that are composed of proteins and those that bind to plasma proteins. Significant amounts of many drugs may reversibly bind to plamsa proteins and, when bound, do not readily diffuse across capillary membranes. Thus, protein-bound drug will essentially become trapped in the bloodstream and will not diffuse into the tissues. If a drug is capable of leaving the capillaries readily, its concentration in the blood will decline extremely rapidly, and the action of that drug might have both a rapid onset and a short duration.

The rate at which drug molecules enter specific body tissues depends on two factors: the rate of blood flow through the tissue and the ease with which drug molecules pass through the capillary membranes. Because blood flow is greatest to the brain and much poorer to the bones, joints, and fat deposits, drug distribution—everything else being equal—should follow a similar pattern. However, some capillaries (such as those in the brain) have special structural properties that may further limit the diffusion of a drug into the brain.

THE BLOOD-BRAIN BARRIER   The brain requires a protected environment in which to function normally, and a specialized structural barrier, called the *blood-brain barrier,* plays a key role in maintaining it.[3] The blood-brain barrier involves specialized cells in the brain that affect nearly all its blood capillaries (see Figure 1.6). In most of the rest of the body, pores are present in the capillary membranes; in the brain, however, the capillaries are tightly joined together and covered on the

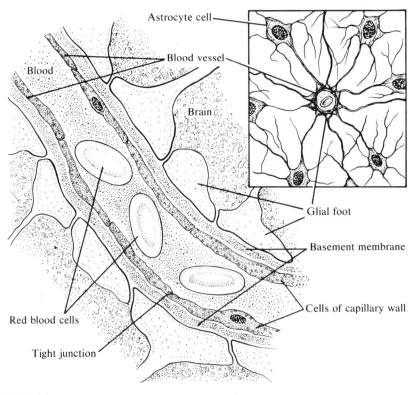

FIGURE 1.6

The blood-brain barrier. Blood and brain are separated both by capillary cells packed tightly together and by a fatty barrier called the *glial sheath,* which is made up of extensions (glial feet) from nearby astrocyte cells (*see inset*). A drug diffusing from the blood to the brain must move through the cells of the capillary wall because there are tight junctions rather than pores between the cells, and it must then move through the fatty glial sheath.

outside by a fatty barrier called the glial sheath, that arises from nearby astrocyte cells.

Thus, a drug leaving the capillaries in the brain has to traverse both the wall of the capillary itself (because there are no pores to pass through) and the membranes of the astrocyte cells in order to reach the cells in the brain. In general, the rate of passage of a drug into the brain is determined by the cerebral blood flow (which is usually quite constant) and the lipid (fat) solubility of the drug (which varies from drug to drug). Highly ionized drugs (penicillin, for example) penetrate poorly, while fat-soluble drugs penetrate rapidly. This decreased permeability of the capillaries in the brain to some substances is frequently described by the term blood-brain barrier, which is used very commonly to distinguish drugs that can penetrate the brain from those that cannot. By definition, drugs that are psychoactive (the drugs discussed in this book) are quite lipid-soluble, since they exert their actions only after crossing the blood-brain barrier in order to reach their target sites in the brain. Drugs whose action is predominantly outside the CNS (vitamins, antibiotics, heart medications, and so on) are usually more highly ionized (less lipid-soluble) and, therefore, CNS actions are not usually a major part of their pharmacology.

THE PLACENTAL BARRIER   Among all the membrane systems of the body, the placenta is unique. It separates two distinct human beings with differing genetic compositions, physiological responses, and sensitivities to drugs. The fetus obtains essential nutrients and eliminates metabolic waste products through the placenta without depending on its own organs, many of which are not yet functioning. This dependence of the fetus on the mother, however, places the fetus at the mercy of the placenta when foreign substances (such as drugs) appear in the mother's blood.

Pregnant women in the United States regularly take both prescription and nonprescription drugs, and they have an undetermined exposure to potentially toxic substances in food, cosmetics, household chemicals, and the general environment. The extent to which these latter substances affect the fetus is not yet known. The consequences of maternal alcohol ingestion and cigarette smoking on fetal growth and development are now well documented and will be discussed in Chapters 4 and 7. The explosive increase in cocaine use has resulted in severe effects on the developing fetus (Chapter 6).

The effects of drugs on the fetus fall into two major categories. First, early in pregnancy, when the limbs and organ systems are forming, drugs   may   induce   structural   abnormalities   (teratogenesis).

Thalidomide was the most dramatic example of a teratogenic compound. This tranquilizer was marketed in several countries during the early 1960s, and, when given to women in the fifth through seventh weeks of pregnancy, produced a high incidence of abnormal limb growth in their fetuses. Second, later in pregnancy and during delivery, drugs may induce respiratory depression in the newborn baby because the baby is unable to metabolize or excrete them.

Schematic representations of the placental network, which transfers substances between the mother and the fetus, are shown in Figures 1.7 and 1.8. In general, the mature placenta consists of a network of vessels and pools of maternal blood, into which protrude tree-like or finger-like villi (projections), which contain the blood capillaries of the fetus (Figure 1.8). Oxygen and nutrients travel from the mother's blood to that of the fetus, while carbon dioxide and other waste products travel from the fetus to the mother's blood.

The membranes that separate fetal blood from maternal blood in

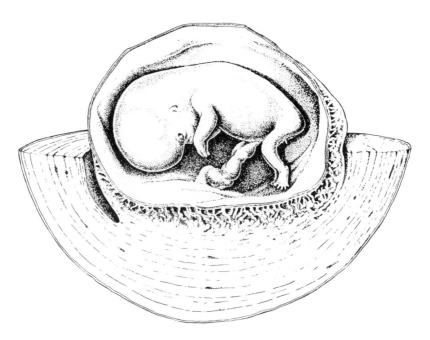

FIGURE 1.7

Placenta, embryo, and section through part of a uterus. [Redrawn from W. J. Hamilton, J. D. Boyd, and H. W. Mossman, *Human Embryology: Prenatal Developmant of Form and Function* (Baltimore: Williams & Wilkins, 1962), fig. 86, p. 85. Courtesy of Professors Hamilton, Boyd, and Mossman and Mr. Heffer.]

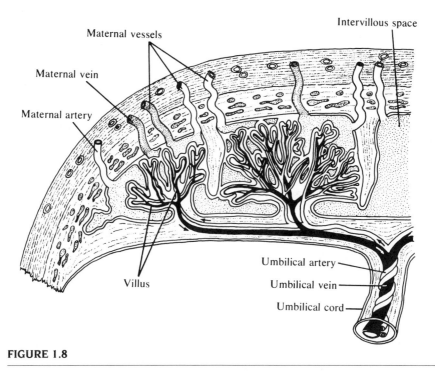

Maternal vessels

Intervillous space

Maternal vein

Maternal artery

Villus

Umbilical artery

Umbilical vein

Umbilical cord

FIGURE 1.8

Placental network separating the blood of mother and fetus. [From C. M. Goss, ed., *Gray's Anatomy of the Human Body*, 29th ed. (Philadelphia: Lea and Febiger, 1973), fig. 2.51, p. 40.]

the intervillous space resemble, in their general permeability, the cell membranes that are found elsewhere in the body. In other words, drugs cross the placenta primarily by passive diffusion. Fat-soluble substances diffuse across readily, while fat-insoluble substances diffuse less well. This pattern is of interest, because late in pregnancy and at the time of delivery most anesthetic liquids and gases and most pain-relieving agents penetrate both the blood-brain barrier and the placenta very readily.

Anesthetics and narcotic analgesics may be found in fairly high concentrations in the newborn infant. There are numerous instances of withdrawal symptoms in infants born of addicted mothers, proving that morphine and other narcotics have free access to, and will affect, the fetus during pregnancy. Tranquilizing and sedating drugs also cross the placenta quite readily. The blood levels of a barbiturate administered intravenously to mothers during labor are plotted in Figure 1.9. The blood concentrations of the drug were determined in both

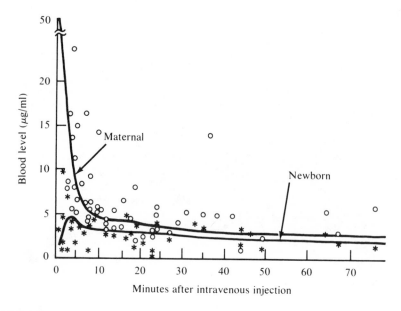

FIGURE 1.9

Effect of barbiturate on mothers in labor. Blood levels of secobarbital in mothers and their newborn infants after intravenous administration of the drug to the mothers . Each point represents one subject (*circles*, mothers; *asterisks*, infants). [From B. Root, E. Eichner, and I. Sunshine, "Blood Secobarbital Levels and Their Clinical Correlation in Mothers and Newborn Infants," *American Journal of Obstetrics and Gynecology* 81 (1961): 948.]

maternal and fetal blood. One can see from this figure that significant amounts of the barbiturate are distributed to the infant and that blood levels in the mother and the newborn baby are almost identical about 10 minutes after injection.

The view that the placenta is a barrier to psychoactive drugs is inaccurate. A more appropriate statement is that the fetus is exposed to any and all psychoactive drugs taken by the mother, with fetal levels of drug approximating those achieved in the mother.

Termination of Drug Action

The main routes through which drugs leave the body are (1) the kidneys, (2) the lungs, and (3) the bile. Excretion through the lungs occurs only with highly volatile or gaseous agents such as inhalation anesthetics (for example, ether and isoflurane) and, in small amounts, alcohol ("alcohol breath"). Excretion through the bile is also unusual, because drugs that are passed through the bile and into the intestine are usually reabsorbed back into the bloodstream from the intestine. Thus, the majority of drugs leave the body in urine.

In general, the same lipid-soluble properties of psychoactive drugs that facilitate rapid transport across cellular membranes into the brain also impair their subsequent excretion by the kidneys. Such impairment is discussed in the following section; it necessitates the metabolic transformation of the drug (by enzymes located in the liver) into a form that may be excreted more rapidly and reliably. Such biotransformation relieves the body of the burden of foreign chemicals and is essential for our survival.[1]

Elimination of Drugs by the Kidneys and Liver

Physiologically, our kidneys perform two major functions. First, they excrete most of the products of body metabolism, and, second, they closely regulate the levels of most of the substances found in body fluids. The kidneys are a pair of bean-shaped organs (see Figure 1.10), each a little smaller than a fist and weighing about a quarter of a pound. They lie at the rear of the abdominal cavity at the level of the lower ribs.

The outer portion of the kidney is made up of some two million functional units, called *nephrons* (Figure 1.11). Each unit consists of a knot of capillaries (the glomerulus) through which blood flows from the

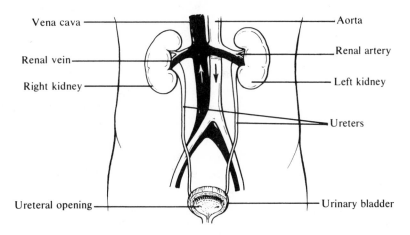

FIGURE 1.10

The architecture of the kidneys.

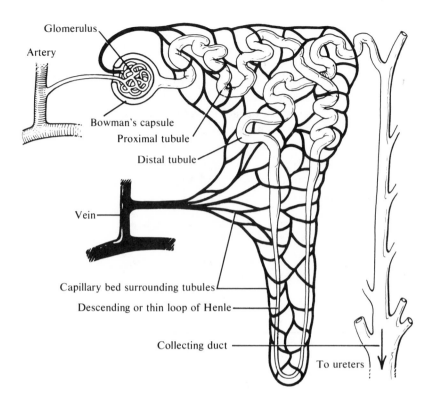

Glomerulus

Artery

Bowman's capsule

Proximal tubule

Distal tubule

Vein

Capillary bed surrounding tubules

Descending or thin loop of Henle

Collecting duct

To ureters

FIGURE 1.11

A nephron within a kidney. Note the complexity of the structure and the intimate relation between the blood supply and the nephron. Each kidney is composed of more than a million such nephrons.

renal artery to the renal vein. The glomerulus is surrounded by the opening of the nephron (Bowman's capsule), into which fluid flows as it filters out of the capillaries. Pressure of the blood in the glomerulus causes fluid to leave the capillaries and flow into Bowman's capsule, from which it flows through the tubules of the kidney and, finally, into a duct that collects fluid from several nephrons. This fluid from the collecting ducts is eventually passed through the ureters and into the urinary bladder, which is emptied periodically.

The basic function of the kidney is to maintain a proper internal environment and, in doing so, to rid the blood of unwanted substances as they pass through. Substances that must be excreted include the products of body metabolism, and the sodium, potassium, and chloride that accumulate in the body in excessive amounts. The kidney must also conserve water, sugar, and the necessary quantities of sodium, potassium, and chloride. The kidney rids the blood of unwanted substances and retains ingredients that are essential to the body in the following manner. First, a large portion of the blood, usually about one-fifth of it, is filtered into the tubules of the kidney. Left behind in the bloodstream are blood cells, plasma proteins, and a small amount of fluid. As the filtered fluid flows through the kidney tubules, the unwanted substances pass into the urinary bladder for excretion later. Substances to be conserved are reabsorbed from the kidney back into the bloodstream by passing through the wall of cells that line the tubules.

Because drugs are small particles that dissolve in the blood, they, too, are usually filtered into the kidneys and then reabsorbed back into the bloodstream. Water is reabsorbed from the tubules into the bloodstream to a much greater extent than are most drugs, so the drugs become more concentrated inside the nephrons than in the blood. Because substances tend to move from areas of high concentration to areas of low concentration, drugs move out of the kidney back into the bloodstream. Thus, the kidney, by itself, is simply not sufficient for the task of eliminating drugs from the body (at least within a reasonable timespan).

In order for the body to hasten the urinary excretion of a drug, it must prevent the drug from being reabsorbed back into the bloodstream from the kidney. The drug must be changed by metabolic processes in the body into a compound that is less fat-soluble and, therefore, less capable of being reabsorbed. This process, the conversion of fat-soluble drugs into water-soluble metabolites that can be excreted by the kidney, is carried out by specialized enzymes that are located in the liver (Figure 1.12).

Free drug (that is, not bound to plasma proteins) is carried to the liver (by the hepatic artery and portal vein) and a portion is "cleared" from the blood by the liver cells and biotransformed (metabolized) to by-products (metabolites), which are returned to the bloodstream (see Figure 1.12). These metabolites are then transported in the bloodstream to the kidneys for excretion.

Usually (but not always) this process of metabolism *decreases* the pharmacological activity of the drug. Thus, even though a metabolite might persist in the body (awaiting excretion), it would usually be in a pharmacologically inactive form, and it would not produce the effects of the parent drug.

The exact mechanisms in the liver that result in the chemical alteration of a drug's structure are beyond the scope of our discussion, but suffice it to state that the reactions are carried out by a special system of enzymes in the liver cells. Many psychoactive drugs have the ability to

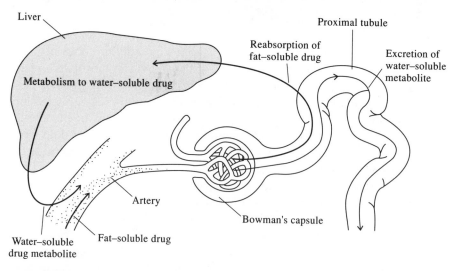

FIGURE 1.12

How liver and kidneys eliminate drugs from the body. Drugs may be filtered into the kidney, reabsorbed into the bloodstream, and carried to the liver for metabolic transformation to a more water-soluble compound that, having been filtered into the kidney, cannot be reabsorbed and is, therefore, excreted in urine.

increase the rate at which this enzyme system metabolizes a variety of such drugs, including themselves, thereby increasing the speed with which drugs are eliminated. Drugs induce an increase both in the enzyme activity of these cells and in the total amount of drug-metabolizing enzymes in the liver. This enzyme-induction process is one mechanism for producing pharmacological *tolerance,* so that increasing doses of a drug must be administered to produce the same effect that smaller doses produced earlier.

Because these enzymes have a low specificity for drugs (that is, one enzyme may metabolize many different types of drugs), an increase in the metabolizing enzymes induced by one drug will increase the enzymes' rate of metabolizing that particular drug as well as a variety of others. This process of cross-tolerance will be elaborated on later in this chapter.

Earlier, we discussed the processes of distribution of drugs from the mother to the fetus through the placenta. While the fetus is attached to the mother, those drugs may be excreted through the umbilical cord back into the mother's bloodstream. The mother can then eliminate the drug through her liver and kidneys. After delivery, however, the newborn baby must get rid of the drug by itself. Unfortunately, the newborn (especially the premature infant) has few drug-metabolizing enzymes in its liver, and its kidneys may not yet be fully functional. Therefore, the infant has great difficulty metabolizing and excreting drugs. If it has received a high concentration of depressants (anesthetics, narcotics, and so on) from the mother, the infant may be depressed for a long time after delivery.

Other Routes of Drug Elimination

As discussed earlier, certain drugs may be absorbed through the lungs, such as many anesthetics, nicotine from cigarettes, cannabinol from marijuana, and the narcotic agents in opium. Although they may be absorbed by this route, nicotine, cannabinol, and opiates are not excreted by the lungs. They are metabolized by the liver, and their metabolites are excreted in the urine in exactly the same way as for orally administered drugs.

Besides the kidneys, bile, and lungs, other possible routes for the excretion of drugs include sweat, saliva, and breast milk. Many drugs and drug metabolites may be found in these secretions; but their concentrations are usually quite low, and these routes are not usually considered to be among the primary paths of drug elimination. Occasionally, however, concern arises over the transfer of drugs (such as nicotine) from mothers to their breast-fed babies. Similarly, concern has been expressed about the secretion of antibiotics, administered to cows, into milk that is ultimately consumed by humans. These topics are of obvious importance to the pharmacologist and to the Food and Drug Administration, especially because guidelines for such uses of drugs are needed to minimize the possible danger to the public.

The Time Course of Drug Distribution and Elimination

The Concept of a Drug Half-Life

Knowledge about the relation between the *concentration* of a drug in the body and the *time* after its administration is essential for (1) predicting the optimal dosages and dose intervals needed to reach a therapeutic effect, (2) maintaining a therapeutic drug level for the desired period of time, and (3) determining the time needed to eliminate the drug. Indeed, it is a fundamental of pharmacology that there is a relationship between the pharmacological or toxic response to a drug and its concentration in a readily measurable site in the body (for example, blood), and, furthermore, that this level correlates with the level of drug at the receptor site that is responsible for the drug's action (Figure 1.1).

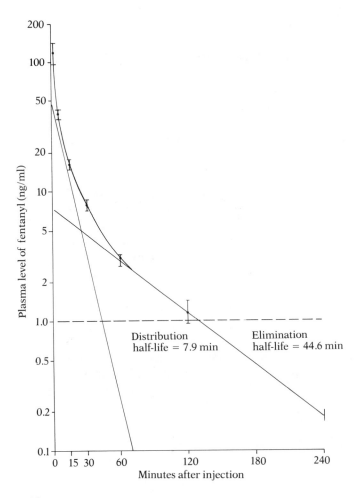

Distribution
half-life = 7.9 min

Elimination
half-life = 44.6 min

FIGURE 1.13

Plasma levels of a narcotic drug (fentanyl) injected intravenously into a rat in a single bolus dose of 50 micrograms per kilogram body weight. The distribution and elimination half-lives are shown as 7.9 and 44.6 minutes, respectively. The horizontal line drawn at 1 nanogram (billionths of a gram) per milliliter plasma concentration is the level needed for analgesic effect. Thus, analgesia would be lost about 130 minutes after drug injection. [Data from C. C. Hug, Jr., and M. R. Murphy, "Tissue Redistribution of Fentanyl and Termination of Its Effects in Rats," *Anesthesiology* 55 (1981):369–375.]

TABLE 1.2

Half-life calculations.

| Number of half-lives | Amount of drug in the body | |
	Percent eliminated	Percent remaining
0	0	100
1	50	50
2	75	25
3	87.5	12.5
4	93.8	6.2
5	96.9	3.1
6	98.4	1.6

Figure 1.13 illustrates this time-concentration relationship for a drug that was administered intravenously to a rat. Note that soon after injection, the drug concentration in plasma peaked and was followed by a rapid and then a slower fall in concentration. The rapid fall reflects distribution of the drug throughout the body after intravenous injection. The steep sloped line in Figure 1.13 (tangent line *A*) represents the blood-flow–independent, rapid distribution phase. The rapid distribution phase is represented by a *distribution half-life* that reflects the time it takes for distribution to reduce the initial peak level of the drug by 50 percent. If the distribution process were to lower the plasma drug level below that required for a pharmacological effect (*dotted horizontal line*), the therapeutic effect would be quite short-lived, and additional amounts of the drug would have to be administered to continue the effect.

The slower decrease (tangent line *B*) represents the time that is required to eliminate the drug from the body as a result of its metabolism (by the liver) and the excretion of metabolites (by the kidneys). The calculated elimination half-life reflects this process and allows calculation of the time course of drug action.

Figure 1.13 shows that the peak levels of pain relief produced by the drug fentanyl (a narcotic analgesic) are reached within seconds after intravenous injection. Fentanyl is highly lipid-soluble and is rapidly redistributed to muscle and fat, reducing blood concentrations of the drug in the process. The elimination half-life is about 45 minutes. As shown in Table 1.2, it takes four half-lives for 90 percent of the drug to be eliminated by the body (3 hours) and six half-lives for 98 percent to be eliminated (4.5 hours). At that point, the patient is, for most practical purposes, drug-free. It is important to remember that even though the analgesia became minimal after 2 hours, the drug persists at low levels in a patient's body for up to 4.5 hours. The so-called drug hangover is a result of such a prolonged elimination half-life. Whenever it is appropriate throughout the text, drug half-lives will be used in referring to the duration of action of psychoactive drugs in the body. Some drug half-lives can be measured in days; thus, recovery from the drug may take a week or more. Diazepam (Valium) is an example of a drug that has a several-day half-life.

Tolerance and Dependence

Drug *tolerance* may be defined as a state of progressively decreasing responsiveness to a drug. A person who develops tolerance requires a larger dose of the drug to achieve the effect originally obtained by a smaller dose.

The mechanisms that are involved in drug tolerance are becoming better understood. One type of tolerance occurs as a result of increased synthesis of drug-metabolizing enzymes that are involved in the metabolism of drugs and other chemicals by the liver. The clinical significance of this *drug-metabolizing* (or *enzyme induction*) *tolerance* is becoming increasingly important. A second type of tolerance, *cellular-adaptive* (or *pharmacodynamic*) *tolerance,* involves the adaptation of receptors in the brain to the continued presence of the drug. As will be discussed in later chapters, neurons can adapt to the presence of drug either by increasing their number of receptors (thereby requiring more drug to occupy them) or by reducing their sensitivity to the continuing presence of the drug. Pharmacodynamic tolerance occurs in people who develop problems with narcotics, barbiturates, and alcohol (although in the latter two, enzyme induction is also involved).

Physical dependence is an entirely different phenomenon, even though it is associated with drug tolerance in most cases. A person who is physically dependent on a drug needs it to function normally. The state of physical dependence is revealed by withdrawing the drug and noting the occurrence of withdrawal symptoms (*abstinence syndrome*) some time after the drug has been withheld. The symptoms of withdrawal can be terminated by readministering the drug.

A more specific example of enzyme-induction tolerance is presented in Table 1.3. In the experiment, rabbits were pretreated with three daily doses of pentobarbital (a short-acting barbiturate), and then

TABLE 1.3

Effect of pentobarbital pretreatment on the duration of pentobarbital action. Rabbits were pretreated with three daily doses of pentobarbital (60 mg/kg) subcutaneously, then given a single challenging dose of 60 mg/kg intravenously.

Pretreatment	Sleeping time (minutes)	Plasma level of pentobarbital on awakening (μg/ml)	Pentobarbital half-life in plasma (minutes)
None	67 ± 4	9.9 ± 1.4	79 ± 3
Pentobarbital	30 ± 7	7.9 ± 0.6	26 ± 2

Source: H. Remmer, "Drugs as Activators of Drug Enzymes," in B. B. Brodie and E. G. Erdos, eds., *Metabolic Factors Controlling Duration of Drug Action* (*Proceedings of the First International Pharmacological Meeting*), vol. 6. (New York: Macmillan, 1962), p. 235.

they were given a single challenging dose of pentobarbital. The length of time that the rabbits slept and the amount of pentobarbital in the animals' bloodstreams at the time of awakening were measured and compared with the sleeping time and the blood levels of pentobarbital in rabbits that were not pretreated but were given an identical dose of the drug. The data indicate that, although the pretreated animals slept less than half as long as the control rabbits, their blood levels of the drug on awakening were approximately the same. Pretreatment had raised the animals' tolerance for the drug-not by affecting the "sleep center" in the brain, but by inducing metabolizing enzymes in the liver, which caused the drug to be metabolized and excreted more rapidly.

This enzyme-induction mechanism of tolerance does not explain the increased tolerance and physical dependence that can develop in persons as a result of using a variety of psychoactive drugs, because it only accounts for the necessity to increase the dosage to produce a given effect. It is not uncommon to see alcoholics and people who are dependent on sedatives increase their dosages by factors of 10 and others who are dependent on narcotic analgesics increase their dosages by factors of between 10 and 20. Therefore, other mechanisms exist in the body that are responsible for inducing tolerance as well as for the withdrawal state that is seen when certain drugs are removed. Such mechanisms are situated within the brain and involve cellular adaptation to the continuous presence of a drug at the receptors. These issues will be discussed further as individual drugs are presented.

DRUG-RECEPTOR INTERACTIONS: PHARMACODYNAMICS

Introduction

Before producing a change in the functioning of a cell, which then leads to a change in body function or behavior, a drug must physically interact with one or more constituents of the cell. The cell component that is directly involved in this initial action of a drug is called the *drug receptor*. One of the most basic concepts in pharmacology is that drug molecules must attach to specific receptors either on a cell membrane or within a cell, and such occupation (of a receptor) by a drug must lead to a change in the functional properties of that cell, thus producing a pharmacological response. Research in this area of pharmacology falls under the general heading of *pharmacodynamics*, which deals with the study of how biochemical and physiological functions are altered by drugs.[4]

A characteristic of the drug receptor is its high (but not absolute) degree of specificity (or *affinity*) for a particular drug molecule. What may appear to be a slight or insignificant variation in the chemical structure of a drug may greatly alter the intensity of a cell's response to it. For example, amphetamine and methamphetamine are both powerful stimulants of the central nervous system (CNS). They differ chemically only very slightly, but methamphetamine is much more potent and, at equal doses of both drugs, produces much greater behavioral stimulation. Both drugs probably affect the same receptors in the brain, but methamphetamine exerts a much more powerful action on them.

The drug molecule with the "best fit" to the receptor will elicit the greatest response from the cell. Thus, methamphetamine might fit the receptor better than amphetamine does. It is currently thought that the cellular response that follows the attachment of a drug to its receptor is followed by a change in the conformation of the cell membrane—a change that is thought to alter the cellular behavior and, ultimately, brain or body function.

In television cartoon advertisements for analgesic tablets, we see a compound being taken orally, dissolving in the stomach, being absorbed into the bloodstream, and then being rapidly (some more rapidly than others, according to the commercial message) distributed exclusively to its receptors in the brain, which are immediately affected so that the headache magically disappears. Thus, a drug is often promoted as being some type of "magic bullet," which, upon being swallowed, immediately knows where its receptor is, streaks to that receptor, and in some mysterious way exerts its effect.

This idea of a drug's being selectively distributed only to specific receptors is, of course, false. Subject to the physical and chemical factors discussed in this chapter, drugs are distributed throughout the body fairly evenly. Selectivity of drug action is not a property of selective distribution; rather, it is a function of selective localization of drug receptors, the specificity of drugs that bind to particular receptors, the strength of the drug's attachment, and the consequences of the interaction between drugs and their receptors.

A major consideration of current drug research is the attempt to characterize, in molecular terms (and in more and more detail), the primary sites and mechanisms of drug action. A drug with a seemingly wide variety of actions can frequently be shown to act quite specifically on a particular type of cell or tissue component (such as an enzyme, a specific neurotransmitter, a DNA molecule, and so on). For example, aspirin exerts a wide variety of effects (analgesic, anti-inflammatory, and fever-reducing), most of which can be explained in terms of inhibition of the action of one or more of the enzymes that are involved in the inflammatory process (discussed later in Chapter 13).[5] Similarly, the benzodiazepine tranquilizers (for example, diazepam) may exert their sedative, antianxiety, and antiepileptic actions by interacting with specific receptor sites in the brain, thereby potentiating the action of an inhibitory neurotransmitter (gamma-aminobutyric acid) (Chapter 5). One goal of this text will be to demonstrate, whenever possible, those single actions that may account for the wide variety of effects that are produced by a drug or specific class of drugs.

Once the actions of a drug can be explained in terms of interaction with a specific type of receptor, we can use that data to develop a classification system (Chapter 2) and to determine a basis for the development of new drugs. For example, we have now identified several subtypes of narcotic receptors (Chapter 9). Research is being carried out in an attempt to develop new analgesics that will act on specific receptor subtypes, possibly leading to increased specificity of analgesia with a concomitant reduction in unacceptable or bothersome side effects.

Several corollaries follow from this recognition that drugs act on specific molecular receptors.[4] First, a drug is potentially capable of altering the rate at which any bodily (or brain) function proceeds. Second, a drug does not create effects but merely modulates ongoing functions. Third, a drug cannot impart new functions to a cell. Finally, in psychopharmacology (the subject of this text), many drugs act to mimic or potentiate the actions of neurotransmitters. Such drugs are termed *agonists*. Other drugs may bind to a receptor but exert *no* intrinsic activity on the cell; the result of such binding may be competitive interference with the effect of the normal neurotransmitter. Such compounds (themselves devoid of intrinsic activity but which cause effects by inhibiting the action of a transmitter) are termed *antagonists*.

The affinity of a drug for its receptor (that is, its ability to "bind" to a receptor), its intrinsic activity (agonist versus antagonist), and its potency (strength in milligrams) are intimately related to the drug's chemical structure. Indeed, in this text, chemical structures are illustrated only to demonstrate that small structural changes can result in profound differences in action. This presumably follows from the supposition that small structural changes can significantly alter the "fit" of a drug for its receptor, thereby producing a significant variation in the drug-induced conformational changes that occur in the three-dimensional structure of a receptor.

Thus, we have stated that the interaction of a drug with its receptor initiates (agonist action) or inhibits (antagonist action) a normal physiological function. It should also be noted that receptors themselves are subject to many regulatory, intrinsic, homeostatic controls, and their sensitivity (and even their absolute numbers) can be modulated (increased or decreased). Such receptor modulation is thought to be involved in the actions of antidepressant drugs, such as imipramine, discussed in Chapter 8).

The Dose-Response Relationship

One way of quantifying the description of drug-receptor interactions (that is, the formation of reversible drug-receptor complexes) is to use what are known as *dose-response curves*. In Figure 1.14, two types of dose-response curves are illustrated. On the left, the dose is plotted against the percentage of persons who exhibit a characteristic effect. On the right, the dose is plotted against the intensity, or the magnitude, of the response in a single person. These curves indicate that a dose exists

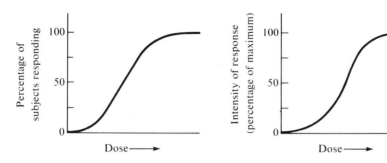

FIGURE 1.14

Two types of dose-response curves. *Left*, the curve obtained by plotting the dose of drug against the percentage of subjects showing a given response at any given dose. *Right*, the dose of drug against the intensity of response observed in any single individual at a given dose. The intensity of response is plotted as a percentage of the maximum obtainable response.

that is low enough to produce little or no effect and, at the opposite extreme, a dose exists beyond which no greater response can be elicited.

All dose-response curves demonstrate four important characteristics: *potency, slope, efficacy* (the maximum effect obtainable), and the *dose* required to produce this maximum effect (Figure 1.14, right). Finally, one can use dose-response curves to estimate *variability* of response and drug *safety*. The latter two factors are discussed in the next section.

The location of the dose-response curve along the horizontal axis is an expression of the *potency* of the drug. If two drugs were capable of producing sedation, but one was capable of exerting this action at half the dose level of the other, the first drug would be considered to be twice as potent as the second drug. Potency, however, is a relatively unimportant characteristic of a drug, because it makes little difference whether the effective dose of a drug is 0.1 gram or 10 grams as long as the drug is administered in an appropriate dose and undue toxicity is not observed at that dose. Thus, there is little justification to say that the more potent drug is the better one. High potency, in fact, is usually a disadvantage, because an extremely potent drug may be much more toxic (or dangerous) and may require much more careful administration to reach a given therapeutic or behavioral endpoint.

Slope refers to the more or less linear, central portion of the dose-response curve. A steep slope on a dose-response curve implies that there is only a small difference between the dose that produces a

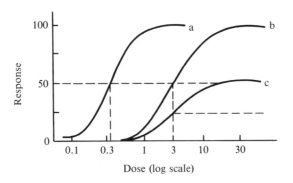

FIGURE 1.15

Dose-response curves for three drugs. See text for discussion.

desired effect and the dose that causes toxicity. The steeper the slope, the smaller the increase in dose that is required to go from a minimum response to a maximum effect.

The peak of the dose-response curve indicates the maximum effect, or *efficacy,* that can be produced by a drug, regardless of further increases in dose. Not all psychoactive drugs are capable of exerting the same level of effect. For example, caffeine, even in massive doses, is incapable of exerting the same intensity of CNS stimulation that is induced by amphetamine. Similarly, aspirin can never achieve the maximum analgesic effect that is exerted by morphine. Thus, the maximum effect is an inherent property of a drug and is one measure of a drug's efficacy. Most psychoactive drugs, however, are not used to the point of their maximum effect, because side effects limit the upper range of dosage. Thus, the usefulness of a compound is correspondingly limited, even though the drug may be inherently capable of producing a greater effect.

To review these concepts, evaluate the three curves in Figure 1.15. Drugs *a* and *b* exhibit the same maximum response, but drug *c* has significantly less *efficacy* (less intrinsic activity). By further comparing drugs *a* and *b*, however, we find that drug *b* is about 10 times less potent than drug *a*, while drug *c* is equally as potent as drug *b*. Drug *c* has a flatter slope than either drug *a* or drug *b*. Thus, drug *c* may be easier to administer, despite its lower intrinsic activity. Note that these curves do not predict safety, side effects, toxicity, or therapeutic superiority.

DRUG SAFETY AND EFFECTIVENESS

Variability in Drug Responsiveness

Variability is another factor to be considered when evaluating drug responses. The dose of a drug that will produce a specific response will vary considerably among subjects. Figure 1.16 illustrates a Gaussian (bell-shaped) distribution of drug variability in a population of animals. Note that, although the *average* dose required to elicit a given response in this population of animals may be calculated easily (illustrated by the *dotted line*), some animals will respond at a dose that is very much lower than the average, and other animals will not respond until extremely large doses have been administered. This occurrence implies that it is *extremely important* that the dose of all drugs be individualized. Generalizations about "average doses" are risky at best. This Gaussian distribution, however, allows us to estimate the dose of a drug that will produce the desired effect in 50 percent of the subjects. This dose is called the ED_{50} for the drug (the effective dose for 50 percent of the subjects). Similarly, we can estimate an LD_{50} (lethal dose for 50 percent of the subjects). The LD_{50} is calculated in exactly the same way as the ED_{50} except that the dose of the drug is plotted against the number of

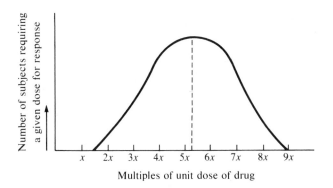

FIGURE 1.16

Biological variation in susceptibility to drugs. This curve is a Gaussian distribution, with the dose of drug plotted against the number of subjects requiring a given dose for a given response to occur. Note that, for a given response, some animals will require only a small amount of the drug while others will require much more than what is considered normal.

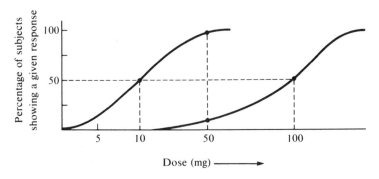

FIGURE 1.17

Two dose-response curves. *Left,* the dose of drug required to induce a given response. *Right,* the lethal dose of the compound.

animals (usually mice) that die following treatment with various doses of the compound. Delineation of both the ED_{50} and the LD_{50} is necessary for public safety to prevent accidental drug-induced deaths in humans. Both the ED_{50} and the LD_{50} are usually determined in laboratory mice, and the ratio of the LD_{50} to the ED_{50} is an index of the relative *safety* of the drug.

In Figure 1.17, two dose-response curves are shown; the one on the left illustrates the dose of drug that is necessary to induce sleep in a population of mice, and the one on the right illustrates the dose of drug that is necessary to kill a similar population. If one extrapolates across the 50-percent point (*dotted lines*), and determines the doses necessary to induce sleep in 50 percent and death in another 50 percent, one could determine a ratio between the median toxic dose and the median effective dose (LD_{50}:ED_{50}). In this case, the ratio would be 100:10, or 10. This figure is referred to as the *therapeutic index* of the drug—that is, the dose that is necessary to kill 50 percent of the mice is 10 times the dose that is necessary to induce sleep in another 50 percent of mice. This may seem like a rather large margin, but note that, at a dose of 50 milligrams, 95 percent of the mice sleep while 5 percent of the mice die. This overlap demonstrates the difficulty we encounter in assessing the relative safety of drugs for use in large populations and serves as an excellent example of biological variation in individual responses to drugs. With this particular compound, a dose could not be administered that would guarantee that 100 percent of the mice would sleep and none would die. Thus, to better predict a more meaningful margin of safety, rather than using the ratio of ED_{50} to LD_{50}, we might consider a ratio of the lethal dose for 1 percent of the population to the effective dose for 99 percent of the population ($LD_1:ED_{99}$). A sedative drug with an $LD_1:ED_{99}$ of 1 would be a safer compound than the drug illustrated in Figure 1.17.

It is important to note, however, that the use of such indices, which are obtained from data in laboratory animals, is limited, because it might miss the occasional unexpected response (discussed next) that might seriously harm a patient.

Variability, either between different persons, or in the same person on different occasions, results from (1) differing concentrations of the drug at its site of action, (2) differing physiological responses to the same drug concentrations, or (3) unusual, idiosyncratic (genetically determined) or allergic (immunologically sensitized) responses that are wholly unanticipated.

Variations of the first kind result from differences in how people handle a dose of drug (pharmacokinetic variation), and they occur because of differences in drug absorption, distribution, metabolism, or excretion. Variations of the second kind result from variations in response to a similar concentration of a drug at the receptor (pharmacodynamic variation). Such might occur if the receptors are desensitized to the presence of a drug or, conversely, if the receptors are hypersensitive to the drug. Age, genetic factors, drug interactions, and certain disease states can all contribute to variability in receptor sensitivity to a drug. Such contributions will be expanded on as individual drugs are discussed.

Drug variability is intimately associated with drug toxicity. Therefore, the side effects that are invariably associated with a drug, as well as its more serious toxicities (including those that may be fatal), must always be considered.

The psychoactive drugs discussed in this book can be classified either according to their most prominent behavioral effect or according to their primary mechanism of action. Most commonly, the former is used, and psychoactive drugs are classified as depressants, stimulants, hallucinogens, narcotics, and so on. However, if such a classification system is used, the behavioral effects produced by a drug should ideally be related to the dose administered. For example, the classification of a drug as a sedative does not adequately describe the actions of the compound, at least not until one understands everything that is implied by the term *sedative*. (The implications are discussed in Chapter 3.)

The time course of a drug's action may be characterized by the latency of onset, the time needed taken to reach maximum effect, and the duration of action. These three characteristics are largely determined by the drug's rates of absorption, distribution, metabolism, and excretion. A drug that is slowly absorbed will have a long latency of onset, whereas a drug administered intravenously may have an almost instantaneous onset of action. The time needed for a drug to reach its peak effect is often determined by its distribution in the body. Psychoactive drugs that cross the blood-brain barrier rapidly and reach nerve tissue quickly usually take a shorter period of time to reach their maximum effect than do drugs that only slowly gain access to the brain. For example, both thiopental and pentobarbital (Nembutal) are sleep-inducing agents. Thiopental is more fat-soluble than pentobarbital and crosses the blood-brain barrier within an extremely short period of time (usually a few seconds). Pentobarbital, because it has some difficulty passing through the blood-brain barrier, may take many minutes to build up concentrations in the brain that are sufficient to induce sleep.

Similarly, rates of redistribution of a drug in the body, metabolism to inactive products, and excretion of the metabolized products determine the duration of drug action. Thiopental, with its high solubility in fat, rapidly leaves brain tissue and is carried to the muscles and fatty areas of the body. Thus, the blood levels of thiopental will be quite low, the patient will awaken (the drug having left the brain but not the body), and then the drug will be slowly metabolized and excreted. Pentobarbital, being less soluble in fat, is not redistributed to the fatty areas. Thus, the blood levels of pentobarbitol will be much more persistent, with the result that the patient is sedated for a prolonged period of time—until the drug is metabolized and excreted. In order for the sedative action of pentobarbital to be terminated, the drug must be metabolized (biotransformed) by the liver and the by-products must be excreted in the urine. As the dosage of the drug is increased, the effects of the drug are usually perceived earlier and the duration of action is prolonged.

Drug Interactions

It is widely appreciated that the effects of one drug can be modified by the concurrent administration of another drug. For example, alcohol, taken after a sleeping pill or a tranquilizer has been ingested (discussed in Chapter 3), will increase sedation and the loss of coordination. This action may have little consequence if the doses of each drug are low (one or two tablets and only one or two drinks), but higher doses of either or both drugs can be dangerous both to the user and to others. Even though a person may normally be able to ingest a limited amount of alcohol and still drive a car without significant loss of control or coordination, the concurrent ingestion of a tranquilizer may profoundly affect his or her driving performance, endangering the driver, the passengers, and other motorists. Literally hundreds of other examples could be given, and one must be aware of the danger of significant interactions that occur when more than one drug is taken at the same time.

We have already discussed two of the primary factors that contribute to drug interactions. First, many drugs bind to plasma proteins, which serve as a reservoir of inactive drugs. If a second drug competes for the same binding site and displaces a drug that has already bound to a protein, more of the previously bound drug will be freed to pass out of the bloodstream and, therefore, be available to the receptor. Thus, a more intense effect may be produced: the second drug (the displacing drug) would increase the effects or the toxicity (or both) of the first drug (the displaced drug).

Second, in our discussion about tolerance we stated that a drug that is metabolized by the liver may induce more enzymes, which can then metabolize any of a variety of other drugs. Thus, an enzyme-inducing drug, such as pentobarbital (see Table 1.3), will decrease the activity of other drugs that are also metabolized in the liver by increasing their rates of metabolism.

As can be seen, a wide variety of factors influence a drug's action in the body, making the use of more than one drug at a time risky, whether they are used separately or mixed in one concoction. As a general rule, mixtures often complicate therapy, because often it has not been established that more than one drug is needed; and if toxic effects should occur, it may be difficult to determine which drug is responsible.

Drug Toxicity

All drugs are capable of producing harmful effects as well as beneficial ones. The nature of these unwanted effects falls into two mechanistic categories:[6] (1) effects that are related to the principal pharmacological action of a drug; and (2) effects that are unrelated to the principal pharmacological action of a drug.

It is important to categorize harmful effects of drugs in terms of their severity and to distinguish between those effects that cause a temporary inconvenience or discomfort and those that can lead to permanent disability or death. Many unwanted effects in the first category are readily predictable from knowledge about the mode of action of a drug. Such effects will be discussed as individual psychoactive drugs are presented.

Virtually all drugs exert effects on several different body functions. These multiple effects occur despite the fact that one is usually interested in obtaining a single, or perhaps a small number of, the drug's many possible effects. The desired effect is usually considered to be the *main effect*, while the unwanted effects are labeled *side effects*. To achieve the main effect, the side effects must be tolerated, which is possible if they are minor but may be a limiting factor in the use of the drug if they are more serious. The distinction between main effects and side effects is relative and depends on the purpose of the drug. What may be one person's side effect may be another person's main effect. With morphine, for example, pain-relieving properties may be sought, but the intestinal constipation that is induced is an undesirable side effect that must be tolerated. However, morphine may also be used to treat diarrhea, so that the constipation induced is then considered to be the main effect, and any relief of pain is a side effect.

In addition to side effects that are merely irritating, drugs may occasionally induce very serious toxicities. Such side effects can include serious allergies, blood disorders, liver or kidney toxicity, or abnormalities in fetal development. The incidence of all these serious toxic effects is fortunately quite low.

Allergies to drugs may take many forms—from mild skin rashes to fatal shock. Allergies differ from normal side effects, which may often be eliminated, or at least made tolerable, by a simple reduction in dosage. A reduction in the dose of a drug may be *useless* for a drug allergy, because exposure to any amount of the drug is hazardous and possibly catastrophic for the patient.

Organ damage, especially to the liver and kidneys, follows from their role in concentrating, metabolizing, and excreting toxic drugs. One example of *drug-induced* liver damage is that caused by alcohol. Similarly, a class of major tranquilizers, the phenothiazines (for example, chlorpromazine [Thorazine]), may induce jaundice by increasing the viscosity of bile in the liver.

Although not side effects of the drug itself, infectious hepatitis or AIDS may accompany drug injection if strict sterility is not observed.

The thalidomide tragedy dramatically illustrated how drugs may adversely influence fetal development. The seriousness of the problem of drug action on the fetus and the wide range of possible consequences was noted as early as 1968:

It is clear that the risks of chemical teratogenesis . . . are accentuated during the first trimester of pregnancy. Until much more information becomes available, the very diversity of known teratogens and mutagens (drugs that alter the structure of chromosomes in the cell) should dictate caution. . . . A woman who is known to be pregnant should not be exposed to drugs at all during the first trimester unless the need is pressing. At least until experimental or statistical investigations show them to be harmless, caffeine, nicotine, and alcohol, to which people are so frequently exposed, should be regarded as possibly hazardous to the fetus during the first three months of pregnancy.[7]

Finally, the chronic toxicity of socially abused drugs should be mentioned. The considerable data compiled since 1968 quite clearly show the adverse effects of nicotine and ethyl alcohol on the fetus. More recently, fetal effects of cocaine abuse are receiving much attention. Indeed, these drugs are thought to be responsible for a majority of preventable fetal toxicities and are three of the major health hazards in the country today. More will be said about the toxicity of these drugs in later chapters.

Placebo Effects

Pharmacology is concerned with the actions of drugs on biological mechanisms. The term *placebo*, however, refers to a pharmacologically *inert* substance that elicits a significant therapeutic response. Because this action is independent of any chemical property of the drug, it arises largely because of what the patient expects, desires, or was told would happen. This placebo response seems to arise from a person's mental set or from the entire environmental situation, or setting, in which the drug is taken. In certain predisposed persons, a placebo may produce extremely strong reactions with far-reaching consequences.

Even more remarkable is the demonstration that placebos may evoke patterns of altered behavior that are similar to and as long lasting as those observed when a pharmacologically active drug is ingested. Thus, in discussing the pharmacology of a psychoactive agent, we must pay particular attention to the mental set of expectations, the social setting, and the predisposition of the subjects taking the placebo if we are to describe the pharmacological effects of a drug accurately.

Responses that closely mimic those produced by pharmacologically active drugs can be learned without drugs or placebos. For instance, meditation techniques can produce states that closely resemble those produced by drugs, especially altered states of consciousness. It may, for example, be possible to use meditation to alter activity in certain centers of the brain in much the same way that a drug would alter the activity. Certainly, the placebo effect is a powerful element in drug-induced responses.

Development of New Drugs

To complete our discussion of the effects of drugs in the body, let us describe briefly the processes and procedures by which new drugs are developed and evaluated before they are released for public use.

The earliest medicinal products were usually natural in origin: crude powders of leaves or roots, or extracts from a variety of plants or animals. One of the great advances of the twentieth century was the development of organic chemistry, which has made it practical to synthesize new drug molecules that, it is hoped, offer more promise than many products obtained from natural sources. Although new drugs are occasionally discovered by accident, they usually result from systematic and tedious laboratory investigation and careful scientific observation.

The development and marketing of new drugs in the United States is rigidly controlled by the federal government through the Food and Drug Administration (FDA). Before it is marketed for general clinical use, a new drug is subjected to thorough laboratory and clinical pharmacological studies that demonstrate its usefulness and safety. Before studies in humans are permitted, the pharmacology of a new drug must be extensively delineated in animals. These studies include the establishment of the range of effective doses, the doses at which side effects occur, and the lethal doses in various animals. The studies on the safety and toxicity of a drug are evaluated after administration of single doses as well as during long-term use. From all these studies, a risk-to-benefit ratio is determined. Because of differences between species of animals, these studies must usually be carried out in at least three different species. In this preliminary testing on animals, neither the mechanism of a drug's action nor the range of its possible clinical usefulness needs to be completely described, but the absorption, distribution, metabolism, and excretion of the drug are carefully documented.

Having been found safe to use in animals, a compound may be taken into an initial clinical trial (phase 1), which is usually conducted

TIME	Phase 1. First Human Administration

Phase 1. First Human Administration

Who? Normal volunteers—small number.
Why? Determine biological effects, metabolism, and safe dosage range in humans
By whom? Clinical pharmacologists.

Phase 2.

a. Early

Who? Selected patients—small number.
Why? Determine potential usefulness and refine therapeutic dosage range.
By whom? Clinical pharmacologists.

Interim review of data by intramural and extramural experts.
Chronic toxicity studies in animals.
Special animal studies for effects on reproduction and fertility.

b. Late

Who? Selected patients—larger number for longer duration.
Why? Determination of final dosage range. More data on elimination, especially by metabolism.
By whom? Clinical pharmacologists.

Phase 3. Broad Clinical Trial

Who? Large sample of specified patients.
Why? Determine safety and efficacy.
By whom? Clinical investigators.

Phase 4. Conditional Approval

a. Monitored Release

Who? Patients under specified supervision.
Why? Monitoring of drug's efficacy and impact under limited marketing.
By whom? Selected medical centers and qualified physicians.

b. Postmarketing Surveillance

Who? Patients under conditions of actual drug use.
Why? Determine patterns of drug utilization and additional efficacy and toxicity after general marketing.
By whom? All physicians agreeing to participate in organized reporting.

ABOUT 4 YEARS / *ABOUT 2 YEARS* / *INDEFINITE*

FIGURE 1.18

The phases of drug development in the United States.. [Adapted from E. M. Ross and A. G. Gilman, "Pharmacodynamics: Mechanism of Drug Action and the Relationship between Drug Concentration and Effect," in A. G. Gilman, L. S. Goodman, T. W. Rall, and F. Murad, eds., *Goodman and Gilman's The Pharmacological Basis of Therapeutics*, 7th ed. New York: Macmillan, 1985), p.59.]

on normal volunteer subjects, as well as on patients, and is aimed at establishing the drug's safety, dose range, and possible problems requiring further study (Figure 1.18). If phase 1 studies indicate safety, the drug may be subjected to a thorough clinical pharmacological evaluation (phase 2). These studies, of necessity, are closely controlled to eliminate such variables as placebo response and investigator bias. Statistical validation is of paramount importance. Finally, if a drug still looks promising, it will enter phase 3 of the human studies—a period of extended clinical evaluation. During this phase, the compound is made available to investigators throughout the country for use in a variety of clinical situations. This procedure is followed to elicit information about the drug's safety, efficacy, side effects, dosage, variability of response, and so on.

If a drug passes all these trials, it may receive conditional approval by the FDA for broad use by physicians and medical centers who agree to a procedure of organized reporting of therapeutic results, limitations, and problems.

Currently, it costs a pharmaceutical manufacturer more than 25 million dollars to take a new compound through laboratory and clinical testing to the marketing stage. Although this attention to detail may seem excessive, it works to the benefit of the public. Most drugs that are currently on the legitimate market have reasonable risk-to-benefit ratios. Although none of the drugs available are completely without risk, most are relatively safe.

STUDY QUESTIONS

1. Differentiate the terms *pharmacokinetics* and *pharmacodynamics*.
2. Why must a psychoactive drug be altered metabolically in the body before it can be excreted?
3. Discuss the advantages and disadvantages of the various methods of administering drugs.
4. List the various membrane barriers that may affect drug distribution.
5. Discuss the placental barrier as it affects the distribution of psychoactive drugs.

6. If a drug has an elimination half-life of 6 hours, how long will it take for the drug to be eliminated from the body after a person has taken a single dose?

7. What is drug *tolerance* and why does it occur?

8. Differentiate the terms *agonist* and *antagonist* as they relate to drug-receptor interactions.

9. Discuss the factors that influence the time course of drug action in the body.

10. Discuss how two drugs might interact with each other in the body.

NOTES

1. L. Z. Benet, J. R. Mitchell, and L. B. Sheiner, "Pharmacokinetics: The Dynamics of Drug Absorption, Distribution and Elimination," in A. G. Gilman, T. W. Rall, A. S. Nies, and P. Taylor, eds., *Goodman and Gilman's The Pharmacological Basis of Therapeutics*, 8th ed. (New York: Pergamon, 1990), pp. 3–32.

2. R. R. Levine, *Pharmacology: Drug Actions and Reactions*, 3d ed. (Boston: Little, Brown, 1983), pp. 211–247.

3. M. W. B. Bradbury, "The Structure and Function of the Blood-Brain Barrier," *Federation Proceedings* 43 (1984): 186–190.

4. E. M. Ross, "Pharmacodynamics: Mechanisms of Drug Action and the Relationship Between Drug Concentration and Effect," in A. G. Gilman, T. W. Rall, A. S. Nies, and P. Taylor, eds., *Goodman and Gilman's The Pharmacological Basis of Therapeutics*, 8th ed. (New York: Pergamon, 1990), p. 33.

5. H. P. Rang and M. M. Dale, *Pharmacology* (Edinburgh: Churchill Livingstone, 1987), p. 5.

6. H. P. Rang and M. M. Dale, *Pharmacology* (Edinburgh: Churchill Livingstone, 1987), p. 692.

7. A. Goldstein, L. Aronow, and S. M. Kalman, *Principles of Drug Action* (New York: Harper & Row, 1968), p. 733.

C H A P T E R   2

Classification of Psychoactive Drugs

A Starting Point for Understanding

Psychoactive drugs are defined as substances that affect mood or behavior, or that are used in the management of neuropsychological illness. Because the management of neuropsychological illness is very complex, the classification of psychoactive drugs is not a straightforward task. Several methods of classification have been formulated, but each has limitations. Certainly, the discussion in Chapter 1 could lead to a method of classification that is based on the mechanisms of action of each drug. However, there are still too many gaps in our knowledge of those mechanisms to present a comprehensive scheme. Another method could be formulated by identifying similarities in the chemical structures of particular drugs on the assumption that drugs with a similar chemical structure may be expected to exert similar effects. However, too many drugs with apparently similar structures exert pharmacological activity that is different; and too many drugs with apparently dissimilar chemical structures exert pharmacological activity that is nearly identical with that of other drugs. Thus, the chemical structure of a drug does not produce a reliable guide to its pharmacological effects. Perhaps the most realistic method of classification uses the most characteristic effects or clinical uses of each drug as a basis for classifying drugs into arbitrary categories, such as those presented in Table 2.1.

Assumptions about the Classification

There are several qualifications to be aware of when you use this table. First, the action of psychoactive drugs is not usually restricted to any one functional or anatomical subdivision of the brain. There are exceptions, of course (such as the use of levodopa for the treatment of Parkinson's disease), but usually a psychoactive drug will affect several processes simultaneously. This factor complicates the classification of drugs because different behavioral actions may predominate at different doses. Some compromises must, therefore, be made.

Second, the ultimate action of any given psychoactive drug may be explained by alterations in the synthesis, release, action, metabolism, and so on of a specific neurotransmitter chemical. (The neurochemical processes that mediate transmission of information between neurons are discussed at some length in Appendix III.) Further, that same neurotransmitter chemical may be involved in many different activities of the brain (norepinephrine, for example, may be involved in temperature regulation, arousal, satiety, rage, and so on). Thus, although a psychoactive drug might ultimately be found to exert a single effect on a specific neurotransmitter chemical, a variety of behavioral effects would be expected to follow, because the neurotransmitter is involved in many different functions.

Third, it is important to understand that psychoactive drugs do not create new behavioral or physiological responses; they simply modify ongoing processes. Current thought holds that the behavioral effects that psychoactive drugs exert are secondary to their blocking or modifying biochemical processes, physiological processes, or both, particularly those processes involved in the various steps of synaptic transmission in the brain.

Fourth, the classification of psychoactive drugs listed in Table 2.1 is not rigid. Different behavioral responses are observed in persons who ingest drugs at different doses. Alcohol, for example, is classified as a general nonselective depressant despite the fact that, at low doses, it may cause behavioral excitation. Thus, classification alone does not clearly describe the pharmacology of a drug. It does, however, serve as

TABLE 2.1

Classification of drugs that alter mood or behavior or that are useful in treating neuropsychological disorders. Only representative agents from each class of drug are listed.

1. Nonselective CNS Depressants
   Barbiturates
      Long-acting: phenobarbital (Luminal)
      Intermediate-acting: amobarbital (Amytal)
      Short-acting: pentobarbital (Nembutal)
      Ultra-short-acting: thiopental (Pentothal)
   Nonbarbiturate hypnotics
      Meprobamate (Miltown, Equanil)
      Glutethimide (Doriden)
      Methyprylon (Noludar)
      Others: methaqualone, chloral hydrate, ethchlorvynol
   Ethyl alcohol
   General anesthetics
      Inhalation anesthetics
      Injectable anesthetics
2. Antianxiety Agents: benzodiazepines
      Long-acting: diazepam (Valium)
      Intermediate-acting: lorazepam (Ativan)
      Short-acting: triazolam (Halcion)
3. Psychomotor Stimulants (Psychostimulants)
   Sympathetic nervous system activators
      d-Amphetamine (Dexedrine)
      Amphetamine derivatives: methylphenidate (Ritalin), pemoline (Cylert)
      Cocaine
   Caffeine
   Nicotine
4. Antidepressants
   Tricyclic antidepressants: imipramine (Tofranil), amitriptyline (Elavil)
   Second-generation antidepressants: fluoxetine (Prozac)
   Monoamine oxidase (MAO) inhibitors: tranylcypromine (Parnate)
5. Mood Stabilizers
   Lithium
   Certain anticonvulsants
6. Narcotic Analgesics: Opioids
   Morphine and its analogues

a starting point from which several compounds may be compared and contrasted.

Fifth, certain factors that predispose persons to compulsive misuse of a drug must be considered in the classification of centrally acting drugs. Such factors include physiological and psychological dependence and tolerance. Psychoactive drugs differ in their potential to induce such hazards. It should be apparent, however, that any drug that is capable of favorably altering a person's mood or behavior or of creating a pleasurable state of consciousness is capable of inducing

TABLE 2.1 (continued)

    Agonists (e.g., morphine, codeine, heroin)
    Partial agonists (e.g., nalbuphine)
    Antagonists (e.g., naloxone, naltrexone)
  Synthetic, structurally unrelated derivatives
    Meperidine (Demerol), fentanyl (Sublimaze), methadone (Dolophine), pentazocine
      (Talwin)
7. Antipsychotic Agents
  Phenothiazines: chlorpromazine (Thorazine)
  Reserpine (Serpasil)
  Butyrophenones: haloperidol (Haldol)
8. Psychedelics and Hallucinogens
  Anticholinergic psychedelics
    Atropine
    Scopolamine
  Norepinephrine psychedelics
    Mescaline
    DOM (STP), MDA, MMDA, TMA, DMA
    Myristin, elemicin
  Serotonin psychedelics
    Lysergic acid diethylamide (LSD)
    Dimethyltryptamine (DMT)
    Psilocybin, psilocin, bufotenine
    Ololiuqui (morning glory seeds)
    Harmine
  Psychedelic anesthetics
    Phencyclidine (Sernyl)
    Ketamine (Ketalar)
  Tetrahydrocannabinol
    Marijuana, hashish, cannabis
9. Neurological Drugs
  Antiepileptic drugs: phenytoin (Dilantin), carbamazepine (Tegretol), valproic acid
    (Depakene), clonazepam (Klonopin)
  Antiparkinsonian drugs: levodopa (Larodopa), amantadine (Symmetrel),
    bromocriptine (Parlodel)
  Drugs for spasticity: baclofen (Lioresal), dantrolene (Dantrium)
  Nonnarcotic analgesics: aspirin, acetaminophen (Tylenol), ibuprofen (Advil, Motrin),
    indomethacin (Indocin), phenylbutazone (Butazolidin)
  Local anesthetics: procaine (Novocain), lidocaine (Xylocaine)

psychological dependence—that is, a compulsion to use the drug for a favorable effect.

The Future Discussion

In subsequent chapters, we will describe specific agents within each of the classes of psychoactive agents listed in Table 2.1. Alcohol and marijuana are discussed separately (in Chapters 4 and 12). Although both agents might well be included in the chapter on sedative-hypnotic compounds (Chapter 3), they deserve a separate discussion because of their wide range of use, ready availability, and social and legal implications. Similarly, the benzodiazepine sedative anxiolytic (antianxiety) compounds (Chapter 5) are not discussed with the other sedatives because they do not exert a nonselective depressant action. Rather, they specifically potentiate the action of the neurotransmitter gamma-aminobutyric acid (GABA) at its synapses.

Chapter 8 presents an expanded discussion of drugs that are used to treat the affective disorders (mania and depression). Those drugs (antidepressants and lithium) have become widely used, and their unique properties clearly separate them from the psychomotor stimulants (Chapter 6).

The drugs discussed in Chapter 13 are useful in treating epilepsy, parkinsonism, spasticity, pain, and inflammation. They are not generally considered to be either drugs of abuse or psychoactive (since they affect neither mood nor behavior). However, they are included to complete this presentation of centrally acting drugs, and to make this text more useful for a comprehensive coverage of neuropsychopharmacology.

Chapter 14 discusses the effects of body hormones on the brain and on behavior (for example, oral contraceptives and fertility agents). Although these compounds are not psychoactive drugs, this material has been retained because of the wide interest in those drugs. Because the limbic system, hypothalamus, and pituitary gland are thought to be important sites of action of these compounds, a discussion of their physiological, pharmacological, behavioral, and sociological effects seems pertinent.

Let us now consider the first category in Table 2.1—general, non-selective CNS depressants.

General Nonselective Central Nervous System Depressants

Drugs That Depress the Central Nervous System

The nonselective central nervous system (CNS) depressants are a group of drugs with diverse chemical structures. They are capable of inducing varying degrees of behavioral depression secondary to a relatively nonselective depression of the CNS.[1] These drugs are divided somewhat arbitrarily into four categories: (1) the barbiturates, (2) the nonbarbiturate hypnotics, (3) the general anesthetics, and (4) ethyl alcohol. Of these drugs, the unique, nonmedical use of alcohol in our culture justifies a separate discussion (Chapter 4).

Each of these agents is capable of inducing progressive, dose-dependent behavioral alterations that vary in a range, including, (at low doses) relief from anxiety, drowsiness, release from inhibition, sedation, sleep, unconsciousness, general anesthesia, coma, and, finally (at very high doses), death as a result of depression of the respiratory and cardiac centers in the brain. This gradation of action is illustrated in Figure 3.1.

The terms *sedative* and *tranquilizer* refer to any of these drugs because each may diminish environmental awareness, spontaneity, and physical activity; higher doses produce drowsiness and lethargy; and

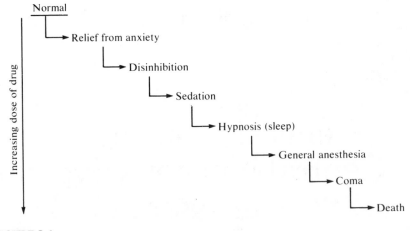

FIGURE 3.1

Continuum of behavioral sedation. How increasing doses of sedative-hypnotic drugs affect behavior.

even higher doses produce sleep and unconsciousness. Individual compounds differ little from one another in their sites of action, uses, or abilities to induce various stages of depression. They do differ in their individual potencies and in the chemical differences that cause them to be handled differently by the body. For example, a much smaller amount of secobarbital (a barbiturate) than of chloral hydrate (an alcohol) may be required to induce sleep. Secobarbital, therefore, is said to be more *potent*. But comparison of these drugs by potency is rather meaningless, because such factors as safety and efficacy may be more important in determining their usefulness.

In past years, low doses of these drugs were used clinically to calm anxious patients. This role in "daytime sedation" is now largely restricted to the benzodiazepines, which are inherently less dangerous. Indeed, because of the availability of the benzodiazepines, the use of barbiturate and nonbarbiturate sedatives is decreasing and becoming more specialized.

Five Principles of CNS Depressants

Five general principles that apply fairly uniformly to all the CNS depressants can be summarized. First, the effects of CNS depressants are *additive* with one another and with the mental set of the user. For example, alcohol will exaggerate the depression induced by barbiturates. Barbiturates will intensify the impairment of the driving ability of a person who has been drinking alcohol. Similarly, a person who is depressed or physically tired may be profoundly affected by a dose of depressant drug that would only slightly affect someone who feels normal or excited. The depressant effects of sedative drugs are also frequently *supra-additive*. Thus, the depression that is observed in a person who has taken more than one drug is greater than would be predicted if the depression caused by each drug were calculated individually. It may be said in this case that the whole is greater than the sum of its parts. Such intense depression is often unpredictable and unexpected, and it can lead to dangerous or even fatal consequences. Depressant drugs should not be used in combination without the advice and guidance of a physician, especially if one of the drugs is ethyl alcohol (Chapter 4).

Second, *antagonism* occurs between the CNS depressants and the behavioral stimulants; and that antagonism is usually nonspecific. When a person is profoundly depressed by a sedative drug, the administration of a stimulant will not *specifically* block the action of the depressant and return the patient to normal, although the stimulant may arouse the patient temporarily. In fact, the stimulant may do more harm than good, because when it wears off, the patient will become even more depressed. Clinically, for these situations we need a specific antagonist to CNS depressants—a drug that actually displaces the depressant from its receptors in the brain, thus immediately terminating the action of the depressant. Such a drug might save thousands of lives each year, for example, in the treatment of persons who have attempted suicide with CNS depressants (sleeping pills). Treatment of those persons is, at present, difficult.

Third, clinical experience indicates that general depressants exert a depressant action on *all neurons* within the brain. However, it is well known that low doses of these compounds induce behavioral excitement—a state that is often sought when a person wants to "get loaded" or "get drunk." The excitement is thought to be caused by a depression of inhibitory neurons within the brain that leaves the person in a state of *disinhibition*. Because alcohol often induces euphoria, we occasionally find alcohol classified mistakenly as a stimulant rather than as a depressant. It is believed that low doses of alcohol (or other depressants) cause inhibitory synapses in the brain to become depressed slightly earlier than are excitatory synapses. If inhibition is depressed, behavioral excitation is observed, because all neurons within the brain are held in a close balance between excitation and inhibition. This mechanism would appear to account for the euphoria induced by low doses of sedative-hypnotic drugs. At higher doses, however, excitatory synapses also become depressed and sleep follows.

Fourth, in general, behavioral depression induced by a single dose of depressant drug is seldom followed by a period of either mental or behavioral hyperexcitability after the drug action is terminated. As the drug is metabolized and excreted, the person slowly reverts from a drug-depressed state to a normal one. However, if large doses of depressants are *repeatedly* administered over a prolonged period of time, the depression induced is followed by a period of hyperexcitability, which, upon withdrawal of the drug, may be quite severe and might even lead to convulsions and death. These agents, therefore, are capable of inducing physiological dependence.

Fifth, use of any CNS depressant carries with it the inherent risk of inducing psychological dependence and tolerance. The tolerance is secondary both to the induction of drug-metabolizing enzymes in the liver (so that the drug is metabolized more rapidly) and to the adaptation of cells in the brain (so that the cells can function in the presence of the drug). In such instances, neurons become tolerant to the presence of the drug, and larger doses must be administered to obtain a given behavioral effect.

In addition, a remarkable degree of *cross-tolerance* may occur. Cross-tolerance is a condition in which tolerance to one drug results in a lessened response to another drug. *Cross-dependence*, too, may be exhibited. Cross-dependence is a condition in which one drug can prevent the withdrawal symptoms that are associated with physical dependence on a different drug. Essentially, any CNS depressant can substitute for any other CNS depressant, regardless of its chemical structure.

Historical Background

The use of depressants is as old as history, and alcohol is the oldest of these agents. It was not until 1912 that phenobarbital was introduced into medicine as a sedative drug. Since that time, approximately 50 other barbiturates have been marketed at one time or another.

The barbiturates (together with older agents, such as bromide and chloral hydrate) were the only sedatives available until the early

1950s, when meprobamate (Equanil) was introduced as a tranquilizer. Then, around 1960, chlordiazepoxide (Librium) became the first available benzodiazepine tranquilizer. This compound and the other benzodiazepine derivatives are similar in many ways to the general depressants. However, they also exert specific effects on inhibitory neurotransmission (discussed in Chapter 5), which are independent of the nonspecific depression that is observed at higher doses.

Site and Mechanism of Action

The barbiturates, the nonbarbiturate sedative-hypnotics, and ethyl alcohol all reversibly depress the activity of all excitable tissue, including that of the CNS, which is exquisitely sensitive.[1] Such sensitivity follows from the observation that *for normal doses* of these compounds, the polysynaptic, diffuse brain stem pathways that are involved in wakefulness are the first to be affected. More specifically, the behavioral-depressant action of these compounds appears to result from depression of the polysynaptic pathways that are located within the arousal centers in the brain: the ascending reticular activating system (the ARAS) of the brain stem and the diffuse thalamic projection system of the medial thalamus. Because these compounds depress synaptic transmission, one would expect that pathways with many synapses would be especially susceptible to drug-induced depression. In fact, physiological studies have demonstrated that the ARAS and the diffuse thalamic projection system are composed of multitudes of such polysynaptic pathways, which accounts for the unusual sensitivity of these areas to depressant drugs[2]. In addition, the inhibition of synaptic transmission within these areas appears to be mediated by the inhibitory neurotransmitter gamma-aminobutyric acid (GABA; discussed in Chapter 5). Barbiturates may thus facilitate GABA activity in these polysynaptic pathways (in a manner similar to, yet distinct from, the action exhibited by the benzodiazepine tranquilizers on GABA neurons.[2,3]

Depression of synaptic transmission processes within these centers appears to account for the various stages of behavioral depression that are induced by the barbiturate and nonbarbiturate sedatives. The mechanism of action of the general anesthetics is, however, quite different (discussed later in this chapter).

Uses

The medical use of both the barbiturates and the nonbarbiturate sedatives has declined rapidly in recent years for several reasons: (1) they lack selective CNS action; (2) they are inherently less "safe" than the benzodiazepine sedatives (Chapter 5); (3) their potential for inducing tolerance and dependence is great; and (4) they interact dangerously with many other drugs. Despite these factors, the barbiturates continue to be used as anticonvulsants (for example, phenobarbital) in the management of epilepsy (Chapter 13), as intravenous anesthetics (for example, thiopental) for the induction of a state of clinical anesthesia, as sedatives in psychiatry (for example, the "amytal interview"), and to help protect the brain after severe head injury (by depressing neuronal activity and by reducing intracranial pressure).

Several limitations restrict the use of sedatives. These compounds are *not* analgesic and, therefore, they are not used for the relief of pain. In addition, their depressant action on the brain stem can interfere fatally with respiration, especially when they are used intravenously or in suicide attempts. These and other problems associated with these drugs (dependence, tolerance, and loss of coordination) are discussed in the following sections.

Drug-Induced "Brain Syndrome"

In certain psychiatric and neurological disorders, such as the dementias, a behavioral pattern that is characteristic of depressed nerve function is observed. To diagnose drug-induced "brain syndrome" and other psychiatric disorders, a mental status examination that encompasses 12 areas of mental function is performed (Table 3.1).

Different psychiatric disorders cause patients to manifest differing deficits in this examination. Schizophrenics, for example, have an intact sensorium, adequate memory and behavior; are cooperative; and may speak with a normal stream of talk. Their mental status examination is characterized by disturbed thought processes with an absence of logic and, frequently, with misperceptions of reality. (The pathological processes that are possibly involved in patients who suffer from schizophrenia are discussed further in Chapter 10).

In instances where a person's neurons are *reversibly* depressed by alcohol (Chapter 4), nonselective depressants or benzodiazepine tranquilizers (Chapter 5), or when a patient's neurons are irreversibly lost

TABLE 3.1

The mental status examination. Twelve areas of mental function.

1. General appearance
2. Sensorium:
   a. orientation to time, place, and person
   b. clear vs. clouded
3. Behavior and mannerisms
4. Stream of talk
5. Cooperativeness
6. Mood: inner feelings
7. Affect: surface expression of feelings
8. Perception
   a. illusions: misperception of reality
   b. hallucinations: not present in reality
9. Thought processes: logical vs. strange or bizarre
10. Mental content: fund of knowledge
11. Intellectual functions: ability to reason and interpret
12. Insight and judgment

(as in dementia), 5 of the 12 functions of the mental status examination are particularly altered (sensorium, affect, mental content, intellectual function, and insight and judgment). The person's sensorium becomes clouded, which causes disorientation in terms of time and place; memory becomes impaired, which is evidenced by forgetfulness and loss of short-term memory; the intellect becomes depressed, and judgment is altered. The person's affect becomes shallow and labile; that is, he or she becomes extremely vulnerable to external stimuli and may be sullen and moody at one moment and exhibit mock anger at the next. When such a mental status is seen, it is diagnosed as a "brain syndrome" secondary to depressed nerve-cell function.

Certain persons (such as the elderly) who already have some natural loss of nerve-cell function are more likely to be adversely affected by these drugs. A person whose sensorium is partially clouded or who is already somewhat disoriented will become even more so when he or she takes these drugs. The net result is increased disorientation and further clouding of consciousness. Frequently, these persons exhibit a state of drug-induced "paradoxical excitement," which is characterized by a labile personality with marked anger, delusions, hallucinations, and confabulations. The treatment of such a drug-induced disorder is discontinuation of the sedative drug.

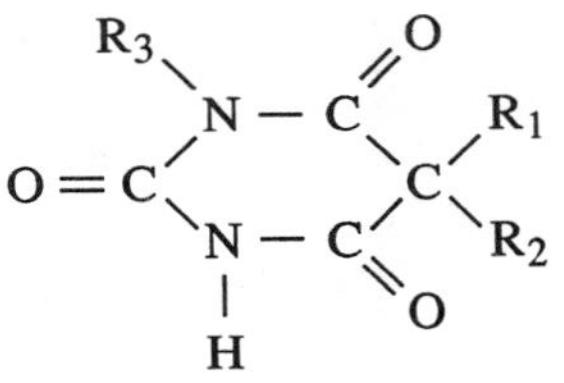

General formula

$$R_3-N-C-C(R_1)(R_2)-...$$

(or S^*=) $O=C$ ... $N-C=O$

Drug name					Half-life		Uses		
Trade	Generic	R_1	R_2	R_3	Distribution (minutes)	Elimination (hours)	Insomnia	Anesthesia	Epilepsy
Amytal	Amobarbital	Ethyl	Isopentyl	H		10–40	X		
Alurate	Aprobarbital	Allyl	Isopentyl	H		12–34	X		
Butisol	Butabarbital	Ethyl	sec-Butyl	H		34–42	X		
Mebaral	Mephobarbital	Ethyl	Phenyl	CH$_3$		50–120			X
Brevital	Methohexital	Allyl	1-methyl 2-pentynyl	CH$_3$		1–2		X	
Nembutal	Pentobarbital	Ethyl	Methyl butyl	H		15–50	X		
Luminal	Phenobarbital	Ellyl	Phenyl	H		24–120	X		X
Seconal	Secobarbital	Allyl	Methyl butyl	H		15–40	X		
Lotusate	Talbutal	Allyl	sec-Butyl	H			X		
Surital	Thiamylal	Allyl	Methyl butyl	H				X	
Pentothal	Thiopental	Ethyl	Methyl butyl	H	3	3–6		X	

*O=, except in thiamylal and thiopental, where it is replaced by S=.

FIGURE 3.2

Structures, half-lives, and uses of some barbiturates

The Barbiturates

The barbiturates comprise a group of compounds (Figure 3.2) that are capable of producing all degrees of behavioral depression, varying from mild sedation, through anesthesia, to coma and death (Figure 3.1). The exact effect depends on several factors: the particular agent in question; the dose; the route of administration; the behavioral state of the person when the drug is administered; and the rates of absorption, distribution, metabolism, and excretion. Thus, the effects will vary over a wide range of doses. Furthermore, the handling of the various barbiturates by the body determines the onset, intensity, and duration of the drug's effect.

Pharmacokinetics

Barbiturates traditionally have been subclassified into compounds that have varying durations of action. As shown in Figure 3.2, their half-lives can be quite short (a 3-minute redistribution half-life for thiopental), longer (a 24- to 48-hour elimination half-life for amobarbital, pentobarbital, and secobarbital), and very long (an 80- to 100-hour elimination half-life for phenobarbital). The reader may recall from Chapter 1 that the action of ultrashort-acting barbiturates (such as thiopental) is essentially terminated by redistribution, while the action of other barbiturates is terminated by the processes of metabolism and excretion.

When taken orally, barbiturates exist in the stomach in a fat-soluble form. Thus, they are rapidly and completely absorbed into the bloodstream. The ultra-short-acting barbiturates (for example, thiopental and methohexital) are administered intravenously as general anesthetics. Note, however, that such injection is only performed by experts and in surroundings where adequate provisions have been made for supporting the patient's respiration and circulation (and, therefore, life), because intravenous doses usually depress breathing for several minutes.

The barbiturates are well distributed to most body tissues. Thiopental and methohexital are very soluble in fat and, therefore, penetrate the blood-brain barrier easily and rapidly. As a result, these compounds induce sleep very quickly (usually within seconds). The longer-acting barbiturates, by contrast, exist in blood in a more water-soluble form. Thus, it is slightly more difficult for them to penetrate the blood-brain barrier. Sleep induction with these compounds, therefore, is delayed, and a drug-induced "hangover" is prominent (especially since the plasma half-lives of most of these drugs vary from 10 to 48 hours). Further, they are unpredictable as a result of individual variation.

The duration of action of barbiturates is determined by three processes: redistribution, metabolism, and excretion. Within a few minutes after thiopental or methohexital is administered, the drug rapidly leaves the brain (so its action is cut short) and is redistributed to muscle and fat deposits, such as adipose tissue. It is then slowly metabolized by specialized enzymes that are located in the liver, and its metabolic by-products are excreted by the kidneys. Thus, people who have been sedated or anesthetized with thiopental or methohexital may find that they are groggy for several hours afterward, even though they awaken within a very few minutes. This grogginess is caused by the low levels of the drug that remain in the bloodstream while it is being slowly metabolized and excreted. Although the drug is still present, its concentration in the brain is not high enough to induce sleep or anesthesia. Because the longer-acting barbiturates are more water-soluble, they remain in plasma in concentrations that are sufficient to keep the person sedated or drowsy until the drug has been metabolized and excreted.

Urinalysis is being used more commonly to screen for the presence of barbiturates and other psychoactive drugs of use and abuse. Depending on the specific barbiturate that a person has taken, positive tests will be found during a period of time that may be as short as 30 hours or as long as several weeks after the drug was ingested. When urinalysis is found to be positive for barbiturates, more specific confirmation is needed to determine the exact drug that was taken.

Thus, in summary, three processes are responsible for the termination of the depressant action of the barbiturates: *redistribution* to the muscle and fat, *metabolism* by the liver, and *excretion* by the kidneys. The process of redistribution has primary importance in terminating the hypnosis that is induced by thiopental and methohexital, while excretion by the kidneys (following metabolism of the drug by the liver) is essential for terminating the hypnotic action of the longer-acting compounds.

Pharmacological Effects

At normal doses, the nonselective depressant action of barbiturates is largely restricted to polysynaptic pathways in the CNS.
According to Rall:

The barbiturates possess a low degree of selectivity and therapeutic index. Thus, it is not possible to achieve a desired effect without evidence of general depression of the CNS. Pain perception and reaction are relatively unimpaired until the moment of unconsciousness, and in small doses the barbiturates increase the reaction to painful stimuli. Hence they cannot be relied upon to produce sedation or sleep in the presence of even moderate pain. In some individuals and in some circumstances, such as the presence of pain, barbiturates cause overt excitement instead of sedation.[2]

This state of overt excitement is caused by the brain syndrome that is induced by the drugs; and the extent of the excitement varies, depending on the person and the circumstances in which the drugs were taken.

Sleep is significantly affected by the use of barbiturates. The initial brain-wave (EEG) alterations that are induced by the barbiturates resemble a high-voltage, low-frequency pattern that is characteristic of slow-wave sleep. Rapid eye movement (REM) sleep is absent. Because dreaming occurs during REM sleep and is largely absent during slow-wave sleep, barbiturate-induced sleep differs from normal sleep. The time spent in REM sleep is greatly reduced and dreaming is suppressed. In fact, some postulate that this absence of REM sleep (with loss of dreaming) may be harmful and may even be capable of precipitating psychotic episodes. Persons who are deprived of REM sleep exhibit an increase in the proportion of time they spend in REM sleep after they have stopped taking barbiturates (one example of a withdrawal effect following prolonged periods of drug ingestion).

As already stated, drowsiness (or a "hangover") usually follows the use of a barbiturate. This condition may appear to last for only a few hours, but more subtle alterations of judgment, motor skills, and behavior may persist for hours or days until the compound is completely eliminated.

The effects of barbiturates on respiration are minimal when they are taken at sedative doses, but they result in death when an overdose is taken. Barbiturates appear to have no significant effects on the cardiovascular system, the gastrointestinal tract, the kidneys, or other organs until toxic doses are reached. In the liver, barbiturates stimulate the synthesis of enzymes that metabolize these as well as other drugs—an effect that produces a degree of tolerance to such drugs.

Psychological Effects
Many of the behavioral effects that are caused by the use of barbiturates are quite similar to those caused by alcohol-induced inebriation and

may even be indistinguishable from them. Barbiturates may initially produce behavioral disinhibition and a mild state of euphoria, presumably by depressing central inhibitory synapses. As with alcohol, however, a person may react by withdrawing, by becoming emotionally depressed, or by becoming aggressive and violent. Higher doses (or low doses combined with another depressant) lead to behavioral depression and sleep.

The person's mental set and his or her physical or social setting can determine whether relief from anxiety, mental depression, aggression, or other unexpected or unpredictable responses are experienced.

An additional behavioral effect of consequence is the ataxia (staggering) and loss of motor coordination that may accompany a person's use of barbiturates or other depressant drugs. For instance, driving skills will be severely impaired by a person's use of barbiturates, and this effect should be considered a predictable and inseparable consequence. The effects of barbiturates are additive with the effects produced by any other depressant compound (including alcohol) that may be in the blood. Thus, the behavior of a person who normally can tolerate a given dose of a barbiturate might be noticeably affected if he or she also ingests alcohol or another depressant. Such additive effects might lead to serious consequences if the person tries to drive a car, for example. When barbiturates are combined with relatively large amounts of alcohol, profound depression is induced. Numerous accidental overdoses, leading to respiratory failure and death, have resulted from such combinations.

Adverse Reactions

SIDE EFFECTS AND TOXICITY.   Drowsiness is one of the primary effects induced by the use of barbiturates, and, obviously, such drowsiness is often the effect a person seeks. Quite frequently, however, persons who take a barbiturate to induce a state of disinhibition or relief from anxiety also find that drowsiness follows.

Another side effect of the barbiturates is impaired motor and intellectual performance and judgment. As one author stated:

> A person need not be rendered staggering drunk before his motor performance and, probably more important, his judgment are significantly impaired. The most common offending agent in this regard is alcohol. . . . At this time it should be emphasized that all

sedatives are equivalent to alcohol in their effects; that all are additive in their effects with alcohol; and that their effects persist longer than might be predicted.[4]

Other side effects are usually minor and include such occurrences as slight decreases in blood pressure and heart rate (as occur during natural sleep) and hangover.

TOLERANCE.   The barbiturates are capable of inducing tolerance by two mechanisms: (1) the induction of metabolizing enzymes in the liver and (2) the adaptation of neurons in the brain to the presence of the drug. As a consequence of the first mechanism, more of the drug would be required to maintain a given level of the drug in the body. In other words, more of the drug would be needed to achieve the same concentration of the drug at the receptor and, therefore, to achieve the same effect. As a consequence of the second mechanism, more of the drug would have to be presented to the receptor in order to interact with it to the same level, because the drug receptors within the brain are capable of adapting to the presence of barbiturates.

A person who takes barbiturates does not develop tolerance to *all* of their effects. The tolerance we have described is primarily restricted to the sedative effects. The respiratory centers in the brainstem apparently *do not* develop tolerance to the presence of barbiturates to the same degree as do the receptors mediating the other effects. Thus, the risks associated with the respiratory depressant effect of the drug would progressively *increase* as tolerance to the behavioral effects develops; in essence, the margin of safety for the person who uses the drug would decrease. Thus, a person who uses increasingly larger doses of barbiturates takes the risk of reaching a dose that may be severely toxic.

PHYSICAL DEPENDENCE.   Barbiturates induce physical dependence. Withdrawal symptoms appear when administration of the drug is stopped. Physical dependence on the barbiturates is in some respects similar to that induced by the opiate narcotics (see Chapter 9), but it differs in two important respects. First, the dose of a barbiturate that is required to induce physical dependence is much higher than the dose usually required to induce sleep. For example, approximately 100 milligrams of pentobarbital (Nembutal) will induce sleep. Serious physical tolerance does not develop until, (as tolerance builds) the patient reaches daily dosages of 800 milligrams or more. Also, it is usually only after such large doses that removal of the drug leads to *serious* and possibly lethal withdrawal symptoms. This is not to say, however, that normal doses of barbiturates do not produce some degree of physical dependence and withdrawal symptoms when discontinued, but such symptoms are not usually serious or life-threatening. One prominent symptom is an increase in the amount of REM sleep, with a concomitant decrease in the time spent in slow-wave sleep. Thus, dreaming increases markedly, and the person experiencing this symptom may have difficulty sleeping. Indeed, vivid dreams and nightmares can result in significant deprivation of restful sleep after the use of barbiturate has been discontinued. In contrast, withdrawal from *high doses* of barbiturates may result in hallucinations, restlessness, disorientation, and life-threatening convulsions.

PSYCHOLOGICAL DEPENDENCE.   Psychological dependence refers to a compulsion to use a drug for a pleasurable effect. All nonselective depressants are apt to be abused compulsively, and the one that is most abused is alcohol. Because they are capable of relieving anxiety, inducing sedation, and producing a state of euphoria, these drugs may be used to achieve a variety of psychological states. Many persons in our society (especially older people) also appear to be psychologically dependent on the hypnotic effect of the barbiturates and the nonbarbiturate sedatives.

EFFECTS IN PREGNANCY.   As discussed in Chapter 1, psychoactive drugs are readily transferred from the mother to the fetus through the placenta. This distribution implies that barbiturates administered to a mother will also depress her fetus at the time of delivery. Drugs taken by mothers within a day or two before delivery are found in the newborn baby in significant concentrations. Also, because the newborn has limited metabolizing and excreting systems, it may be depressed for a significant period of time after delivery. Thus, it is prudent to avoid the use of barbiturates and other sedatives within a few days of delivery. One exception involves the administration of ultrashort-acting barbiturates to induce general anesthesia when an emergency cesarean section must be performed.

Aside from the depressant effects of sedatives when they are administered to mothers near the time of delivery, we must also be concerned about drug administration throughout the entire nine months of pregnancy. The congenital malformations that can occur when drugs are used during the first trimester of pregnancy are especially important. Data concerning the barbiturates are controversial because congenital problems have been reported in the offspring of epileptic mothers who take antiepileptic medications (including barbiturates) during pregnancy. In this situation, however, it is felt that the benefit to the pregnant epileptic mother continuing her medication during pregnancy outweighs the rare occurrence of congenital abnormalities. Unless strictly indicated, though, these drugs should be avoided during pregnancy.

Nonbarbiturate Hypnotics

During the early 1950s, two nonbarbiturate sedatives, *glutethimide* (Doriden) and *methyprylon* (Noludar), were introduced as new drugs to produce sedation and sleep. Their chemical structures were virtually identical to those of the barbiturates, they exhibited few advantages, and they had little to justify their widespread use.

Although structurally dissimilar to glutethimide and methyprylon, *ethchlorvynol* (Placidyl) was a third nonselective depressant in widespread use. It had an intermediate duration of action, with a 1- to 3-hour distribution half-life and a 10- to 24-hour elimination half-life. Drug interactions were common and withdrawal from the drug was difficult. None of these agents is used much today.

Methaqualone (Quaalude) was another nonbarbiturate depressant that had little to justify its widespread use. During the late 1970s and early 1980s, use of methaqualone rose dramatically until it became one of the leading drugs of abuse, trailing only marijuana and alcohol in its level of abuse. Such attention was due to its undeserved reputation as an aphrodisiac, which reputation created such illicit use and so many fatalities that the manufacturer stopped its production and removed it from the market in 1984. Pharmacologically, methaqualone was similar to the barbiturates in its effects and, as might be expected, was actually an anaphrodisiac. It appeared that the effects of mental set, physical setting, and personal expectation were more potent than the drug's pharmacological effects. Methaqualone, far from being a "love drug," was merely one of several nonselective depressants that were thought to affect the user favorably when they were taken in the right setting and with a particular set of expectations.[5]

Meprobamate (Equanil, Miltown) was introduced as an antianxiety agent in 1955, offering a therapeutic alternative to the barbiturates for daytime sedation and relief from anxiety. Around it developed the term *tranquilizer* to distinguish meprobamate from the barbiturates, a distinction that, with meprobamate, appeared to be more theoretical than real. It produces long-lasting daytime sedation, mild euphoria, and relief from anxiety; higher doses induce sleep. Unlike the benzodiazepines (Chapter 5), it is not a selective antianxiety agent and it exhibits no striking clinical advantages. Meprobamate has a long duration of action and the sedation it induces lasts for 10 hours or longer. Its half life is between 6 and 17 hours. Unfortunately, meprobamate may exert untoward effects on fetal development. Therefore, it should be avoided during pregnancy, especially during the first trimester.

In general, meprobamate and the barbiturates induce the same pharmacological and toxicological effects. Tolerance, physical dependence, and psychological dependence can be induced to approximately the same extent. Because meprobamate is not as potent as a respiratory depressant as the barbiturates, its margin of safety may be greater. Successful suicide following the ingestion of meprobamate is rare. Despite a continued reduction in clinical use, abuse and dependency continue to be widespread and difficult to treat.[6]

Chloral hydrate is a drug that is rapidly metabolized to trichlorethanol (a derivative of ethyl alcohol). Trichlorethanol, which is a nonselective CNS depressant, is the pharmacologically active form of chloral hydrate. It has been noted that REM sleep is not greatly depressed by chloral hydrate, and REM rebound does not occur when its use is discontinued. Chloral hydrate appears to be a relatively safe and effective sedative-hypnotic, with a plasma half-life of about 4 to 8 hours. Hangover is less likely to occur than with compounds that have longer half-lives. Its liability in producing tolerance and dependence is similar to that of the barbiturates. One interesting side note about chloral hydrate is the popular belief that its combination with alcohol results in a supra-additive effect, leading to a loss of consciousness. Thus, adding chloral hydrate to alcohol produces a "Mickey Finn." Certainly the two drugs are additive in their effects and, indeed, a supra-additive effect is not beyond possibility and is even likely.

General Anesthetics

General anesthesia, a behavioral state on the continuum of depression illustrated in Figure 3.1, is the most severe state of intentional drug-induced depression. Beyond general anesthesia in this continuum, only coma and death occur. Thus, the induction of general anesthesia with depressant drugs is a serious undertaking and should be performed only by competent persons.

The agents that are used as general anesthetics differ widely in physical properties and chemical structure. They vary in a range from gas (nitrous oxide), to volatile liquids (isoflurane, halothane, and enflurane), to drugs in solutions that are intended for intravenous administration (thiopental, methohexital, propofol, and etomidate). The gases and volatile liquids are administered by inhalation through the lungs; the other anesthetics are injected directly into the bloodstream.

General anesthetics (like the other nonselective depressants) produce a generalized, graded, dose-related depression of all functions of the CNS. Thus, their pharmacological effects are similar to those observed with the barbiturates: an initial period of sedation, relief from anxiety, and disinhibition, followed by the onset of sleep. As anesthesia deepens, the patient's reflexes become progressively depressed and analgesia is induced. At that point, a patient is said to be anesthetized. Deepening of anesthesia results in loss of reflexes, depression of both respiration and brain excitability—a state of deep anesthesia.

Of the injectable anesthetics, thiopental and methohexital (ultra-short-acting barbiturates) are the most widely used. Propofol (Diprovan) and etomidate (Amidate) are used as alternatives in special situations. The mechanism of action of the latter two anesthetics is probably the same as that of the barbiturates, that is, nonselective CNS depression produced secondary to depression of synaptic transmission in polysynaptic pathways in the brain.

The mechanism of action of the inhalation anesthetics is quite different from the synaptic depressant actions of either injectable anesthetics or the barbiturates. The inhaled general anesthetics appear to act directly on nerve membranes rather than acting at synaptic junctions between cells. Theories about the action of these drugs correlate anesthetic action with the lipid (fat or oil) solubility of each drug (Figure 3.3). In Figure 3.3, anesthetic potency correlates directly with the oil-to-gas partition coefficient (with a higher figure representing increased solubility in lipid). This correlation means that anesthetic gases are highly soluble in nerve membranes, because nerve membranes are high in lipid content. Anesthetic theory holds that when one of these drugs dissolves in the nerve membranes, the structure of the lipid matrix of the membranes becomes distorted, thereby perturbing the function of the ion channels and the membrane proteins. Thus, nerve function is depressed and a state of clinical anesthesia is produced. Upon discontinuation of anesthesia, the anesthetic leaves the nerve membranes (the

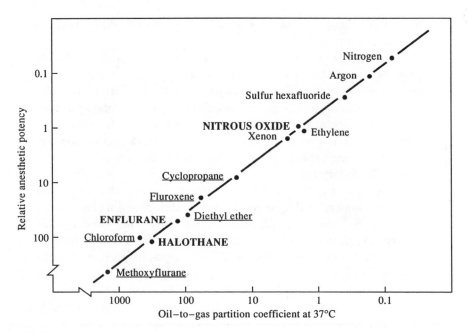

FIGURE 3.3

The correlation of anesthetic potency with the oil-to-gas partition coefficient. The correlation is shown for a number of general anesthetic agents and for other inert gases that are not usually used for anesthesia. Note the log scales and the excellent correlation over a very wide range of fat solubilities and potencies. Agents that are used today in anesthesia are shown in **boldface** capital letters. Agents that were used *formerly* as anesthetics are underscored. [Modified from S. K. Kennedy and D. E. Longnecker,[1] p. 282.]

anesthetic is absorbed back into the bloodstream and is exhaled through the lungs), and normal membrane structure and function return.

Occasionally, certain anesthetic agents become misused drugs. Nitrous oxide, a gas of low anesthetic potency, is an example. At a 50-percent concentration, nitrous oxide induces a state of behavioral disinhibition, analgesia, and mild euphoria. Since at least 50 percent of the inhaled gas mixture must consist of nitrous oxide for it to be effective, extreme caution must be exercised. Unless at least 21 percent oxygen is inhaled (room air is 21 percent oxygen), hypoxia (decreased oxygen content of the blood) will result. In order to achieve a 50-percent concentration of nitrous oxide, room air is inadequate as a diluent; the nitrous oxide must be mixed in an air-oxygen blender so that a minimum oxygen concentration of 21 percent is maintained. If the nitrous oxide were to be mixed with room air only, hypoxia would result, which would produce irreversible brain damage.

Within the last few years, other forms of recreational anesthesia with accompanying hypoxia, that are induced by the inhalation of such substances as glue, gasoline, and so on, have been encountered. The volatile hydrocarbons in these products are capable of inducing a general anesthesia. Thus, when these products are administered by people who are not aware of the dangers, hypoxia or depression of respiration from too deep a level of anesthesia may occasionally result in death. Other toxicities that involve the liver as well as as other vital body organs have also been reported.

STUDY QUESTIONS

1. List the various classes of nonselective CNS depressants, and give examples of each class.
2. Describe the gradation of action that occurs in a person as a result of taking progressively increasing doses of a nonselective CNS depressant.
3. Describe what is meant by *supra-additive CNS depression*.
4. Describe the two types of drug tolerance that can develop as a result of repeated use of barbiturates.
5. Describe the mechanism of action of nonselective CNS depressants.
6. What is meant by *drug-induced, reversible brain syndrome?*
7. What mechanisms are responsible for the differing durations of action (and, therefore, classification by duration) of various barbiturates?
8. Describe the effects of barbiturates on sleep patterns both acutely and during drug withdrawal.
9. Compare the effects of barbiturates and chloral hydrate on the elderly.
10. Compare the mechanism of action of barbiturates with that of an inhaled general anesthetic.

NOTES

1. T. W. Rall, "Hypnotics and Sedatives: Ethanol," in A. G. Gilman, T. W. Rall, A. S. Nies, and P. Taylor, eds., *Goodman and Gilman's The Pharmacological Basis of Therapeutics*, 8th ed. (New York: Pergamon, 1990), p. 345.

2. T. W. Rall, "Hypnotics and Sedatives: Ethanol," in A. G. Gilman, T. W. Rall, A. S. Nies, and P. Taylor, eds., *Goodman and Gilman's The Pharmacological Basis of Therapeutics*, 8th ed. (New York: Pergamon, 1990), p. 358–360.

3. R. W. Olsen, "GABA-Drug Interactions," *Progress in Drug Research* 31(1987): 224–238.

4. H. Meyers, E. Jawetz, and A. Goldfien, *Review of Medical Pharmacology*, 3d ed. (Los Altos, Calif.: Lange Medical Publications, 1972), p. 219.

5. C. V. Wetli, "Changing Patterns of Methaqualone Abuse," Journal *of the American Medical Association* 249 (1983): 621.

6. J. D. Roache and R. R. Griffiths, "Lorazepam and Meprobamate Dose Effects in Humans: Behavioral Effects and Abuse Liability," *Journal of Pharmacology and Experimental Therapeutics* 243 (1987): 978.

Alcohol

The Most Popular Drug

When we use the term *alcohol* we mean ethyl alcohol (ethanol)—a psychoactive drug that is similar in most respects to the sedative-hypnotic compounds (discussed in Chapter 3). Thus, ethyl alcohol is classified as a general nonselective CNS depressant. It differs from the other depressants in that it is used primarily for social or recreational purposes rather than for medical reasons. Because it is one of the most widely used of all drugs, alcohol has created special problems both for individual users and for society in general.

How Alcohol Is Handled by the Body: Pharmacokinetics

Alcohol is absorbed, distributed, metabolized, and excreted in certain specific ways by the body.

Absorption

Alcohol is a simple molecule that contains two carbon atoms; a hydroxyl (OH) group is attached to one of those carbons (Figure 4.1). The molecule is very soluble in both water and fat, and it diffuses easily through biological membranes. Thus, it is rapidly and completely ab-

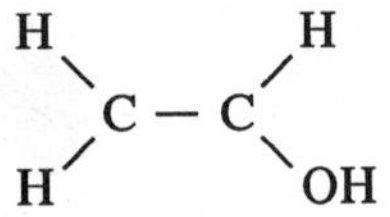

FIGURE 4.1

Structure of ethanol.

sorbed from the entire gastrointestinal tract. Because it is already in liquid form, alcohol does not have to dissolve in the stomach (as does a drug that is in tablet form).

The rate of absorption can be modified in various ways. In a person who has an empty stomach, approximately 20 percent of a single dose of alcohol is absorbed directly from the stomach, usually quite rapidly. The remaining 80 percent is absorbed rapidly and completely from the upper intestine; the only limiting factor is the time it takes to empty the stomach. If a person drinks alcohol on a full stomach, gastric emptying is delayed, and the rapid absorption that usually occurs in the upper intestine is slowed. Thus, blood levels of alcohol will increase much faster in a person who has fasted than in someone who has just eaten a large meal. In either case, however, the alcohol will still be completely absorbed eventually.

Distribution

Because alcohol is a small molecule that is soluble in both water and fat, it is evenly distributed throughout all body fluids and tissues. This feature forms the basis for breath analysis tests, because alcohol equilibrates rapidly across the membranes of the lungs, which separate air from the blood. Thus, small amounts of alcohol are excreted from the body through the lungs. Most of us are familiar with the "alcohol breath" that results from this exhalation of alcohol.

The blood-brain barrier is freely permeable to alcohol. Indeed, entry rates that are as high as 90 percent have been found in persons who drink alcohol. In other words, when alcohol that is consumed appears in the blood and reaches the person's brain, 90 percent of it crosses the blood-brain barrier immediately. This high rate of entry implies that there is little hindrance to the penetration of alcohol into the brain.

Alcohol is also freely distributed from a pregnant woman's blood to the fetus. It crosses both the placenta and the infant's blood-brain barrier rapidly and easily. Fetal alcohol levels become the same as those of the drinking mother. Alcohol can be detected on a baby's breath at birth, in amniotic fluid during pregnancy, and in the baby's blood. Research on the impact of maternal alcohol consumption on human infants has demonstrated the occurrence of a *fetal alcohol syndrome*, which consists of serious birth defects in 30 to 50 percent of babies who are born to alcoholic mothers. The fetal alcohol syndrome can result when alcohol is ingested by a pregnant woman at critical times during embryonic development.[1] This syndrome is discussed more completely in the section on side effects and toxicities of alcohol.

Metabolism

Approximately 95 percent of the alcohol that a person ingests is metabolized before it is excreted. Most metabolism of alcohol (about 85 percent) occurs in the liver, but a small, variable amount (up to 15 percent) occurs in the stomach.[2] Indeed, gastric (stomach) metabolism significantly decreases the amount of alcohol that is available to be absorbed, which attentuates its systemic toxicity. Recently, Frezza and coworkers[3] reported that when women and men consume comparable amounts of alcohol in terms of their respective body weights, the women have higher blood ethanol concentrations than do the men. Such elevations are caused by reduced alcohol metabolism and gastric alcohol dehydrogenase enzyme activity in both alcoholic and nonalcoholic women. These factors may contribute to the enhanced vulnerability of women to both acute intoxication and chronic complications of alcoholism.

Once alcohol is absorbed, the metabolism of alcohol in the liver occurs by a two-step process. The first step is initiated by the enzyme *alcohol dehydrogenase*, which converts alcohol to acetaldehyde. Acetaldehyde is converted to acetyl-CoA by the enzyme *aldehyde dehydrogenase*, and it is ultimately broken down into carbon dioxide and water, with the release of energy (calories). Other than providing calories, alcohol has no nutritional value. The small amount (5 percent) that is not metabolized is excreted unchanged, primarily in the urine and through the lungs.

The rate of metabolism of alcohol in the liver is unusual because it is independent of the concentration of alcohol in the blood, and it is linear with time. In an adult, the metabolic rate is approximately 10 milliliters (one-third ounce) of 100-percent ethanol per hour. In other words, it would take an adult 1 hour to metabolize the amount of alcohol that is contained in a 1-ounce glass of 80-proof whiskey (about 40 percent ethanol), a 4-ounce glass of wine, or a 12-ounce bottle of beer. Alcohol is metabolized slowly, constantly, and independently of the amount that a person ingests. Consumption of 4 ounces of wine, 12 ounces of beer, or 1 ounce of whiskey per hour would keep the blood levels of alcohol in a person fairly constant. Thus, if a person ingests more alcohol in any given hour than is metabolized, his or her blood concentrations will increase. This occurrence demonstrates that there is a limit to the amount of alcohol that a person can consume in an hour without becoming drunk as a result of the accumulation of alcohol in the blood.

Factors that may alter this predictable rate of metabolism of alcohol are usually not clinically significant. With long-term use, however, alcohol is capable of inducing drug-metabolizing enzymes in the liver, thereby increasing its own rate of metabolism (*inducing tolerance*) as well as the rate of metabolism of other compounds that are similarly metabolized by the liver (*cross-tolerance*).

Mention should be made here of disulfiram (Antabuse), a drug that is frequently used to treat chronic alcoholism. Disulfiram inhibits aldehyde dehydrogenase, the enzyme responsible for the metabolism of acetaldehyde to acetyl-CoA. As a result of such enzyme inhibition, acetaldehyde accumulates in the body, making the patient extremely uncomfortable, with headache, nausea, vomiting, drowsiness, hangover, and so on. Disulfiram makes alcoholics feel so dreadful when they drink that they are discouraged from drinking. According to Rall:

> Disulfiram is not a cure for alcoholism; it merely affords a volunteer a crutch by which the sincere desire to stop drinking can be fortified. The rationale for its use is that the patients know that if they are to avoid the devastating experience of the "acetaldehyde syndrome" they cannot drink for at least 3–4 days after taking disulfiram.[4]

Excretion

Approximately 95 percent of alcohol that is ingested is metabolized to products that, eventually, are converted to carbon dioxide and water. The remaining 5 percent is excreted unchanged by the kidneys and lungs. Thus, severe alcohol intoxication cannot be treated by increasing the alcoholic's rate of urinary excretion, because so little alcohol is removed from the body by that route. Therefore, it appears that the slow, steady rate of metabolism of the drug by the liver is the only way to detoxify and remove alcohol from the body.

Sites and Mechanism of Action: Pharmacodynamics

Like the sedative-hypnotics, alcohol depresses all the neurons in the brain, producing disorientation, mental clouding, impaired memory, decreased judgment, and labile affect. Such a state, which is often misinterpreted as behavioral stimulation, is similar to the loss of inhibition and induction of euphoria that is characteristic of low doses of all nonselective CNS depressants. It is postulated that neurons in the ARAS are exquisitely sensitive to depression by alcohol, thus inducing a state of disinhibition or mild euphoria.[5,6] Presumably, as a result, the higher centers in the cerebral cortex are released from the inhibitory controls that are exerted on them from the brain stem, which results in impaired thought, impaired organization, and impaired motor processes. A low dose of alcohol may produce mild euphoria, but it also produces a loss of discrimination, fine muscle movement, memory, concentration, control, and so on. The drinker may experience wide fluctuations in mood with frequent emotional outbursts. As the levels of alcohol in the brain are increased, the cerebral cortex becomes depressed and the state of disinhibition or euphoria is progressively lost. Objective testing has clearly demonstrated that alcohol does not increase or improve performance (intellectual, motor, or sexual).

The mechanism of action of alcohol is becoming better understood. Many years ago, it was postulated that alcohol (like the general anesthetics) produced its CNS effects as a result of perturbing neuronal membrane lipids. Such disruption occurs because alcohol readily dissolves in cell membranes (that is, it enters the internal structure of the membranes) and thus distorts their anatomy. More recently, this disordering of membranes has been confirmed, and it is now referred to as *membrane fluidization*. Indeed, the degree of alcohol-induced intoxication can be correlated with the extent of such fluidization of the neuronal membranes.[7,8] The distortion of the fluidized membranes reduces the efficiency of axonal conduction of nerve impulses, reducing the amplitude of the action potential that reaches the synapse, thus indirectly inhibiting both the release of neurotransmitter and synaptic transmission (see Appendix II).

Research interest has been focused on the possibility of a specific action on GABA-, dopamine-, enkephalin-, or serotonin-mediated transmission at the synapse (Appendix III). Although a multitude of actions have been demonstrated, our knowledge in this area remains far from complete.[9]

Pharmacological Effects

The graded, reversible, nonselective depression of CNS function is the primary pharmacological effect of alcohol. Respiration, though transiently stimulated at low doses, becomes progressively depressed and, at very high blood concentrations of alcohol, is the cause of death.

Also like the other sedative-hypnotic compounds, alcohol is an anticonvulsant; it may suppress epileptic convulsions. When an epileptic patient stops drinking alcohol, however, this antiepileptic action may be followed by a prolonged period of hyperexcitability. An alcoholic (whether or not he or she is also epileptic) may have seizures when the drug is withdrawn, with the seizures peaking approximately 8 to 12 hours after the last dose of the drug was taken. Finally, it should be stressed that the effects of alcohol are additive with those of other sedative-hypnotic compounds, resulting in more sedation, greater impairment of driving, or greater impairment of other types of performance than might be expected.

Other sedatives (especially the benzodiazepines) and marijuana are the drugs that are most frequently combined with alcohol, and they increase its deleterious effects on a person's motor and intellectual skills as well as alertness. The combination of alcohol and sedatives may produce supra-additive effects that cause fatal depression of cardiac and respiratory functions. Thus, these combinations can be hazardous and, occasionally, fatal. The combined use of alcohol and other sedatives during the performance of such tasks as driving is extremely dangerous, especially when the hazards are not recognized. Alcohol is a leading cause of acute drug-related deaths.

The effects of alcohol on the circulation and the heart are significant. Alcohol dilates the blood vessels in the skin, producing a warm flush and a decrease in body temperature. Thus, if it is vital to conserve body heat, it is pointless and might even be dangerous to drink alcohol to keep warm when one is exposed to cold weather. Long-term use of alcohol is also associated with diseases of the heart muscle, which result in heart failure. Several reports have noted that low doses of alcohol consumed daily (up to 2.5 ounces) may reduce the risk of coronary artery disease. This protective effect occurs because of an alcohol-induced increase in high-density lipoprotein in blood with a corresponding decrease in low-density lipoprotein. (The higher the concentration of high-density lipoprotein and the lower the concentration of low-density lipoprotein, the lower the incidence of coronary heart disease.)

Unfortunately, the protective effect of low doses of alcohol is lost in persons who also smoke cigarettes.

Liver damage is the most serious long-term consequence of excessive alcohol consumption. Irreversible changes in both its structure and function are common. The significance of alcohol-induced liver dysfunction is illustrated by the fact that 75 percent of all deaths that are attributed to alcoholism are caused by cirrhosis of the liver,[10] and cirrhosis is the seventh most common cause of death in the United States.[11] The mechanism through which alcohol causes cirrhosis appears to be a reflection of alcohol-induced interference with normal body immune functions. Indeed, cirrhosis is a clear indication of the immunosuppressive effect of alcohol.[12]

Alcohol exerts a diuretic effect on the body by increasing the excretion of fluids as a result of its effects on the function of the kidney, by decreasing the secretion of an antidiuretic hormone and by the diuretic action that is simply produced as a result of the large quantities of fluid ordinarily ingested in the form of alcoholic beverages. Alcohol, however, does not appear to harm either the structure or the function of the kidney.

Alcohol (like all depressant drugs) is not an aphrodisiac. In fact, the behavioral disinhibition that is induced by low doses of alcohol may appear to cause some loss of restraint, but alcohol depresses body function and actually interferes with sexual performance. As Shakespeare wrote, "it provokes the desire, but it takes away the performance" (*Macbeth*).

Psychological Effects

The psychological and behavioral effects of alcohol are similar to those of other nonselective CNS depressants. Figure 4.2 correlates the effects of alcohol with levels of the drug measured in the blood. In general, the short-term effects are primarily restricted to the CNS. The behavioral reaction to disinhibition, which occurs at low doses, is unpredictable. It is determined, to a large extent, by the person, his or her mental expectations, and the setting in which the drinking occurs. In one setting a person may become relaxed and euphoric; in another, he or she may become withdrawn or violent. Mental expectations and the physical setting become progressively *less* important at increasing doses, because the sedative effects will increase and behavioral activity will decrease. At low doses, a person may still function (although in a

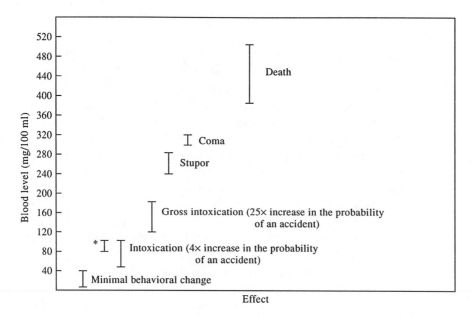

FIGURE 4.2

Correlation of the blood level of ethanol with degrees of intoxication. The legal level of intoxication (*) varies by state; the range of values is shown.

less-coordinated fashion) and attempt to drive or otherwise endanger himself and others. Memory, concentration, and insight are progressively dulled, and then lost. As the dose is increased, the drinker becomes progressively incapacitated.

Convincing data now show that alcohol intoxication, with its resulting disinhibition, plays a major role in a large percentage of violent crimes, including rape, sexual assault, and certain kinds of deviant behaviors.[13] More than 50 percent of crimes and highway accidents are alcohol related.[14]

Long-term effects of alcohol may involve many different organs of a person's body, depending on whether the drinking is *moderate* or *heavy*. It appears that long-term ingestion of moderate amounts of alcohol (approximately two martinis a day) produces few physiological, psychological, or behavioral changes in a person. But long-term ingestion of larger amounts of alcohol leads to a variety of disorders that are associated with serious neurological, mental, and physical deficits. These disorders are included in the description of *alcoholism*. Alcoholism is a multifaceted syndrome that is characterized by chronic, excessive ingestion of alcohol, accompanied by the development of tolerance and dependence.

As stated previously, alcohol is quite caloric but has little nutritional value. Thus, a person may survive for years on a diet of alcohol and not much else, but he or she will suffer slowly, developing vitamin deficiencies and nutritional diseases, which may result in gradual physical deterioration. Indeed, alcohol abuse has been suggested as the most common cause of vitamin and trace element deficiencies in adults.[11]

Tolerance and Dependence

The patterns and mechanisms for the development of tolerance, physical dependence, and psychological dependence on alcohol are similar to those for all the depressant compounds. The extent of tolerance depends on the amount, pattern, and extent of alcohol ingestion. Persons who ingest alcohol only intermittently (on sprees), or more regularly, but in moderation, develop little or no tolerance; persons who regularly ingest large amounts of alcohol develop marked tolerance.

The physical dependence that develops as a result of chronic ingestion of alcohol is such that withdrawal of the drug results in a period of rebound hyperexcitability that may lead to convulsions and even death. Concomitant with this hyperexcitability is a period of tremulousness, with hallucinations, psychomotor agitation, confusion and disorientation, sleep disorders, and a variety of associated discomforts—a syndrome that is sometimes referred to as *delirium tremens* (DTs, rum fits).

Psychological dependence on alcohol also occurs and, indeed, frequently appears to be socially acceptable. This psychological dependence appears to result from the state of disinhibition, relief from anxiety, and euphoria, so that the use of alcohol becomes a compulsive pleasure. Certainly, this psychological attraction to the drug is a major problem to be considered in the treatment of alcoholics or, more widely, in attempts to discourage the recreational misuse of alcohol.

Side Effects and Toxicity

Many of the side effects and toxicities that are associated with the use of alcohol have already been mentioned, but let us summarize and expand on them here. In the acute cases involving use of alcohol, a person's behavior is altered as a result of depression of the function of the CNS, and a reversible drug-induced "brain syndrome" is induced. This syndrome is manifested as a clouded sensorium with disorientation, impaired insight and judgment, amnesia ("blackouts"), and diminished intellectual capabilities. The person's affect may be labile, with vulnerability to external stimuli and expressions of anger. In persons who ingest high doses of alcohol, delusions, hallucinations, and confabulations may occur. Socially, these alterations result in an unpredictable state of disinhibition (drunkenness), alterations in driving performance, and uncoordinated motor behavior.

A variety of chronic toxicities are observed in persons who exhibit chronic alcohol ingestion. Whereas acute intoxication produces a *reversible* brain syndrome that is secondary to a reversible depression of the nerve cells, long-term alcohol ingestion may *irreversibly* destroy nerve cells, producing a permanent "brain syndrome" with dementia (Korsakoff's syndrome). The liver may become infiltrated with fat and, over a period of time, become cirrhotic (scarred). The digestive system may also be affected and pancreatitis (inflammation of the pancreas) and chronic gastritis (inflammation of the stomach), with development of peptic ulcers, may be seen.

A great deal of epidemiological evidence now exists, showing that chronic excessive alcohol consumption is a major risk factor for cancer in humans. Although ethanol alone may not be carcinogenic, heavy drinking increases a person's risk of developing cancer of the tongue, mouth, throat, voice box, and liver.[15] This cancer-potentiating effect can be explained by the role of alcohol in modifying the action of other cancer-causing agents. Indeed, alcohol clearly exerts a synergistic action with tobacco. For example, the risk of head and neck cancers for heavy drinkers who smoke is 6 to 15 times greater than for those who abstain from both. The risk of throat cancer is 44 times greater for heavy users of both alcohol and tobacco than for nonusers (Figure 4.3). Thus, alcohol may promote tumor growth—an effect that may follow from its immunosuppressive action and the resultant reduction in body defense mechanisms against tumor cells.[12]

During the mid-1980s, data appeared that linked a minimal-to-moderate alcohol intake in women with increases in the incidence of breast cancer.[16,17] More recent data dispute this claim,[18] leading to the current impression that the data are inconsistent and, most likely, a strong correlation or causation does not exist.

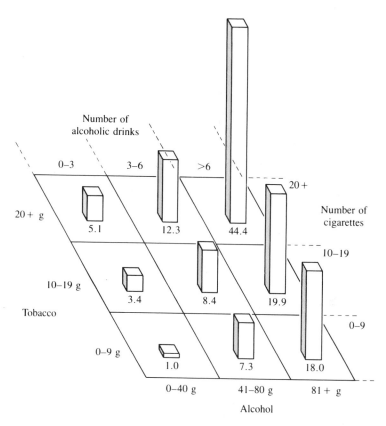

FIGURE 4.3

Relative risks of esophageal cancer in relation to the daily consumption of alcohol and tobacco. The risk is 44.4 times greater for persons who consume 20 grams or more of tobacco and 80 grams or more of alcohol per day (upper right block) than for persons who consume little or none of either drug (lower left block). One ounce of ethyl alcohol is approximately 23.4 grams; thus 40 grams is 1.7 ounces, or approximately equivalent to three drinks. [From *Third Special Report to the* U.S. *Congress on Alcohol and Health.*[19] Data from A. J. Tuyns, G. Pequignot, and O. M. Jenson, "Le cancer de l'oesophage en Ille et Vilaine en fonction des niveaux de consommation d'alcool et de tabac: Des risques qui se multiplient," *Bulletin du Cancer* 65(1)(1977): 45–60.]

Teratogenic Effects

As mentioned earlier, a fetal alcohol syndrome occurs in the offspring of mothers who demonstrated high blood levels of alcohol during critical stages of fetal development. In 1977, the National Institute on Alcohol

Abuse and Alcoholism released the following statement relevant to this syndrome:

> Heavy use of alcohol by women during pregnancy may result in a pattern of abnormalities in the offspring, termed the fetal alcohol syndrome, which consists of specific congenital and behavioral abnormalities. Studies undertaken in animals corroborate the initial observation in humans and also indicate an increased incidence of stillbirths, resorption, and spontaneous abortions. Both the risk and the extent of abnormalities appear to be dose-related, increasing with higher alcohol intake during pregnancy. In human studies, alcohol is an unequivocal factor when the full pattern of the fetal alcohol syndrome is present.[19]

Information gathered since 1977 more clearly characterizes the syndrome. Factors include[20] (1) CNS dysfunction, including low intelligence and microcephaly (reduced cranial circumference), mental retardation, and behavioral abnormalities (often presenting as hyperactivity and difficulty with social integration); (2) retarded body growth rate; (3) facial abnormalities (short palpebral fissures, short nose, wideset eyes, and small cheek bones); (4) other anatomical abnormalities (for example, congenital heart defects and malformed eyes and ears).

The mechanism by which alcohol produces these problems may be direct; either ethanol or its metabolite, acetaldehyde, may inhibit embryonic cell division and proliferation early in pregnancy. Effects on facial development are produced during early pregnancy (up to 4 to 6 weeks), while the effects on brain development are produced during later pregnancy. There is also evidence of fetal malnutrition, which is caused by injury to the placenta. Finally, some children with fetal alcohol syndrome exhibit marked deficits in their immune systems, increasing their susceptibility to infections.

To cause this syndrome, the average daily alcohol consumption may not be as important as the maximum concentrations that are obtained during binge drinking at critical periods. Infants who are born to moderately heavy drinkers exhibit at least twice the incidence of congenital anomalies as infants born to nondrinking mothers. Not all features are necessarily present in any given infant. At the present time, the projected incidence of fetal alcohol syndrome makes it the third leading cause of birth defects with associated mental retardation, following only Down's syndrome and spina bifida—and fetal alcohol syndrome is the only one of these conditions that is preventable. Indeed, alcohol is the most frequent cause of teratogen-induced mental deficiency that is known in the Western World.[21]

A study of more than 31,000 pregnancies shows that the consumption of only one or two drinks daily can cause a substantially increased risk of producing a growth-retarded infant.[22] Less than one drink per day has minimal effect, but it could not be considered "safe." The incidence of the full-blown fetal alcohol syndrome ranges from 1 in 300 to 1 in 2000 live births; it occurs in 1 out of 3 infants of alcoholic mothers.

Despite these statistics, 20 percent of pregnant women continue to consume alcohol.[23] The highest rates of alcohol use during pregnancy occur in women who also smoke (37 percent) and in women who are not married (28 percent). It has been concluded that special efforts are needed to convince pregnant women who are smokers, unmarried, less educated, or younger to avoid alcohol—these are women who may already be at high risk of having a poor pregnancy outcome.

The effects of *paternal* drinking or alcoholism on the fetus are unknown. More than 25 percent of pregnant women who are moderate-to-heavy drinkers report that their infants' fathers are also heavy drinkers. This factor may or may not be significant.

Chronic Excessive Alcohol Ingestion

Of the 160 million Americans who are old enough to drink legally, 112 million drink and 48 million do not.[24,25] As many as 12 million Americans may have serious alcohol problems, and about half that number (6 million) are considered to be alcoholic. The daily consumption of about ½ pint of 80-proof liquor is thought to place a person's health at risk. Approximately 10 percent of the drinking population ingests this quantity of alcohol in the form of beer, wine, or "hard" liquor.

As stated by Jaffe:

> If cigarette smoking is excluded, alcoholism is by far the most serious drug problem in the United States and most other countries. Measured in terms of accidents, lost productivity, crime, death, or damaged health, the combined social costs of problem drinking in the United States were estimated for 1980 to exceed 89 billion dollars annually. The cost in broken homes, wasted lives, loss to society, and human misery is beyond calculation.[26]

Effects of chronic alcoholism include psychological problems (anxiety, depression, loss of control over drinking), social problems (work, family life), and pathological problems (tremors, periods of amnesia and memory loss, poor motor control, liver disease, and so on).

In long-term alcoholics, malnutrition and chronic physiological degeneration may occur. This condition causes a bloated look, flabby muscles, fine tremors, decreased physical capacity and stamina, and increased susceptibility to infections. Although this state of chronic degeneration is not present in the majority of alcoholics who receive adequate nutrition, nutrition alone does not fully protect the brain, the liver, or the digestive tract from damage.[27]

When does alcohol produce a state of physical dependence? When might one say that alcohol harms the body? Clearly, long-term maintenance of high concentrations of alcohol in the body produces a state of physical dependence.[28] Since the body metabolizes about 10 cc, or one-third of an ounce, of absolute alcohol (95 percent or 190 proof) per hour, ingestion of more than that amount will result in alcohol accumulation.

There is a reasonably good correlation between drinking habits, maximum blood concentrations, and the intensity of a withdrawal syndrome. With a low level of dependence, alcohol withdrawal consists of altered sleep patterns, nausea, anxiety, wakefulness, and mild tremors that may only last for a day or so. At higher levels of dependence, an *alcohol withdrawal syndrome* is seen, which consists of intensification of those signs, combined with vomiting, cramps, nightmares, and transient hallucinations. If the hallucinations persist, the syndrome is called *alcoholic hallucinosis*.[28] With progression of the dependence, withdrawal may include confusion, disorientation, agitation, persecutory hallucinations, and severe tremors or seizures. This late stage is termed *alcoholic withdrawal delirium*, or *delirium tremens*.

After recovery, depression, sleep deficits, cognitive and memory deficits, and other alterations of brain function may persist for months.

Aids to Withdrawal of Alcohol

It is now apparent that the pharmacological effects of alcohol closely resemble those of the nonselective CNS depressants. These effects also closely resemble those of the benzodiazepines (Chapter 5). Thus, one should not be surprised that administration of either a

CNS sedative or a benzodiazepine will substitute for alcohol in its absence.

One might question, however, why we would use one drug to substitute for another one that we want to withdraw from someone. The short duration of action of alcohol and its narrow range of safety makes it an extremely dangerous drug. When alcohol ingestion is stopped, it is rapidly metabolized (within hours), and withdrawal symptoms are precipitated. Once dependence has developed, substituting a longer-acting drug (usually a benzodiazepine) in sufficient doses will prevent or suppress the withdrawal symptoms.[29-31] The longer-acting drug is then either maintained at a level low enough to allow the person to function or else it is withdrawn gradually. In general, the longest-acting agents are preferred [especially those with pharmacologically active metabolites, for example, chlordiazepoxide (Librium) or diazepam (Valium)].

The substitution of a long-duration drug (usually a benzodiazepine) for a short-acting drug (alcohol) is analogous to the use of methadone as an aid in withdrawing a person from a dependence on opioid analgesics (Chapter 9).

Drugs Used to Treat Alcoholism

Disulfiram (Antabuse) has been used in the treatment of alcoholism for a long time. As stated previously, it alters the metabolism of alcohol, allowing acetaldehyde to accumulate. This accumulation results in an *acetaldehyde syndrome* if the patient ingests alcohol within several days of taking disulfiram. Patient cooperation in taking disulfiram is essential, and the efficacy of treatment correlates only with the patient's willingness to take the disulfiram.

Haloperidol (Haldol) and other antipsychotic agents (Chapter 10) may be used to treat the hallucinations that are associated with severe delirium tremens. If seizures occur, haloperidol cannot be used (because it lowers the seizure threshold) and antiepileptic agents (Chapter 13) must be used instead.

Conditioned-avoidance techniques that include the use of emetic (vomiting) agents (*apomorphine or Ipecac*) have, in past years, been used in the treatment of alcoholism. The patient takes the emetic agent and, shortly thereafter, drinks a dose of alcohol. When nausea and vomiting occur, the patient associates the drinking of alcohol with the unpleasant reaction. Alcohol thus becomes a conditioned stimulus for the production of nausea and vomiting. Although this technique is decreasing in popularity, treatment with low doses of apomorphine is being tried in an attempt to possibly reduce the craving for alcohol.[30]

As noted previously, persistent depression can follow alcohol withdrawal. Thus, *antidepressants* (Chapter 8) have been widely used to treat alcoholics during the months following withdrawal. Evidence for the efficacy of this approach is lacking.[30]

More recently, antidepressants that selectively inhibit serotonin reuptake (Chapter 8) have been shown to reduce daily alcohol intake in persons who are in the early stages of alcoholism.[32,33] Two such agents are currently available, one of which, *fluoxetine* (*Prozac*), is the safer and better studied. Indeed, increased levels of the neurotransmitter serotonin in the CNS correlate with a reduction in the spontaneous consumption of alcohol by problem drinkers. Thus, at present, drug-induced inhibition of serotonin reuptake (which increases serotonin availability) suggests an innovative approach for modulating ethanol intake in problem drinkers.[34] Such reduction in alcohol intake by persons who take fluoxetine appears to be an effect of the drug that is independent of its antidepressant effect.

Treatment of Alcoholism

In a text that is devoted to the basic principles of drug action, discussion of the treatment of persons who have drug problems is a secondary objective. However, because the use and abuse of alcohol are so widespread in our society, it seems pertinent to delineate briefly some of the newer concepts that relate to alcoholism and its treatment.

Prior to about 1960, alcoholism was seldom considered a medical problem. Alcoholics were routinely arrested for public drunkenness, denied medical services, and allowed to go through a withdrawal syndrome in the local jail. It was not until the late 1950s that the American Medical Association recognized the syndrome of alcoholism as an illness. In his book *The Disease Concept of Alcoholism*, E. M. Jellinek presented the hypothesis that alcoholism is a disease.[35] Such labeling served to reduce much of the social stigma of alcoholism, and it helped to form the concept that alcoholics have a deficiency in the ability to tolerate the effects of alcohol. To be free of the disease, therefore, the person with this problem must abstain totally from alcohol. This concept also implies that no matter how a person becomes alcoholic, all alcoholics are the same because they all have the same disease. This concept is the basis of nearly all alcoholism treatment programs today. As M. Mann puts it, "alcoholism is a disease which manifests itself chiefly by the uncontrollable drinking of the victim, who is known as an alcoholic."[36]

In contrast to this uniform concept, others postulate that no single entity can be defined as alcoholism and that alcoholism is not a unitary concept but a collection of various signs, symptoms, and behaviors.[37-41] Alcohol dependence is a health problem (rather than a disease) that affects five areas of health: (1) acute intoxication (drinking health), (2) emotional health, (3) vocational health, (4) social and family health, and (5) physical health. Not all alcohol-dependent persons are impaired in every area of life health, nor does impairment in one area necessarily imply impairment in other areas.

One person may drink to excess without much alteration in his or her physical or vocational health—for example, an executive who is an alcoholic but maintains an adequate diet and has social and family supports. On the other hand, as a result of treatment, an alcoholic's physical health may be improved by embracing total abstinence, yet other life problems, such as social, family, and emotional difficulties may not be remedied or may even be worsened. Therefore, different kinds of persons with alcohol problems will exhibit different profiles of impairment in their lives. As such, different prescriptions for treatment and different levels of expectation for success must be employed for each individual. For example, sobriety may be a reasonable expectation for a person whose impairment in life is minimal, while attenuated drinking with modest improvements in health may be all that can be reasonably expected for a more severely impaired alcoholic.

Such individualism of treatment may be some distance off, however, because society has only recently begun to look less scornfully on the alcoholic and is just beginning to recognize that each alcoholic should have an individual set of therapeutic objectives. The goal of future treatment programs may not *necessarily* be total abstinence from alcohol for every alcoholic but, rather, a reduction in life problems that are associated with drinking. It has been estimated that alcohol abuse and alcoholism cost various segments of the American economy some $90 billion every year. Business and industry sustain some $20 billion of that total cost in lost productivity.[41] More than 2400 organizations have functioning programs that are designed to identify employees who have alcohol-related problems and to provide them with counseling.

Finally, in a recent report[42] evaluating more than 20,000 persons for the lifetime prevalence of any substance abuse disorder, 13.5 percent experienced alcohol dependence or abuse. Those classified as alcoholic had a sevenfold increase in the probability of having another addictive disorder, and a large percentage displayed generalized anxiety (19 percent), antisocial personalities (14 percent), affective disorders (13 percent), or schizophrenia (3 percent). Overall, mental dysfunction appeared in 37 percent of persons who suffer from alcoholism. Obviously, then, one must recognize the high incidence of alcohol (and other substance) abuse among those persons who have severe mental disorders. Similarly, in treating persons for alcohol abuse, one must recognize the presence of this 37-percent incidence of mental dysfunction.

STUDY QUESTIONS

1. Describe the relation between alcohol and nonselective CNS depressants.
2. Describe the metabolism of alcohol and how it is altered by disulfiram. How is this alteration applied in the treatment of alcoholism?
3. Describe how alcohol exerts its effect on the CNS.
4. List several of the major physiological and societal problems that are associated with alcohol.
5. Describe the fetal alcohol syndrome. What is a "safe" level of alcohol intake by a pregnant woman?
6. If a person has developed a physical dependence on alcohol, why might he or she be treated with a benzodiazepine to substitute for the alcohol?
7. Summarize some of the drugs and techniques used to aid in the treatment of alcoholism.
8. What drug offers promise for reducing daily alcohol intake in some alcoholics? Why?
9. Describe the disease concept of alcoholism.
10. How is alcohol involved in the genesis of certain cancers?

NOTES

1. J. W. Hanson, K. L. Jones, and D. W. Smith, "Fetal Alcohol Syndrome," *Journal of the American Medical Association* 235 (5 April 1976): 1458–1460.

2. J. Caballeria, M. Frezza, R. Hernandez-Munoz, C. DiPadova, M. A. Korsted, E. Baraona, and C. S. Lieber, "Gastric Origin of the First-Pass Metabolism of Ethanol in Humans: Effect of Gastrectomy," *Gastroenterology* 97(1989): 1205–1209.

3. M. Frezza, C. DiPadova, G. Pozzato, M. Terpin, E. Baraona, and C. S. Lieber "High Blood Alcohol Levels in Women. The Role of Decreased Gastric Alcohol Dehydrogenase Activity and First-Pass Metabolism," New England Journal of Medicine 322(1990): 95–99.

4. T. W. Rall, "Hypnotics and Sedatives: Ethanol," in A. G. Gilman, T. W. Rall, A. S. Nies, and P. Taylor, eds., *Goodman and Gilman's The Pharmacological Basis of Therapeutics*, 8th ed. (New York: Pergamon, 1990), p. 379.

5. E. Majchrowicz and E. P. Noble (eds.), *Biochemistry and Pharmacology of Ethanol*, vols. 1–3 (New York: Plenum Press, 1979).

6. R. Room and G. Collins (eds.), *Alcohol and Disinhibition: Nature and Meaning of the Link,* National Institute on Alcohol Abuse and Alcoholism, U. S. Department of Health and Human Services (Washington, D. C.: U. S. Government Printing Office, 1983).

7. W. G. Wood and F. Schroeder, "Membrane Effects of Ethanol: Bulk Lipid versus Lipid Domains," *Life Sciences* 43(1988): 467–475.

8. T. W. Rall, "Hypnotics and Sedatives: Ethanol," in A. G. Gilman, T. W. Rall, A. S. Nies, and P. Taylor, eds., *Goodman and Gilman's The Pharmacological Basis of Therapeutics*, 8th ed. (New York: Pergamon, 1990), pp. 374–375.

9. B. Tabakoff and P. L. Hoffman, "Biochemical Pharmacology of Alcohol," in H. Y. Meltzer, ed., *Psychopharmacology: The Third Generation of Progress* (New York: Raven, 1987), pp. 1521–1526.

10. C. S. Lieber, "Alcoholism: Medical Implications," in R. B. Millman, P. Cushman, Jr., and J. H. Lowinson, eds., *Research Developments in Drug and Alcohol Use, Annals of the New York Academy of Sciences* 362(1981): 132–135.

11. M. J. Edkardt, T. C. Harford, C. T. Kaelber, et al., "Health Hazards Associated with Alcohol Consumption," *Journal of the American Medical Association* 246(1981): 648–666.

12. S. I. Mufti, H. R. Darban, and R. R. Watson, "Alcohol, Cancer, and Immunomodulation," *Critical Reviews in Oncology/Hematology* 9(1989): 243–261.

13. S. C. Woods and J. G. Mansfield, "Ethanol and Disinhibition: Physiological and Behavioral Links," in R. Room and S. Collins, eds., *Alcohol and Disinhibition: Nature and Meaning of the Link*, National Institute on Alcohol Abuse and Alcoholism, U. S. Department of Health and Human Services (Washington, D. C.: U. S. Government Printing Office, 1983), pp. 4–23.

14. R. G. Niven, "Alcoholism—A Problem in Perspective," *Journal of the American Medical Association* 252(1984): 1912–1914.

15. S. Palmer, "Diet, Nutrition and Cancer," *Progress in Food and Nutrition Science* 9(1985): 283–341.

16. A. Schatzkin, Y. Jones, R. W. Hoover, et al., "Alcohol Consumption and Breast Cancer in the Epidemiologic Follow-Up Study of the First National Health and Nutrition Examination Study," *New England Journal of Medicine* 316(1987): 1169–1173.

17. W. C. Willett, M. J. Stampfer, G. A. Colditz, et al., "Moderate Alcohol Consumption and the Risks of Breast Cancer," *New England Journal of Medicine* 316(1987): 1174–1180.

18. R. E. Harris, N. Spritz, and E. L. Wynder, "Studies of Breast Cancer and Alcohol Consumption," *Preventive Medicine* 17(1988): 676–682.

19. U.S. Department of Health, Education, and Welfare, *Alcohol and Health: Third Special Report to the U.S. Congress* (Washington, D.C.: U.S. Government Printing Office, 1978).

20. National Institute on Alcohol and Alcoholism, *Alcohol and Birth Defects: The Fetal Alcohol Syndrome and Related Disorders*, U. S. Department of Health and Human Services Publication Number ADM 87-1531 (Washington, D. C.: U. S. Government Printing Office, 1987), pp. 6–10.

21. T. W. Rall, "Hypnotics and Sedatives: Ethanol," in A. G. Gilman, T. W. Rall, A. S. Nies, and P. Taylor, eds., *Goodman and Gilman's The Pharmacological Basis of Therapeutics*, 8th ed. (New York: Pergamon, 1990), p. 373.

22. J. L. Mills, B. I. Granbard, E. E. Harley, et al., "Maternal Alcohol Consumption and Birth Weight," *Journal of the American Medical Association* 252(1984): 1875–1879.

23. M. Serdula, D. F. Williamson, J. S. Kendrick, R. F. Anda, and T. Byers, "Trends in Alcohol Consumption by Pregnant Women," Journal of the American Medical Association 265(1991): 876–879.

24. S. Blume, "National Patterns of Alcohol Use and Abuse," in *Research*

Developments in Drug and Alcohol Use. Annals of the New York Academy of Science 362(1981): 4–15.

25. G. B. Cloninger, S. H. Dinwiddie, and T. Reich, "Epidemiology and Genetics of Alcoholism," *Annual Reviews of Psychiatry* 8(1989): 331:346.

26. J. H. Jaffe, "Drug Addiction and Drug Abuse," in A. G. Gilman, L. S. Goodman, T. W. Rall, and F. Murad, eds., *Goodman and Gilman's The Pharmacological Basis of Therapeutics*, 7th ed. (New York: Macmillan, 1985), p. 548.

27. U.S. Department of Health and Human Services, *Fifth Special Report to the U.S. Congress on Alcohol and Health. (Washington, D.C.: U.S. Government Printing Office, 1984).*

28. J. H. Jaffe, "Drug Addiction and Drug Abuse," in A. G. Gilman, T. W. Rall, A. S. Nies, and P. Taylor, eds., *Goodman and Gilman's The Pharmacological Basis of Therapeutics*, 8th ed. (New York: Pergamon, 1990), pp. 538–539.

29. J. H. Jaffe, "Drug Addiction and Drug Abuse," in A. G. Gilman, T. W. Rall, A. S. Nies, and P. Taylor, eds., *Goodman and Gilman's The Pharmacological Basis of Therapeutics*, 8th ed. (New York: Pergamon, 1990), p. 562.

30. H. R. Kranzler and B. Orrok, "The Pharmacotherapy of Alcoholism," *Annual Reviews of Psychiatry* 8(1989): 397–417.

31. O. Nutt, B. Adinoff, and M. Linniola, "Benzodiazepines in the Treatment of Alcoholism," *Recent Developments in Alcoholism* 7(1989): 283–313.

32. D. A. Gorelick, "Serotonin Uptake Blockers and the Treatment of Alcoholism," *Recent Developments in Alcoholism* 7(1989): 267–281.

33. C. A. Naranjo, K. E. Kadlee, P. Sanjueze, and D. Woodley-Remus, "Fluoxetine Differentially Alters Alcohol Intake and Other Consummatory Behaviors in Problem Drinkers," *Clinical Pharmacology and Therapeutics* 47(1990): 490–498.

34. C. A. Naranjo and E. M. Sellers, "Serotonin Uptake Inhibitors Attenuate Ethanol Intake in Problem Drinkers," *Recent Developments in Alcoholism* 7(1989): 255–266.

35. E. M. Jellinek, *The Disease Concept of Alcoholism* [New Haven: Hillhouse Press, 1960).

36. M. Mann, *New Primer on Alcoholism*, 2d ed. (New York: Holt, 1968).

37. E. M. Pattison, L. Sobel, and L. C. Sobel, *Emerging Concepts of Alcohol Dependence* (New York: Springer-Verlag, 1977).

38. S. Cohen, *The Alcoholic Problem: Selected Issues* (New York: Haworth Press, 1983).

39. H. J. Harwood, D. M. Napolitano, P. L. Kristiansen, et al., *Economic Costs to Society of Alcohol, Drug Abuse, and Mental Illness* (Rockwell, Md.: Alcohol, Drug Abuse, and Mental Health Administration, June 1984).

40. J. E. Peachey and C. A. Naranjo, "Role of Drugs in Treatment of Alcoholism," *Drugs* 27(1984): 171–182.

41. H. A. Skinner, "Primary Syndromes of Alcohol Abuse: Their Measurement and Correlates," *British Journal of Addiction* 76(1981): 63–76.

42. D. A. Regier, M. E. Farmer, D. S. Rae, B. Z. Locke, S. H. Keith, L. L. Judd, and F. K. Goodwin, "Comorbidity of Mental Disorders with Alcohol and Other Drug Abuse," *Journal of the American Medical Association* 264(1990), pp. 2511-2518.

Benzodiazepines

Today's Tranquilizers

Throughout the 1950s, the only drugs that were available for the treatment of anxiety were the CNS depressants: alcohol, barbiturates, meprobamate, and the other nonbarbiturate sedatives. In 1960, the first benzodiazepine, chlordiazepoxide (Librium), was introduced. It was met with almost immediate acceptance. The subsequent history of the benzodiazepines can be divided into two phases.[1] The first phase began in 1960 and lasted until 1977. That period of time was characterized by an exponential increase in the clinical use of benzodiazepines, by the introduction of a dozen competing benzodiazepines, and by the recognition of limitations to their use, their side effects and toxicities, and their potential for abuse. During that period of time, it was thought that the benzodiazepines acted (in the absence of any clear evidence to the contrary) in the same way as the nonspecific depressants and, therefore, that they did not differ much from the older drugs.

The second phase in benzodiazepine history began in 1977, when researchers in Denmark and Switzerland independently established the

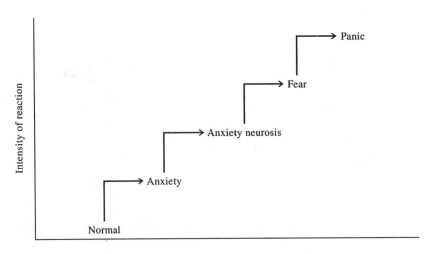

FIGURE 5.1

Continuum of anxiety through fear as progressively more intense emotional states.

fact that diazepam (Valium) binds specifically and with high affinity to a distinct population of receptors in the brain. Since 1977, there has been little increase in the clinical use of benzodiazepines, but there has been a dramatic increase in our understanding of their mechanism of action and, indeed, our understanding of the neurochemistry of anxiety, fear, and panic disorders.

Anxiety: Search for a Neurochemical Basis

Anxiety can be described as apprehension, tension, or uneasiness that stems from the anticipation of danger, which may be internal or external. It may be a response to stress that is associated with external stimuli, or it may be devoid of any apparent precipitating stimulus.[2]

Anxiety is a fundamental emotion and a normal response to an experience that mimics a past experience that caused a problem of significant magnitude. However, when the degree of anxiety is disproportionate, when it occurs without an object stimulus, or when it disrupts normal function, it becomes an anxiety neurosis. Anxiety is characterized by any of the following symptoms: helplessness, apprehension, faintness, headaches, pain, sweating, rapid heart rate, rapid breathing, nausea, dry mouth, and so on. As shown in Figure 5.1, a continuum can be drawn that relates anxiety, anxiety neurosis, fear, and panic in a progressive manner. Thus, severe anxiety is a state that is similar to, but milder than, fear. Certainly, both anxiety and fear are important for survival in a hostile world (serving as the cognitive and emotional concomitant of a behavioral alarm system), while panic may be a more extreme reaction.

The hypothesis in this discussion is that an understanding of the mechanism of action for a given psychoactive drug (or class of drugs) will provide insight into the neurochemistry of the disorder for which the drug is used. Several examples of this hypothesis will be used in this text. Indeed, when we identify receptors that are specific for the actions of benzodiazepines, we are provided with insight about the cause of those disorders for which benzodiazepines are clinically effective.

Anxiety disorders (for example, panic, generalized anxiety, phobias, and obsessive-compulsive disorders) are characterized by tension, hyperactivity of the autonomic nervous system, apprehension, expectation, and increased vigilance. As a group, anxiety disorders are the most common of all psychiatric disorders, with a lifetime prevalence rate that is between 10 and 25 percent. Morbidity is significant, especially evidenced by a high rate of suicide. Anxiety disorders are also prominent components of almost all other psychiatric disorders. As stated by Breier and Paul:

> Given the high population prevalences and significant levels of morbidity associated with anxiety, it is not surprising that anti-anxiety drugs are among the most widely used of all medications. Anti-anxiety agents are the fourth most frequently prescribed class of medication, with over 55 million prescriptions written for benzodiazepines alone in 1989.[3]

Benzodiazepines markedly decrease the symptoms of anxiety, which supports the view that:

> Anxiety that is sensitive to benzodiazepines is not unique or confined to a specific anxiety disorder but is present, to a certain extent, in many of us. In this context, pathological anxiety can be viewed as an inappropriate or exaggerated response rather than a qualitatively unique state.[1]

In essence, therefore, analysis of the receptors on which benzodiazepines act to relieve anxiety provides us with insight about the neurochemical mechanisms that are involved in normal anxiety responses as well as in the more pathologic states of anxiety neurosis, fear, and

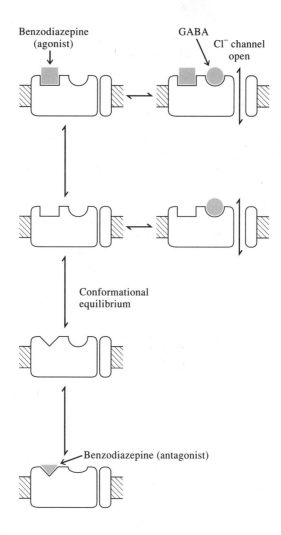

FIGURE 5.2

Benzodiazepine-GABA receptor interaction. Benzodiazepine agonists (e.g., diazepam) and antagonists (e.g., flumazenil) are believed to bind to a site on the GABA receptor that is distinct from the GABA binding site. A conformational equilibrium exists between states in which the benzodiazepine receptor exists in its *agonist binding* conformation (*above*) and in its *antagonist binding* conformation (*below*). In the latter state, the GABA receptor has a much reduced affinity for GABA, so the chloride channel remains closed. [Modified from H. P. Rang and M. M. Dale,[4] Figure 21.6.]

panic. Let us now examine those receptors which underlie both the action of the benzodiazepines and the chemistry of the anxieties.

The Benzodiazepine-GABA Receptor

It is now clear that all of the major pharmacological actions of the benzodiazepines are mediated through a specific action on identifiable benzodiazepine receptors. The affinity of the various types of benzodiazepines for specific receptors correlates closely with their individual pharmacological potencies. Within the brain, benzodiazepine receptors are specifically located in the cerebral cortex (the most), the limbic system and midbrain (fewer), and the brain stem and spinal cord (the least). This distribution roughly agrees with the distribution of GABA (gamma-aminobutyric acid) receptors.

As discussed in Appendix III, GABA is one of the most important inhibitory neurotransmitters in the brain. It inhibits neuronal excitability by selectively increasing the trans-membrane conductance of chloride ions; that is, GABA opens chloride channels in the nerve membrane. Recent studies demonstrate that the benzodiazepine binding site is located next to the site where GABA binds (Figure 5.2); both sites actually exist on the same protein subunit.[1,4] Indeed, the benzodiazepine binding site, the GABA binding site, and the chloride channel form a large macromolecular receptor complex, the function of which is to inhibit neuronal activity. The benzodiazepine does not cause the neuronal inhibitory action; rather, it potentiates and facilitates GABA-induced increases in chloride conductance, which, in turn, inhibits synaptic action. Thus, benzodiazepines increase GABA-mediated inhibitory neurotransmitter activity. The benzodiazepine and GABA bind to separate sites on the same receptor–ion-channel complex, and each increases the activity of the other. A benzodiazepine *antagonist* (flumazenil, discussed later in this chapter) can occupy the benzodiazepine binding site; this binding distorts the GABA binding site in such a way that membrane binding of GABA is reduced and the chloride channels cannot open (Figure 5.2). Of interest is the speculation that a pure GABA antagonist might induce a state of anxiety (as would be predicted by this model). Indeed, there is some evidence that such might be the case. Pentylenetetrazol (a convulsant) is a GABA antagonist (much like flumazenil), and low, subconvulsant doses of pentylenetetrazol do produce anxiety in humans.[1] Thus, a decrease in GABA activity can be associated with a drug-induced anxiety state.

Whether an endogenous benzodiazepine agonist or antagonist exists is unclear. (This concept would be analogous to that of endorphins in relation to the narcotic receptor that is discussed in Chapter 9 and in Appendix III.) A substance (beta-CCEE) that was proposed in 1980 to be an endogenous "anxiogenic" compound has been rejected, and the search for such an anxiogenic compound (to block GABA activity) is continuing.[3,4]

In summary, benzodiazepines reduce anxiety by increasing GABA-receptor–coupled chloride conductance. Conversely, anxiety-producing agents may exert an opposite effect on the complex that contains receptors for benzodiazepines and GABA, and the chloride channel. Thus, this receptor complex may be involved in the mechanism for normal and pathological states of anxiety, fear, and panic.

Pharmacokinetics

The benzodiazepines are considered to be the drugs of choice for the pharmacological treatment of anxiety. They are also useful in the management of panic disorders, certain types of epileptic seizures, certain sleep disorders, and aggression, and as "muscle relaxants" (especially when anxiety or tension are also present), and preanesthetic sedatives.[2,4–6]

The basic structure of the benzodiazepines is shown in Figure 5.3 along with a list of currently available derivatives. Note that all these drugs share the same basic structure and differ only in terms of their substituent groups. As might be expected, the actions of all the benzodiazepines are very similar: major differences primarily occur in their pharmacokinetic behavior (for example, metabolic breakdown and durations of action).

Absorption and Distribution

Benzodiazepines are all completely absorbed when they are administered orally; peak plasma concentrations are achieved in about one hour. Three of them are also available for use by injection (Table 5.1). After absorption, all benzodiazepines become highly bound to plasma proteins. Some (for example, diazepam) undergo extensive excretion in bile and are subsequently reabsorbed back into the blood from the intestine. This is one reason that several benzodiazepines have extremely long half-lives (Table 5.1). Furthermore, most are very fat-soluble and, therefore, tend to accumulate gradually in body fat. These two processes prolong the half-lives of

General structure / Chlordiazepoxide (Librium)

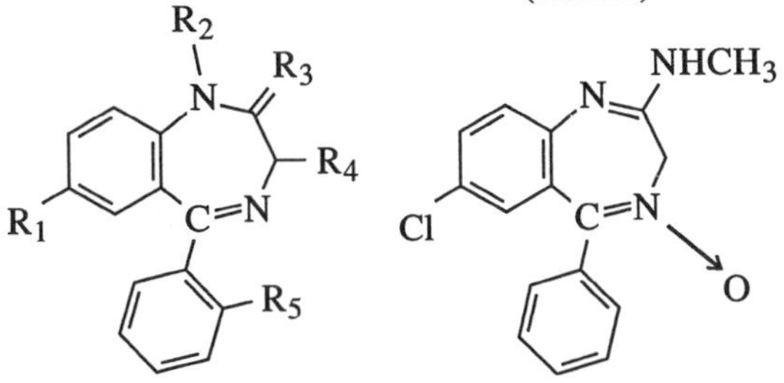

Drug	R_1	R_2	R_3	R_4	R_5
Diazepam	Cl	CH_3	=O	H_2	H
Nitrazepam	NO_2	H	=O	H_2	H
Flurazepam	Cl	$(CH_2)_2N(C_2H_5)_2$	=O	H_2	H
Flunitrazepam	NO_2	H	=O	H_2	F
Oxazepam	Cl	H	=O	OH	H
Temazepam	Cl	CH_3	=O	H_2	H
Clonazepam	NO_2	H	=O	H_2	Cl
Lorazepam	Cl	H	=O	OH	Cl
Clorazepate	Cl	H	=O	COOH	H
Nordiazepam	Cl	H	=O	H_2	H

FIGURE 5.3

Structures of some benzodiazepines.

many of these compounds. In addition, as we will see next, metabolism to pharmacologically active intermediate products also prolongs the time of course of drug action.

Metabolism and Excretion

In Chapter 1, we stated that most psychoactive drugs must be metabolized to pharmacologically inactive, water-soluble products, which are excreted in urine. While this holds true for several benzodiazepines, some of them are first biotransformed to intermediate products that are pharmacologically *active;* these, in turn, must be detoxified by further metabolism before they can be excreted (Figure 5.4). As we can see from Table 5.1 and Figure 5.4, several long-acting compounds are biotransformed into a long-lasting pharmacologically active metabolite, such as nordiazepam, the half-life of which is about 60 hours. The short-acting benzodiazepines are metabolized directly into inactive products. Figure 5.5 demonstrates the buildup

TABLE 5.1

Benzodiazepines

| Drug name | | Dosage form | | | | Elimination half-life (hours) (mean range) |
Trade	Generic	Oral	Parent-eral	Active metabolite	Active compounds in blood	
Long-acting agents						
Valium	Diazepam	X	X	Yes	Diazepam Nordiazepam	24 (20–50) 60 (50–100)
Librium	Chlordiazepoxide	X		Yes	Chlor- diazepoxide Nordiazepam	10 (8–24) 60 (50–100)
Dalmane	Flurazepam	X		Yes	Desalkyl- flurazepam	80 (70–160)
Paxipam	Halazepam	X		Yes	Halazepam Nordiazepam	14 (10–20) 60 (50–100)
Centrax	Prazepam	X		Yes	Nordiazepam	60 (50–100)
Tranxene	Chlorazepate	X		Yes	Nordiazepam	60 (50–100)
Intermediate-acting agents						
Ativan	Lorazepam	X	X	No	Lorazepam	15 (10–24)
Klonopin	Clonazepam	X		No	Clonazepam	30 (18–50)
Dormalin	Quazepam	X		Yes	Quazepam Desalkyl- flurazepam	35 (25–50) 80 (70–160)
Short-acting agents						
Versed	Midazolam		X	No	Midazolam	2.5 (1.5–4.5)
Serax	Oxazepam	X		No	Oxazepam	8 (5–15)
Restoril	Temazepam	X		No	Temazepam	12 (8–35)
Halcion	Triazolam	X		No	Triazolam	2.5 (1.5–5)
Xanax	Alprazolam	X		No	Alprazolam	12 (11–18)

and slow disappearance of nordiazepam from the plasma of a human volunteer who was given diazepam daily for 15 days.

The elderly have a severely reduced ability to metabolize these long-acting benzodiazepines. Thus, they stay in the body of an elderly person even longer, which often results in an elimination half-life (for both the parent drug and the active metabolite) of more than 10 days. Since it takes about six half-lives to totally rid the body of a

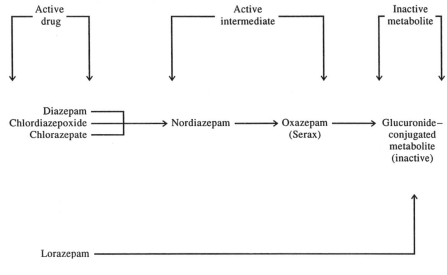

FIGURE 5.4

Metabolism of benzodiazepines. The intermediate metabolite, nordiazepam, is formed from many agents. Oxazepam (Serax) is commercially available and is also an active intermediate in the metabolism of nordiazepam to its inactive products.

drug (Chapter 1, Table 1.2), it would take an elderly patient about 60 days to become drug-free after even a single dose. Because these drugs can induce a "brain syndrome" (or reversible, drug-induced dementia) that is similar to the one caused by nonselective CNS depressants (see the following discussion), elderly patients can become profoundly demented as a result of using these drugs. In general, *no* long-acting benzodiazepine should be administered to an elderly patient.

Because of the long elimination time of the benzodiazepines, a person who has been using a drug for prolonged periods of time may maintain detectable urinary concentrations of the drug for many weeks after discontinuing its use.

Pharmacodynamics

Low doses of benzodiazepines bound to the complex containing the benzodiazepine and GABA receptors and the chloride channel alleviate anxiety, agitation, fear, or panic without necessarily producing bar-

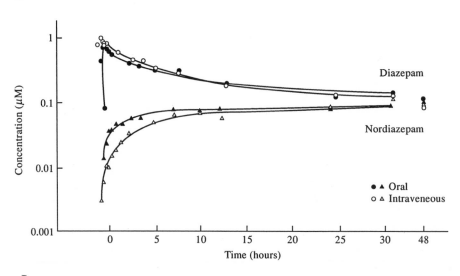

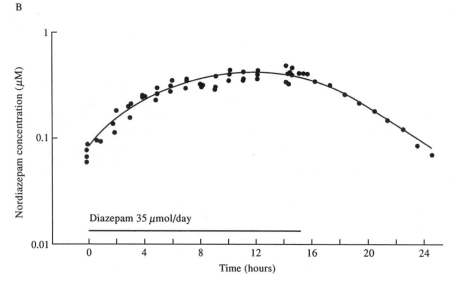

FIGURE 5.5

Pharmacokinetics of diazepam in man. (A) Concentrations of diazepam and its active metabo-lite, nordiazepam, following a single oral or intravenous dose. Note the negligible disap-pearance of both substances after the first 20 hours. (B) Accumulation of nordiazepam during two weeks of daily administration of diazepam, and slow decline (half-life about 3 days) after cessation of diazepam administration. (From H. P. Rang and M. M. Dale,[4] Figure 21.8, p. 495.)

biturate-like sedation or hypnosis. The antiepileptic and muscle-relaxant effects are probably also produced by this mechanism. Higher doses of benzodiazepines cause the characteristic barbiturate-like syndrome of sedation, hypnosis, dementia, or anesthesia. Tolerance appears to build to the barbiturate-like effects (for example, sedation and drowsiness) but not to the antianxiety effects.[5]

The major indication for benzodiazepine therapy is to help patients who experience anxiety that is so debilitating that their lifestyle, work, and interpersonal relationships are severely hampered. However, the absolute necessity for concurrent psychological support and counseling cannot be overemphasized.

Benzodiazepines have been called *minor tranquilizers* to differentiate them from the *major tranquilizers* (the antipsychotic compounds discussed in Chapter 10). Benzodiazepines do not substitute for antipsychotic agents, and they are not effective in treating psychotic depression. However, they are often used along with antidepressant drugs (Chapter 8) in patients who are suffering from depression accompanied by severe anxiety.

Alprazolam (Xanax) has been used in the treatment of panic disorders and phobic disorders, apparently because of its rapid onset of action and relatively low incidence of side effects.[2] However, withdrawal from alprazolam has posed a significant clinical problem for many patients. Further, emerging evidence indicates that alprazolam is not unique in its effective treatment of panic disorders; other benzodiazepines are probably just as effective.[7] Currently, the antidepressant drugs are usually considered to be the most effective, and a benzodiazepine may be added in combination with them.[8]

Unlike the hypnotics, REM sleep is not suppressed by the benzodiazepines (as it is with the barbiturates). Therefore, REM rebound is not usually a significant problem when the drug is discontinued, although rebound insomnia may and does occur. As mentioned in Chapter 4, benzodiazepines can substitute for alcohol, especially the ones that are long acting. Therefore, they are widely used both as the treatment of choice for patients who are experiencing acute alcohol withdrawal and for long-term maintenance. However, their use in long-term maintenance is risky in patients with a history of alcohol dependence because dependence on the benzodiazepines can develop.[9]

All benzodiazepines exert antiepileptic actions because they raise the threshold for seizure generation. This action is exerted through augmentation of GABA activity in the limbic system, the midbrain, and, perhaps, the cerebellum.

Side Effects and Toxicity

Acute side effects that are commonly encountered during benzodiazepine therapy include sedation, drowsiness, light-headedness, ataxia, and lethargy. Tolerance develops to most of these effects as a result of continued use. Less frequent side effects (usually at higher doses) include impaired mental and psychomotor function, confusion, reduced reaction time, and other signs of organic brain dysfunction. Unlike the effects of using barbiturates, respiration is not seriously affected, even at high doses, and, as a result, successful suicides are rare following a benzodiazepine overdose.

Significant drug interactions can occur during benzodiazepine therapy. Perhaps the most common and the most serious interaction is the additive (or supra-additive) combination that occurs when alcohol is also used.[9] In this instance, the person consuming the drugs can experience respiratory depression that can be severe or even fatal. More commonly, an additive impairment of motor abilities occurs—especially a person's ability to drive an automobile.

Administered intravenously, benzodiazepines are very effective in causing temporary, reversible amnesia. This effect is useful in medicine when unpleasant diagnostic or therapeutic procedures must be performed on a patient and it is desired that the patient not remember what happened.

Tolerance and Dependence

When benzodiazepines are taken for long periods of time, a pattern of dependence develops. Even in therapeutic dosages, long-term, daily use of the drugs followed by discontinuation can cause a predictable abstinence (withdrawal) syndrome.[10,11] The first withdrawal signs that are observed include a return of the symptoms for which the drug originally was given, possibly in a more intense form. Second, there is a gradual appearance of rebound increases in insomnia, restlessness, agitation, irritability, and muscle tension as the blood level of the drug falls. The shorter acting the drug, the quicker the onset of withdrawal symptoms. Uncommonly, hallucinations, psychosis, and seizures can occur. Most of these withdrawal symptoms ameliorate within 1 to 4 weeks, depending on the half-life of the drug that is being used. Treatment involves gradual tapering of the dose and substitution of a long-acting benzodiazepine when the patient has developed a dependence on a drug of short duration. Recent research on possible neuroreceptor mechanisms that underlie benzodiazepine withdrawal symptoms when the drug is discontinued postulate that there is both an unmasking of the formerly drug-occupied benzodiazepine receptors and, as a result of chronic drug use, an increased number of receptors formed.[11]

Tolerance can develop, which can necessitate small increases in dose. Such development of tolerance, however, is not nearly as marked as that which occurs as a result of using nonselective CNS depressants. The mechanism of tolerance is receptor adaptation ("down-regulation" of the binding activity and the function of benzodiazepine-GABA receptors)[11]; it is not caused by metabolic pharmacokinetic changes, because benzodiazepines do not induce their own metabolism.[12]

Fetal Effects

Rarely, benzodiazepines have been reported to cause fetal abnormalities, including cleft lip and cleft palate, when they were taken by mothers during the first trimester of pregnancy. What could not be determined in these reports was whether the mothers had taken other drugs. The results given in these case reports have not been confirmed and more recent data suggest that there is no increased risk of congenital malformations in children whose mothers take only benzodiazepines during pregnancy.[13] It does appear, however, that a fetus can develop benzodiazepine dependence; and withdrawal may occur in the newborn following delivery. Overall, data that are currently available cannot assess the safety of using benzodiazepines during pregnancy. Thus, unless it is absolutely necessary (as in an epileptic mother who takes a benzodiazepine as an anticonvulsant), benzodiazepines should be avoided during pregnancy.

Finally, benzodiazepines can be detected in breast milk. Maternal intake and infant behavior should be carefully monitored in any situation that involves breast feeding.

Nonmedical Use and Abuse of Benzodiazepines

Benzodiazepines were introduced during the 1960s, and their popularity peaked during the mid-1970s, when 100 million prescriptions for these drugs were written each year. Recognizing overuse, physicians wrote only 65 million prescriptions in 1981, and, currently, about 55 million perscriptions are written each year.[14] This level of use represents conservative treatment of anxiety, with short term or occasional use far outdistancing long-term use. More women use benzodiazepines than do men, but such a distribution appears to be appropriate, because men are both more reluctant to seek medical care and more likely to use alcohol to relieve anxiety.[2] Most clinicians appear to recognize that long-term use of benzodiazepines is undesirable.

The nonmedical use (that is, abuse) of benzodiazepines peaked from 1975 through 1977 and has been decreasing ever since. It appears that the only abuse of benzodiazepines that is occurring now involves polydrug abusers rather than persons who use one drug alone in an abusive pattern. As part of a polydrug pattern, benzodiazepines (especially diazepam and alprazolam) may be taken for a euphoriant effect or to enhance the euphoriant effect of narcotics.[15] In patients who take methadone (Chapter 9), benzodiazepines augment euphoria, reducing the anxiety occurs when the blood level of the opiate falls. Many alcohol and cocaine abusers take benzodiazepines, presumably for their reinforcing and anxiolytic properties.

Benzodiazepine Receptor Antagonist

Flumazenil is a benzodiazepine derivative that binds with high affinity to the benzodiazepine receptor (Figure 5.2), where it competitively antagonizes the binding of pharmacologically active benzodiazepines.[16] Flumazenil is an antagonist at these receptors because it has affinity for the benzodiazepine receptor but exerts little intrinsic activity after it has become bound. Thus, it inhibits GABA-mediated increases in chloride conductance across membranes. Flumazenil is, therefore, a specific benzodiazepine antagonist; in the same manner, naloxone (Narcan) and naltrexone (Trexan) are specific narcotic antagonists at opiate receptors (Chapter 9). Flumazenil is capable of reversing the antianxiety effects and most of the sedative effects of the benzodiazepines.

Clinically, flumazenil is being used to reverse benzodiazepine-induced anesthesia and, in emergency rooms, to treat benzodiazepine overdose toxicity. Only about 40 percent of flumazenil becomes bound to plasma proteins; it is metabolized quite rapidly in the liver; and it has a short half-life (about 50 to 70 minutes). Because this half-life is much shorter than that of diazepam and other long-acting benzodiazepines, the effect of diazepam and other long-acting benzodiazepines can reappear as flumazenil is lost. Thus, the flumazenil must be reinjected or administered by continuous intravenous infusion, usually in an intensive-care facility.

If flumazenil were a pure antagonist at the benzodiazepine receptor (that is, if it had *no* agonist activity), and if a "natural benzodiazepine anxiolytic" does exist in the body, then one would expect to see precipitation of anxiety when flumazenil is injected into someone who has not received a benzodiazepine. In fact, flumazenil, given alone does not affect a person's behavioral response to emotional stress, nor does it cause anxiety or induce cardiovascular or other autonomic changes.[16] It appears that flumazenil may not be pure antagonist; rather, it may have a very small amount of agonist activity.[17] Thus, it is not a definitive compound that can be used to assess whether a substance exists that acts as a naturally occurring anxiolytic at the benzodiazepine-GABA receptor. It is, however, a valuable clinical addition for the treatment of benzodiazepine overdose.

STUDY QUESTIONS

1. Describe the progression of thought concerning the mode of action of the benzodiazepines.
2. Describe evidence for and against the existence of a "natural anxiolytic" in the brain.
3. Describe the structure and function of the benzodiazepine receptor.
4. How might you describe anxiety or panic in terms of receptors or neurochemicals?
5. List some of the clinical uses of benzodiazepines.
6. List three processes that might prolong the half-life of a benzodiazepine.
7. Why should the elderly avoid using long-acting benzodiazepines?
8. Describe the most significant drug interaction that involves benzo–diazepines.
9. Discuss benzodiazepine withdrawal and its treatment.
10. What is flumazenil and for what purpose might it be used?

NOTES

1. D. W. Hommer, P. Skolnick, and S. M. Paul, "The Benzodiazepine/GABA Receptor Complex and Anxiety," in H. Y. Meltzer, ed., *Pharmacology: The Third Generation of Progress* (New York: Raven, 1987), pp. 977–983.

2. American Medical Association, "Drugs Used for Anxiety and Sleep Disorders," in Drug Evaluations Annual 1991 (Milwaukee, Wis.: American Medical Association, 1990), p. 212

3. A. Breier and S. M. Paul, "The GABA-A/Benzodiazepine Receptor: Implications for the Molecular Basis of Anxiety," *Journal of Psychiatric Research* 24, Supplement 2(1990): 91–104.

4. H. P. Rang and M. M. Dale, *Pharmacology* (Edinburgh: Churchill Livingstone, 1987), pp. 486–496.

5. G. J. DiGregorio, "Antianxiety Drugs," in J. R. DiPalma and G. J. DiGregorio, eds., *Basic Pharmacology in Medicine*, 3d ed. (New York: McGraw-Hill, 1990), pp. 222–229.

6. T. W. Rall, "Hypnotics and Sedatives: Ethanol," in A. G. Gilman, T. W. Rall, A. S. Nies, and P. Taylor, eds., *Goodman and Gilman's The Pharmacological Basis of Therapeutics*, 8th ed. (New York: Pergamon, 1990), pp. 346–358.

7. J. C. Ballenger, "Efficacy of Benzodiazepines in Panic Disorder and Agoraphobia," *Journal of Psychiatric Research* 24, Supplement 2 (1990): 15–24.

8. D. D. Gold, "Management of Panic Disorder: Case Reports Support a Potential Role for Amoxapine," *Hospital Formulary* 25(1990): 1178–1184.

9. M. I. Linnoila, "Benzodiazepines and Alcohol," *Journal of Psychiatric Research 24, Supplement 2(1990): 121–128.*

10. R. L. DuPont, "A Practical Approach to Benzodiazepine Discontinuation," *Journal of Psychiatric Research* 24, Supplement 2(1990): 81–90.

11. D. J. Greenblatt, L. G. Miller, and R. L. Shader, "Benzodiazepine Discontinuation Syndromes," *Journal of Psychiatric Research* 24, Supplement 2(1990): 73–80.

12. American Psychiatric Association, "Clinical Pharmacology of Benzodiazepines," in *Benzodiazepine Dependence, Toxicity, and Abuse* (Washington D.C.: American Psychiatric Association, 1990), pp. 3–6.

13. L. S. Cohen, V. C. Heller, and J. F. Rosenbaum, "Treatment Guidelines for Psychiatric Drug Use in Pregnancy," *Psychosomatics* 30 (1989): 25–33.

14. R. R. Griffiths and C. A. Sannerud, "Abuse of and Dependence on Benzodiazepines and Other Anxiolytic/Sedative Drugs," in H. Y. Meltzer, ed. *Pharmacology: The Third Generation of Progress* (New York: Raven, 1987), pp. 1535–1566.

15. American Psychiatric Association, "Abuse Liability of Benzodiazepines," in *Benzodiazepine Dependence, Toxicity, and Abuse,* (Washington, D.C.: American Psychiatric Association, 1990), pp. 49–53.

16. A. Nilsson, "Autonomic and Hormonal Responses After the Use of Midazolam and Flumazenil," *Acta Anaesthesiologica Scandinavica,* Supplement, 92 (1990): 51–54.

17. W. Haefely, "The Preclinical Pharmacology of Flumazenil," *European Journal of Anaesthesiology,* Supplement 2 (1988): 25–36.

Psychostimulants: Cocaine and the Amphetamines

The Powerful Behavioral Stimulants

Overview

Cocaine and the amphetamines are powerful psychostimulants which markedly affect the mental function and behavior of persons who use them. Their effects include excitement, alertness, euphoria, a reduced sense of fatigue, and an increase in motor activity.

Before describing the pharmacology of these drugs, we must first distinguish them from other compounds that also stimulate the CNS, elevate mood, or alleviate depression. This can be done most conveniently by using a simple classification scheme (Table 6.1).

These powerful behavioral stimulants (cocaine, amphetamines, and amphetamine derivatives) acutely and rapidly augment or potentiate the action of at least three of the major CNS neurotransmitters: norepinephrine, dopamine, and serotonin. The time that is needed to accomplish a drug-induced potentiation of the transmitter effect parallels the time that is needed to observe the clinical effects.

Examples of psychostimulants include cocaine, *d*-amphetamine, methamphetamine, methylphenidate (Ritalin), pemoline (Cylert), and phenmetrazine (Preludin). Cocaine, methamphetamine, and d-amphetamine are commonly abused drugs. Methylphenidate and pemoline are used to treat hyperkinetic disorders in children. Phenmetrazine (as well as the amphetamines and methylphenidate) have, in past years, been used as appetite suppressants to treat obesity.

The clinical antidepressants (Chapter 8) also appear to act by reinforcing the same neurotransmitters, but they have important differences: (1) clinical antidepressants do not elevate mood or produce euphoria in normal persons; (2) their antidepressant effect in depressed patients is of slow onset, usually several weeks in duration, (3) mechanistically, such action seems to follow from a long-term reduction in receptor sensitivity or number rather than through acute potentiation of transmitter action, and (4) they may act preferentially on serotonin receptors rather than on dopamine neurons (discussed next).

The other CNS stimulants (cellular stimulants) include two widely used compounds. The first compound is caffeine, which acts by blocking adenosine receptors; and the second compound is nicotine, the principal ingredient in tobacco. Nicotine exerts its action as a secondary effect, following the stimulation of certain acetylcholine synapses that are both within the brain and in the peripheral nervous system. These two drugs are discussed in Chapter 7.

TABLE 6.1

Classification of CNS stimulants.

Class	Mechanism of action	Examples
Behavioral stimulants	Augmentation of norepinephrine and dopamine neurotransmitter	Cocaine Amphetamines Methylphenidate (Ritalin) Pemoline (Cylert) Phenmetrazine (Preludin)
Clinical antidepressants	Blockade of norepinephrine reuptake Increased norepinephrine secondary to MAO inhibition Blockade of serotonin reuptake	Imipramine (Tofranil) Amitriptyline (Elavil) Tranylcypromine (Parnate) Fluoxetine (Prozac)
Caffeine*	Blockade of adenosine receptors	
Nicotine*	Acetylcholine receptor stimulation	

*See Chapter 7

Psychostimulants and the Fight/Flight/Fright Syndrome

Cocaine and the amphetamines elevate mood, induce euphoria, increase alertness, reduce fatigue, provide a sense of increased energy, decrease appetite, improve task performance, and relieve boredom. Anxiety, insomnia, and irritability are common side effects of cocaine and the amphetamines. At higher doses, irritability and anxiety become more intense, and a pattern of psychotic behavior may appear. Indeed, cocaine and the amphetamines produce remarkably similar behavioral effects: in both animals and humans there is difficulty differentiating between the two when they are injected intravenously. At low doses, these drugs evoke an alerting, arousal, or behavioral-activating response that is not unlike a normal reaction to an emergency or to stress. These effects occur because both compounds can augment or potentiate the action of dopamine and norepinephrine in the brain. Interestingly, our own biological amines (such as adrenaline) are involved in the alerting or activating response that we experience in normal fight/flight/fright situations (see Appendix II). Thus, one would predict that psychomotor stimulation would occur when there is drug-induced augmentation of amine neurotransmission within the brain. Indeed, it is an exaggerated mobilization of this normal function that accounts for the psychomotor stimulation that is caused by these drugs.

COCAINE

History

Cocaine is a naturally occurring alkaloid that is obtained from the leaves of *Erythroxylon coca*—trees that are indigenous to Peru, Columbia, and Bolivia. In these countries, the *E. coca* leaves are used for religious, mystical, social, stimulant, and numerous medicinal purposes—most notably to increase endurance, promote a sense of well-being, and alleviate hunger.

Pharmacologically, cocaine has three prominent actions: (1) it is a potent local anesthetic; (2) it is a powerful constrictor of blood vessels (a vasoconstrictor); and (3) it is a powerful psychostimulant that has strong reinforcing qualities. It is the psychostimulant property that contributes to the compulsive abuse of the drug.[1]

The active alkaloid in *E. coca* was isolated in 1859 and was named *cocaine*. In 1884, Freud advocated the use of cocaine to treat depression and to alleviate chronic fatigue. Freud described cocaine as a "magical drug;" he even wrote a "Song of Praise" to it. In the same year, Koller demonstrated cocaine's local anesthetic properties and introduced the drug for use in ophthalmologic surgery. Freud, while using cocaine to relieve his own depression, described cocaine as inducing "exhilaration and lasting euphoria, which in no way differs from the normal euphoria of the healthy person."[2] However, he did not immediately perceive its side effects—tolerance, dependence, a state of psychosis, and withdrawal depression.[2] By 1891, at least 200 reports of cocaine intoxication and 13 deaths were reported. In 1924, the American Medical Association reviewed 43 deaths that occurred in patients who had been under local anesthesia induced by cocaine and attributed 26 of those deaths to cocaine toxicity. Guidelines for the safe use of cocaine were then established.[3]

The use of cocaine rose during the 1920s and then decreased during the 1930s, when amphetamines became available, presumably because amphetamines cost less and produced effects that lasted longer. Thus, cocaine was not used much again until the late 1960s, when tight federal restrictions on amphetamine distribution raised the cost of amphetamines, at which point cocaine became attractive once again. Because their net effects are nearly indistinguishable, cocaine and the amphetamines can be used almost interchangeably as euphoriants. Therefore, the use and popularity of cocaine and amphetamines in the future will probably be determined by availability, price, and social-cultural considerations.

It is now estimated[4,5] that 20 to 30 million people in the United States have used cocaine—5 million people use it regularly, and each day 5000 people try it for the first time. The intense, recent campaign against cocaine is beginning to decrease the number of people who use cocaine. However, the potency of currently popular cocaine products is much greater than in the past, as increasing numbers of people use injected or smoked forms ("crack" cocaine). In addition, more people are using illicit amphetamines (especially methamphetamine), which may be substituting for any reduction in the use of cocaine.

Chemistry

In South America, the leaves of *E. coca* are soaked and mashed, and cocaine is extracted in the form of coca paste (60 to 80 percent cocaine). Persons who smoke coca paste may experience the occurrence of psychopathological states, extreme toxicity, and severe dependence. Coca paste, therefore, is usually treated to form a hydrochloride salt before it is exported. Then it is diluted (to increase its bulk and decrease its potency) and sold illicitly. Until recently, this type of preparation was used most frequently. However, with the desire for increased effective potency, the diluted drug is now commonly extracted either in ether (for "freebasing") or in alkaline water (to make crack). Following either method of extraction, the concentrated drug can produce effects of utmost intensity and danger to the user. People who use these preparations do not experience the low-dose behavioral effects but, rather, the high-dose, high-intensity effects dominate. The incidence of acute panic states, toxic psychosis, and paranoid schizophrenia is greatly magnified by use of these preparations.

Pharmacokinetics

Absorption

Cocaine is rapidly absorbed when it is placed on a person's mucus membranes, such as those that line the nose, larynx, or upper respiratory tract. Following nasal application, drug levels in plasma will peak within 30 to 60 minutes (Figure 6.1) and decline over about 6 hours. Only a modest proportion of the amount of drug administered is absorbed, presumably because the resulting potent vasoconstriction, which is caused by the drug, limits its own rate of absorption.[3] When the drug is administered orally, absorption is delayed and is incomplete, presumably because a significant amount of the drug is broken down in the stomach by enzymes (*esterases*) that are located there. When cocaine is smoked, some particles probably become trapped in the nose while others pass through the nasal pharynx into the trachea and onto lung surfaces, from which absorption is rapid and quite complete.

Distribution

Cocaine penetrates the brain rapidly; initial brain concentrations far exceed those in plasma. After it penetrates into the brain, it is redistributed to other tissues. As stated by Jaffe:

It is thought that the sharp contrast between these high but brief concentrations in the brain and the subsequent rapid decline

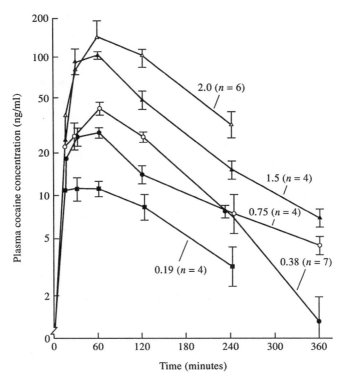

FIGURE 6.1

Time course of plasma cocaine levels following various doses (0.38–2.0 mg/kg) of intranasal cocaine. Points are mean ± S.E. [From J. A. Fleming, R. Byck, and P. G. Barash,[3] Figure 2, p. 520.]

generates the intense drive to use more drug within a very brief period. Crack users may progress from experimentation to dependence in a matter of weeks.[5]

Elimination

Cocaine has a biological half-life of 30 to 90 minutes, and it is almost completely metabolized (in plasma and in the liver) before its metabolites are excreted in urine. After a single intravenous dose, the drug becomes undetectable in about 6 to 8 hours. Its inactive metabolites, however, are detectable for a much longer period of time in urine. Some persons genetically lack the plasma enzyme that metabolizes cocaine, so the duration of action can be prolonged. There is some question as to whether cocaine metabolites can be toxic to the liver under certain circumstances.[3]

Cocaine is rapidly and freely distributed to the fetus; and the fetus, in turn, can metabolize cocaine, presumably to substances that can be feto-toxic.[6]

Because only about 1 percent of a dose of cocaine is excreted unmetabolized in urine, laboratory detection techniques instead look for urinary metabolites. Metabolites of cocaine can be detected for about 2 days after a person has used cocaine. However, long-term, high-dose users seem to sequester unmetabolized cocaine in their bodies, in which case metabolites can sometimes be detected for up to a week after they have stopped using the drug.

Pharmacodynamics

Mechanism of Action

Cocaine exerts two distinct actions on the nervous system. First, it is a potent local anesthetic and, like all other local anesthetics (Chapter 13), it blocks the conduction of nerve impulses down axons by reversibly blocking sodium channels that are located in nerve membranes (it prevents the flow of transmembrane sodium that is essential for the propagation of nerve impulses; see Appendix II). In this action, cocaine is virtually indistinguishable from other local anesthetics (for example, lidocaine). Cocaine is now seldom used clinically as a local anesthetic—not because it is ineffective, but because of its effects on the CNS and its adverse social connotations. Occasionally, however, it is still used in nasal surgery when both its local anesthetic effects and its vasoconstrictive properties are desired.

Second, cocaine is a powerful potentiator of dopamine and (less so) of norepinephrine neurotransmission in the CNS. This action of cocaine is unique among all other local anesthetics. During the period from 1959 through 1961, it was demonstrated that cocaine blocks the active presynaptic neuronal reuptake of both norepinephrine and dopamine, especially in those portions of the brain that underlie behavioral reinforcement, or reward, mechanisms.[1,7] Indeed, the augmentation of dopamine neurotransmission as a result of inhibiting its active reuptake appears to account for virtually all of the behavioral reinforcing effects of cocaine (discussed further in Chapter 15).

What is perplexing is the fact that the tricyclic antidepressants (Chapter 8) also block biological amine reuptake (and relieve depression), but they are neither euphoriants nor psychostimulants. Although we have not yet solved this dilemma at the synaptic level, there is much speculation that cocaine may also act postsynaptically to produce a change in the postsynaptic neurons, which would make them capable of generating an increased maximum response.[3] Thus, cocaine may also somehow alter the sensitivity of postsynaptic dopamine receptors. Eventually, a cohesive theory may emerge that will resolve the dichotomy between the actions of cocaine and those of the antidepressants. This topic is discussed further in Chapter 8.

Behavioral Effects

As stated previously, cocaine inhibits the active reuptake of dopamine and norepinephrine from the synaptic cleft back into presynaptic nerve terminals in the brain as well as in the peripheral nervous system. Such a blockade of uptake increases the amount of transmitter that remains in the synaptic cleft, which (along with a possible sensitization of the postsynaptic membrane) results in intense stimulation of postsynaptic receptors in the CNS as well as in the peripheral nervous system.

In the peripheral nervous system, the potentiation of norepinephrine neurotransmission initiates responses in a person that are characteristic of the fight/flight/fright syndrome. Cocaine increases a person's heart rate, constricts blood vessels, increases blood pressure, produces bronchodilation in the lungs, increases body temperature, dilates the pupils, and shifts blood flow from the stomach and intestine to the muscles. The intense vasoconstriction that occurs after "snorting" cocaine can produce marked hypoxia (oxygen deprivation) of the nasal tissues, with eventual necrosis (tissue death) and perforation of the nasal septum.

Cocaine is a brief but powerful CNS stimulant and euphoriant, which affects both the cortex and the brain stem. It is a potent behavioral reinforcer.[1,5] It increases mental awareness and alertness, and these effects are accompanied by a feeling of well-being and euphoria. Although the user's sense of fatigue is decreased and his or her motor activity is increased, coordination decreases rapidly when higher doses are taken, because the brain stem centers that control the coordination of movement are affected. At even higher doses, a progressive loss of coordination is followed by tremors and, eventually, seizures. CNS stimulation is followed by depression, dysphoria, anxiety, somnolence, and drug craving. Deaths due to cocaine usually result from respiratory failure, seizures, stroke, or cardiac arrhythmias and cardiac arrest.

As stated by Jaffe:

> In the early stages of use, the increased energy and sociability may elicit positive responses from friends and associates. These positive experiences tend to lead to frequent use of the drug in increasing doses. Eventually, the socially reinforcing experiences are supplanted by a focus on drug-induced euphoria.[5]

A person's sexual interest may be heightened by using cocaine, and high doses of cocaine that are injected or smoked may be described as "orgasmic," leading to the impression that the drug is an aphrodisiac. However, sexual dysfunction is common in persons who use cocaine. Further, when that dysfunction is combined with the isolation that addicts experience when they are taking high-doses, normal interpersonal, sensual, and sexual interactions are compromised.

Although low doses of cocaine cause CNS stimulation that is mostly pleasurable or euphoric, higher doses produce toxic symptoms, including anxiety, sleep deprivation, hypervigilance, suspiciousness, paranoia, and persecutory fears. One's perception of reality can become markedly altered in person's who use cocaine, and they can become aggressive or homicidal against imagined persecution.[5] These behaviors comprise what is called a *toxic paranoid psychosis*.

Rounsaville and coworkers[8] recently studied 300 cocaine abusers seeking treatment for their substance abuse problem. They found that 56 percent met *current* criteria and 73 percent met *lifetime* criteria for the presence of a neuropsychological disorder (major depression, anxiety disorder, bipolar affective disorder, antisocial personality, or history of childhood attention-deficit–hyperactivity disorder). Thus, appearance of toxic symptoms (discussed previously) may indicate either high-dose drug toxicities or the onset of symptoms of a coexisting neuropsychological disorder.

The most notable (and most notorious) property of cocaine is its intense reinforcing property, which is the source of most of the confusion and controversy that surround use of the drug.[9] No current theory adequately explains the euphoria—an action that is not caused by the clinical antidepressants and both resembles and is distinctly different from that of the opioid narcotics. Indeed, this euphoria and activation of functional reward systems may relate to dopamine receptor mechanisms, or it may involve other neuronal systems altogether.

Side Effects and Toxicity

Undesired side effects are not common for recreational users of *low doses* of cocaine. When acute anxiety reactions occur, they are manifested by increased blood pressure and heart rate, sweating, anxiety, and paranoia. Hallucinations and delusions are rare. More common are the feelings of irritability and lassitude that occur in the user after the effects subside, together with a desire for more of the drug. Withdrawal after a longer period of using even modest doses of cocaine is followed by profound physical and emotional depression, which is similar to that occasioned by amphetamine withdrawal (discussed in the following text).

More serious *high-dose, long-term* toxicities include a toxic paranoid syndrome, sleep disorders, sexual dysfunction, acquisition of needle-transmitted diseases (hepatitis and AIDS) in intravenous users, interpersonal conflicts (resulting from the isolation and the paranoia), and severe depression and dysphoria that occur when a person stops using the drug.

The acutely toxic dose of cocaine has been estimated to be about 1 to 2 mg per kilogram of body weight. Thus, 70 to 150 milligrams of cocaine is a toxic, one-time dose for a 150-pound (70-kg) person. Doses that are higher than that are extremely dangerous to the heart, the respiratory system, and the brain, causing death following respiratory or cardiac arrest, pulmonary edema, or seizures. Unfortunately, when a person is using an illicit drug, her or she is seldom aware of the dose, in milligrams, that is being taken. Toxic doses for persons who use the drug for prolonged periods of time cannot be predicted with any degree of safety. Long-term users must consider not only the acute toxicity to the cardiovascular system, the respiratory system, and the brain, but also the toxicity to social, health, and cultural well-being (already noted).

Fetal Effects

One of the great tragedies of the late 1980s and early 1990s is the birth of thousands of "crack babies." For some time, we have known that women who take cocaine during pregnancy are much more likely to have spontaneous abortions, to experience placental detachment or placental insufficiency, and to have fetal death late in pregnancy. Premature labor and precipitous delivery are common in women who use cocaine. Cocaine reduces infant birth weight and increases the incidence of stillbirths. All of these effects are presumed to follow from the intense vasoconstriction that is induced by cocaine; that is, the fetus suffers from a lack of oxygen because the uterine and placental arteries become severely constricted, subsequently reducing blood flow to the fetus.[6,10]

New on the scene is the epidemic of babies that have been born of mothers who used high doses of cocaine during pregnancy. Some are born with visible birth defects, but, in most, the defects are neurological and more difficult to detect. Nearly all these infants are irritable, tremulous, and difficult to soothe. Returned to a drug environment and possibly to poverty, newborns experience little physical or emotional nurturing, so bonding is incomplete or absent. These crack babies are just now beginning to enter the school system, and they seem to have difficulty developing attachments to anyone or dealing effectively with multiple stimuli. They may become either aggressive or withdrawn when they are overstimulated. They have difficulty with unstructured play; they have a low tolerance for frustration; and they structure input and information poorly. Probably all these difficulties are the combined effects of prenatal drug exposure (with abnormal CNS development), fetal hypoxia, and an early growth period in difficult homes or institutions. As stated by Besharov:

> These children form a *"bio-underclass"*—a cohort of children whose combined physiological damage and extrinsic socio-economic disadvantage could foredoom them to a life of inferiority. In other words, a generation of children so damaged neurologically and environmentally that their inferiority is determined from birth.[11]

What kind of numbers are we talking about? Certainly, 30,000 to 50,000 births per year is a low estimate; 200,000 per year is probably a high estimate. Perhaps 2 percent of infants born annually are born to women who have used cocaine during pregnancy. With these numbers and with the severe degree of impairment that occurs in the children, the societal costs will be enormous, especially since intensive care and nurturing are needed from the moment of birth, through schooling, and into the early adult years, when deviance or social inferiority will become more obvious.

AMPHETAMINES AND RELATED DRUGS

Amphetamine (Fig. 6.2), the more potent active form *dextroamphetamine*, the methyl derivative (*methamphetamine*), and several derivatives (*methylphenidate, fenfluramine,* and *pemoline*) comprise a group of drugs

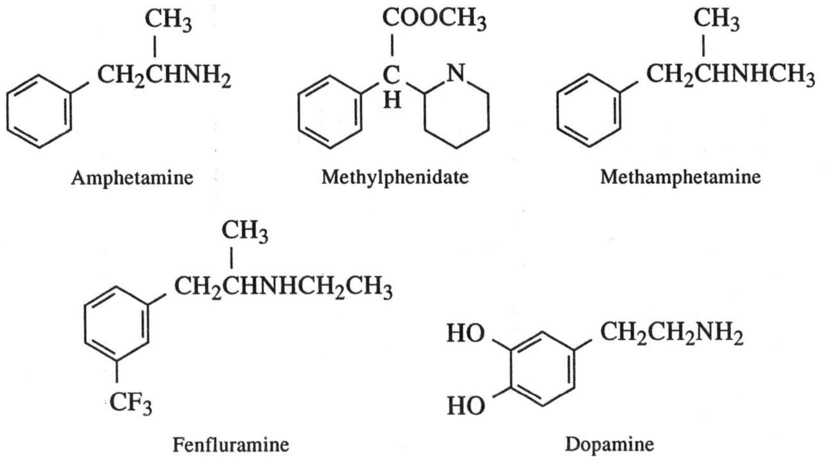

FIGURE 6.2

Structures of amphetamines and dopamine.

that exert psychostimulant effects through similar mechanisms and, therefore, share similar pharmacological properties that closely resemble the psychostimulant properties of cocaine.

Amphetamine was first synthesized in the early 1900s, but it was not used for medicinal purposes until the early 1930s, when it was found that it increased blood pressure, stimulated the CNS, and caused bronchodilation. Amphetamine was used to treat narcolepsy, a disorder in which the patient repeatedly lapses into sleep. Since then, amphetamines have been used both licitly and illicitly for a wide variety of clinical and recreational purposes. Despite variances in potency (compensated for by an adjustment in dose), the effects of most of the amphetamine derivatives are similar to those of amphetamine itself; therefore, amphetamine is discussed at length and the derivatives are compared with it.

Pharmacological Effects

The pharmacological responses to amphetamine vary markedly in persons, depending on the dose of the drug that they are taking. In general, however, they may be categorized as those observed at low-to-moderate doses (5 to 50 milligrams of amphetamine, usually administered orally) and those observed at high doses (doses higher than approximately 100 milligrams, often administered intravenously).

These dose ranges are not the same for all amphetamines. For example, dextroamphetamine is three to four times more potent than amphetamine. Low-to-moderate doses of dextroamphetamine are in a range from 2.5 to 20 milligrams, while high doses are considered to contain 50 milligrams or more. Methamphetamine ("speed") is even more potent, so doses must be lowered even further.

At normal oral doses, all of the amphetamines induce a significant increase in blood pressure, with a reflex slowing of heart rate, a relaxation of bronchial muscle, and a variety of other responses that follow from the body's chemical preparation for our fight/flight/fright response (that is, increased blood sugar, increased blood flow to muscles, decreased blood flow to internal organs, dilation of pupils, increased rate of respiration, increased heart rate and blood pressure, and so on).

In the CNS, amphetamine is a potent psychomotor stimulant, producing increased alertness, euphoria, excitement, wakefulness, a reduced sense of fatigue, loss of appetite, mood elevation, increased motor and speech activity, and an increased feeling of power. Although task performance is improved, dexterity may deteriorate, which is evidenced by the increased number of errors that a user can make as a result of irritability and nervousness. When short-duration, high-intensity energy output is desired, such as during an athletic competition, a user's performance may be enhanced, despite the fact that his or her dexterity and fine motor skills may be reduced. Amphetamines are excreted in the urine and are easily detected for up to 48 hours after use.

At moderate doses (5 to 50 milligrams), the further effects of amphetamine include stimulation of respiration, production of a slight tremor, restlessness, a greater increase in motor activity, insomnia, and agitation. In addition, amphetamine prevents fatigue, suppresses appetite, promotes wakefulness, and causes sleep deprivation. The biological need for sleep cannot be postponed indefinitely, and deep sleep follows when use of the drug is discontinued. Complete recovery of normal sleeping patterns may take many weeks. Indeed, both the prolonged use of low doses of amphetamine and the single use of high doses of amphetamine are characteristically followed by an intensity of mental depression and fatigue that mirrors the behavioral stimulation and euphoria that were produced by the initial dose of the drug.

In persons who use high doses of amphetamine chronically, a state of amphetamine psychosis may develop, which may be indistinguishable from an acute attack of schizophrenia. These persons experience visual and auditory hallucinations, which are accompanied by paranoid symptoms and aggressive behavior. As stated by Rang and Dale:

The close similarity of this condition to acute paranoid schizophrenia and the effectiveness of neuroleptic drugs [the antipsychotic drugs discussed in Chapter 10] in controlling it, is consistent with the dopamine theory of schizophrenia.[12]

An intravenous injection of amphetamine provides a sudden "flash," or "rush," which is described by users as being extremely pleasurable and even "orgasmic." These pleasurable effects, however, are offset by the state of manic paranoia that follows. When the drug is withdrawn and the "spree" is subsequently terminated, fatigue and deep sleep occur. Upon awakening, the user is lethargic, emotionally depressed, and usually intensely hungry.

Mechanism of Action

Amphetamine and related drugs exert virtually all of their CNS effects by causing the release of biological amines (dopamine, norepinephrine, serotonin, or all of these) from presynaptic storage sites that are located in nerve terminals.[12]

Controversy enters, however, when we attempt to decide which of these transmitters is the most important to the action of amphetamine. Hoffman and Levkowitz state:

> The alerting effect, . . . its anorectic [appetite-suppressing] effect, and at least a component of its locomotor-stimulating action are presumably mediated by release of *norepinephrine* from central norepinephrine neurons. . . . Some aspects of locomotor activity and the stereotyped behavior . . . are probably a consequence of the release of *dopamine* from dopaminergic nerve terminals. . . . With still higher doses, disturbances of perception and overt psychotic behavior . . . may be due to release of *serotonin* from serotonin neurons as well as of dopamine.[13]

In contrast, Rang and Dale state:

> The behavioral effects of amphetamine are probably due mainly to release of dopamine rather than norepinephrine. [Furthermore,] the anorectic actions may depend more on serotonin release than on the release of norepinephrine or dopamine.[12]

The relation between serotonin and appetite suppression will be discussed further in Chapter 8.

Gold, Gold, and Koob argue for a *dopamine* release mechanism that includes the rewarding effects of both the locomotor and the psychomotor stimulant properties of amphetamine, where

> disinhibition of the dopamine neurons from serotonin modulation may be involved in the stimulant and psychostimulant (hallucinogenic) effects.[14]

Despite these conflicting views, there appears to be a consensus that all three transmitters (with dopamine probably being the most dominant) are released by the amphetamines from the many sites of transmitter storage in the CNS, and such release underlies most, if not all, of the effects of the amphetamines (from behavioral stimulation and anorexia to toxic psychosis). Exactly how these transmitters interact with each other to cause all the effects of amphetamines is far from clear.[15]

Side Effects and Toxicity

The side effects of *low doses* of amphetamines include increased irritability, restlessness, insomnia, blurred vision, increased blood pressure, cardiac palpitations, and anxiety. Occasionally, aggression, hallucinations, and psychosis may occur, but usually these are seen only at higher doses.

As already stated, *high-dose intravenous* use induces a pattern of psychosis or schizophrenia that is characterized by confused and disorganized behavior, compulsive repetition of meaningless acts, irritability, fear, suspicion of everything and everyone, hallucinations, and delusions. The user may become aggressive and extremely antisocial. Persons who inject amphetamines either dissolve oral tablets or crystalline methamphetamine ("crystal") that is manufactured illegally. When they are used intravenously, the amphetamines are known as "speed." Users of injectable amphetamines (or cocaine) often attempt to antagonize high-dose toxic symptoms by adding an opioid analgesic (such as morphine or heroin] to the stimulant. Such a concoction is called a "speedball." Amphetamine abusers also usually consume significant amounts of other CNS depressants such as barbiturates, benzodiazepines, or alcohol. The depression and lethargy that follow amphetamine use are accentuated by depressant drugs, which serve to intensify fatigue, lethargy, and mental depression. Reinitiation of amphetamine use eliminates this state, but it starts a new cycle of abuse.

Severe toxicities are seen in the deteriorating, high-dose user. Psychosis and abnormal mental conditions, weight loss, skin sores, infections resulting from neglected health care, and a variety of other consequences occur because of the actions of the drug itself or because of poor eating habits, lack of sleep, and the use of unsterile equipment for intravenous injections. Most high-dose users show progressive social, personal, and occupational deterioration; and their course is often characterized by intermittent periods of hospitalization for episodes of toxic psychosis.

The toxic dose of amphetamine varies widely. Severe reactions can occur as a result of using very low doses (that is, 20 to 30 mg). On the other hand, persons who do not have tolerance have survived doses of 400 to 500 milligrams. Even larger doses are tolerated by chronic users. The slogan "speed kills" not only refers to a direct fatal effect of single doses of amphetamine but also to the deteriorating mental and physical condition that occurs in the user as well as the destructive, aggressive behavior that is induced by prolonged high-dose amphetamine sprees.

Of interest and concern are several reports that amphetamine, methamphetamine, or the psychedelic amphetamines MDMA and MDA (Chapter 11), can be neurotoxic to dopamine (and possibly serotonin) neurons when they are administered in high doses to rodents and non-human primates.[16,17] An experimental, structurally similar neurotoxin, termed *MPTP* (1-methyl-4-phenyl-tetrahydro-pyridine) causes a parkinsonism-like syndrome by irreversibly destroying dopamine neurons in the brain (through a mechanism that is not yet known).

At present, there is no clear evidence that amphetamine or any of its derivatives cause neurotoxicity (neuronal death) in humans. However, since MPTP can destroy dopamine neurons and can produce conditions that are a laboratory model for Parkinson's disease, a conservative view might include the notion that abuse of amphetamine, methamphetamine, MDMA, or MDA may predispose humans to neurotoxicity. Long-term, high-dose use of these drugs (where signs and symptoms of toxic psychosis or paranoid schizophrenia are present) might increase the likelihood of neuronal damage.

Dependence and Tolerance

Dependence is twofold: psychological and physiological. Psychological dependence is described as a compulsion to use a drug repeatedly for its enjoyable effects. The euphoric or pleasurable state that follows even moderate doses of amphetamines and the drug-induced "rush" and orgasmic sensations that may be induced by intravenous use can lead to a compulsion to misuse the drugs.

Physiological dependence to a nonselective CNS depressant compound was described in Chapter 3 as being characterized by a period of rebound hyperexcitability following withdrawal of the sedative. In contrast, withdrawal of amphetamine (a psychostimulant) produces behavioral depression that is characterized by fatigue, profound and prolonged sleep, EEG changes that are characteristic of sleep, severe emotional depression, and increased appetite. These withdrawal symptoms are certainly not unexpected; one would predict that if the body and the brain were continually stimulated by amphetamine, such stimulation would be followed by depression when the drug was removed.

Tolerance to the many effects of amphetamines develops in different people at different rates and to different degrees. Tolerance to the appetite-suppressing effect of amphetamines develops invariably and rapidly, which accounts for the failure of these compounds to produce effective long-term treatment for obesity. Although the mood-elevating action of amphetamines is subject to tolerance, it is not as pronounced as the tolerance to the appetite-suppressant effect. There are also some effects of amphetamines to which only minimal tolerance develops. For instance, in the treatment of attention-deficit, hyperactivity problems in children (discussed in the next section), once an adequate controlling dose is achieved, there may be little need to increase the dose further.

Therapeutic Uses and Status

The primary medical uses of amphetamines are restricted today. Amphetamines were first found to be useful and specific in the treatment of narcolepsy, and, to some degree, this use continues. Amphetamines also are useful in treating attention-deficit–hyperactivity disorder in children. This disorder affects up to 6 percent of school-aged children. It is characterized by inattentiveness and impulsiveness, usually with impaired learning and behavioral hyperactivity.

There is some evidence that the disorder may be inherited[18] and that symptoms may persist into adulthood in a large percentage of persons with the childhood disorder.[19] Recently, Zametkin and coworkers[20,21] studied the rates of glucose metabolism in selected areas of the brains of adults who had histories of hyperactivity in childhood and who continued to have these symptoms as adults (each patient was also the parent of a hyperactive child). Areas of the brain that are known to be involved in attention and motor activity (especially the prefrontal cortex) were shown to have low rates of glucose metabolism. If this result can be reproduced by others, it may offer intriguing insights into a biological cause of attention-deficit–hyperactivity disorder.

Pharmacologically, stimulant drugs have long been the mainstay of treatment for attention-deficit–hyperactivity disorder. Amphetamine, and more recently the amphetamine derivatives methylphenidate (Ritalin) and pemoline (Cylert), improves behavior and learning ability in 50 to 75 percent of children who are correctly diagnosed. However, indiscriminate use of these behavioral stimulants for "problem children" and sole dependence on drug therapy for attention-deficit disorders should be discouraged. The family situation of a child who is diagnosed as hyperkinetic should be investigated to rule out external causes for his or her behavior. Adjunctive treatments, such as remedial education, behavior modification, and counseling with parents and teachers are indicated. The treatment of children with attention-deficit–hyperactivity disorder was recently critically reviewed.[22]

Why stimulants calm hyperactive children is becomong better understood.[22] If one postulates that attention-deficit–hyperactivity disorder is a reflection of depression, use of a stimulant or an antidepressant drug might alleviate the behavioral symptoms. On the other hand, by increasing attention, vigilance, memory performance, and learning abilities, a child's anxieties may be relieved, and the anxious state may be replaced by a more pleasant and productive one. Indeed, adults in certain anxiety states (such as studying for final examinations) often find that they become calmer, more alert, and can work more efficiently after taking amphetamine or other psychostimulants. Finally, if prefrontal cortical hypometabolism is involved, the CNS stimulation afforded by psychostimulants would increase oxygen utilization and improve the disorder.

The amphetamines have, in the past, been used widely in the treatment of obesity; however, today such use is considered unwise and has been abandoned. Weight loss following amphetamine use is caused by a depression of appetite that is secondary to the drug's action on feeding and satiety centers in the hypothalamus. Tolerance to this effect develops rapidly, and weight loss is not usually maintained. Because the amphetamines were the first drugs widely prescribed to suppress appetite, they remain the standard to which newer drugs are compared (despite the fact that they are no longer recommended, because the risk of drug dependence is so great). Newer drugs that are currently promoted as appetite suppressants include diethylpropion (Tenuate,

Tepanil), mazindol (Mazanor, Sanorex), fenfluramine (Pondimin), and phentermine (Ionamin). Formerly, phenmetrazine (Preludin) was used widely, but a high incidence of drug abuse and dependence has rendered it obsolete. All these drugs closely resemble amphetamine both structurally and pharmacologically. Although none of these drugs is superior to the amphetamines as appetite suppressants, few of them are currently associated with significant drug-abuse problems. Therefore, they are preferred in those rare instances when drug supplementation may be beneficial in appetite-suppression programs.

Phenylpropanolamine (available in multiple over-the-counter diet aids) is a mild stimulant that is promoted as an aid in weight reduction. It has low potency and, as a result, exerts only mild CNS effects. At doses that are as effective as those of amphetamine, phenylpropanolamine probably would be equally euphoric, but the drug has not yet been abused widely.

Specific Agents

Dextroamphetamine is the pharmacologically active form of amphetamine (which is a mixture of dextroamphetamine and levoamphetamine; amphetamine is one-third to one-fourth as active as dextroamphetamine as a psychostimulant).

Methamphetamine is somewhat more potent than dextroamphetamine, and it is easier to manufacture in illicit laboratories. It has been implicated as a neurotoxic agent, although such toxicity has not been demonstrated in humans.

Methylphenidate (Ritalin) is a mild CNS stimulant that is structurally related to amphetamine. It has a short half-life (1 to 2 hours) and, therefore, it must be administered in divided daily doses. This is sometimes a problem when it is taken by school-age children for the treatment of attention-deficit disorders. A long-acting, sustained release preparation is available to minimize this problem.

Pemoline (Cylert) exerts effects that are similar to those of methylphenidate. Pemoline has a long half-life and can be administered once daily. Treatment for several weeks might be necessary before clinical effects are seen.

Fenfluramine (Pondimin) reduces appetite, apparently with little or no behavioral stimulation. This anorectic action may result from the drug-induced release of serotonin rather than from the release of norepinephrine or dopamine. This action is consistent with the results of trials of antidepressants that block serotonin uptake (Chapter 8) in the treatment of obesity (where they decrease the spontaneous intake of food).

Nasal decongestants are structurally related to amphetamine. They can alter the synaptic actions of norepinephrine both in the brain and in the peripheral nervous system. Most nasal decongestants are more potent in the peripheral nervous system than in the brain. Representative products include ephedrine, tetrahydrozoline (Tyzine), metaraminol (Aramine), phenylephrine (Neo-Synephrine), pseudoephedrine (Sudafed), xylometazoline (Otrivin), nylidrin (Arlidin), propylhexedrine (Benzedrex), phenmetrazine (Preludin), naphazoline (Privine), and oxymetazoline (Afrin). These compounds differ from one another primarily in terms of the intensity of their effects on the body (heart rate, breathing, and the like) and in the degree to which they stimulate behavior. In general, the responses to these drugs are similar to those observed for amphetamine, except that most have very few CNS effects. Many are used as nasal decongestants, and cessation of use may result in rebound increases in nasal stuffiness, a response that is similar to the stuffy nose that follows the use of cocaine. Ephedrine is found as the active ingredient in many illicit preparations that are alleged to be amphetamine.

STUDY QUESTIONS

1. Compare and contrast cocaine and amphetamine.
2. Explain the actions of cocaine and amphetamine in light of the fight/flight/fright syndrome.
3. What is "crack"?
4. Describe the three major actions of cocaine.
5. Discuss the effects of cocaine on the fetus.
6. Describe the behavioral states that are observed in high-dose amphetamine users.
7. Describe the effects of amphetamine on neurotransmitters.
8. Why might amphetamine-like drugs be useful in the treatment of children who have attention-deficit–hyperactivity disorder?
9. Compare and contrast the psychostimulants with the clinical antidepressants.
10. What is meant by the term "speed kills"?

NOTES

1. D. Clouet, K. Asqhar and R. Brown, eds. *Mechanisms of Cocaine Abuse and Toxicity*, NIDA Research Monograph 88, U.S. Department of Health and Human Services (Rockville, Md.: National Institute on Drug Abuse, 1988).

2. S. Freud, *Cocaine Papers* (New York: Stonehill, 1974).

3. J. A. Fleming, R. Byck, and P. G. Barash, "Pharmacology and Therapeutic Applications of Cocaine," *Anesthesiology* 73 (1990): pp. 518–531.

4. R. H. Cravey, "Cocaine Deaths in Infants," *Journal of Analytical Toxicology* 12 (1988): 354–355.

5. J. H. Jaffe, "Drug Addiction and Drug Abuse," in A. G. Gilman, T. W. Rall, A. S. Nies, and P. Taylor, eds., *Goodman and Gilman's The Pharmacological Basis of Therapeutics*, 8th ed. (New York: Pergamon, 1990), pp. 539–545.

6. I. J. Chasnoff, W. J. Burns, S. H. Schnoll, and K. A. Burns, "Cocaine Use in Pregnancy," *New England Journal of Medicine* 313 (1985): 666–669.

7. R. A. Wise, "Neural Mechanisms of the Reinforcing Action of Cocaine," in J. Grabowski, ed., *Cocaine: Pharmacology, Effects, and Treatment of Abuse*, National Institute on Drug Abuse, Research Monograph No. 50, Department of Health and Human Services (Washington, D. C.: U. S. Government Printing Office, 1984), pp. 15–33.

8. B. J. Rounsaville, S. F. Anton, K. Carroll, D. Budde, B. A. Prusoff and F. Gawin, "Psychiatric Diagnoses of Treatment-Seeking Cocaine Abusers," *Archives of General Psychiatry* 48(1991), 43–51.

9. R. Byck, "Cocaine Use and Research: Three Histories,"in S. Fisher, A. Raskin, and E. H. Uhlenhuth, eds., *Cocaine: Clinical and Biobehavioral Aspects* (New York: Oxford, 1987), pp. 3–20.

10. I. J. Chasnoff, C. E. Hunt, and D. Kaplan, "Prenatal Cocaine Exposure as Associated with Respiratory Pattern Abnormalities," *American Journal of Diseases of Childhood* 143 (1989): 583–587.

11. M. C. Rist, "The Shadow Children," *The American School Board Journal* (January 1990): 19–24.

12. H. P. Rang and M. M. Dale, *Pharmacology* (Edinburgh: Churchill Livingstone, 1987), pp. 571–575.

13. B. B. Hoffman and R. J. Lefkowitz, "Catecholamines and Sympathomimetic Drugs," in A. G. Gilman, T. W. Rall, A. S. Nies, and P.

Taylor, eds., *Goodman and Gilman's The Pharmacological Basis of Therapeutics*, 8th ed. (New York: Pergamon, 1990), p. 211.

14. L. H. Gold, M. A. Gold, and G. F. Koob, "Neurochemical Mechanisms Involved in Behavioral Effects of Amphetamines and Related Designer Drugs," in K. Asqhar and E. DeSouza, eds., *Pharmacology and Toxicology of Amphetamine and Related Designer Drugs*, NIDA Research Monograph 94, U.S. Department of Health and Human Services (Rockville, Md.: National Institute on Drug Abuse, 1989), pp. 101–126.

15. P. M. Groves, L. J. Ryan, M. Diana, S. Y. Young, and L. J. Fisher, "Neuronal Actions of Amphetamine in the Rat Brain," in K. Saqhar and E. DeSouza, eds., *Pharmacology and Toxicology of Amphetamine and Related Designer Drugs*, NIDA Research Monograph 94, U.S. Department of Health and Human Services (Rockville, Md.: National Insitute on Drug Abuse, 1989), pp. 127–145.

16. R. W. Fuller, "Recommendations for Future Research on Amphetamines and Related Designer Drugs," in K. Asqhar and E. DeSouza, eds., *Pharmacology and Toxicology of Amphetamine and Related Designer Drugs*, NIDA Research Monograph 94 (Rockville, Md.: National Insitute on Drug Abuse, 1989), pp. 341-357.

17. L. S. Seiden and G. A. Ricaurte, "Neurotoxicity of Methamphetamine and Related Drugs," in H. Y. Meltzer, ed., *Psychopharmacology: The Third Generation of Progress* (New York: Raven, 1987), pp. 359–366.

18. J. Biederman, K. Munir, D. Knee, et al., "A Family Study of Patients with Attention Deficit Disorder and Normal Controls," *Journal of Psychiatry Research* 20 (1986): 263–274.

19. G. Weiss, L. Hechtman, T. Milroy and T. Perlman, "Psychiatric Status of Hyperactives as Adults: A Controlled Prospective 15-Year Follow-Up of 63 Hyperactive Children," *Journal of the American Academy of Child and Adolescent Psychiatry* 24 (1985): 211–220.

20. A. J. Zametkin and G. G. Borcherding, "The Neuropharmacology of Attention-Deficit Hyperactivity Disorder," *Annual Review of Medicine* 40 (1989): 447–451.

21. A. J. Zametkin, T. E. Nordahl, M. Gross, A. C. King, W. E. Semple, J. Rumsey, S. Hamburger, and R. H. Cohen, "Cerebral Glucose Metabolism in Adults with Hyperactivity of Childhood Onset," *The New England Journal of Medicine* 323 (1990): 1361–1366.

22. D. Jacobvitz, A. Sroufe, M. Stewart, and N. Leffert, "Treatment of Attentional and Hyperactivity Problems in Children with Sympathomimetic Drugs: A Comprehensive Review," *Journal of the American Academy of Child and Adolescent Psychiatry* 29(1990): 677–688.

Caffeine and Nicotine
Our Most Casually Used Drugs

CAFFEINE

Caffeine, the most popular and widely consumed drug in the world, is found in significant concentrations in coffee, tea, cola drinks, chocolate candy, and cocoa.[1] As shown in Table 7.1, the average cup of coffee contains about 80 to 120 milligrams of caffeine, and a 12-ounce bottle of a cola drink contains between 35 and 55 milligrams of caffeine, much of which is added as a supplement by the manufacturer. The caffeine content may be as high as 25 milligrams per ounce in chocolate. The annual consumption of caffeine in the United States in the form of coffee alone is estimated at about 15 million pounds, with the *daily* per-capita intake of caffeine averaging between 170 and 200 milligrams.[2] Eighty percent of adults consume an average of three to five cups of coffee every day.

Pharmacokinetics

After oral ingestion, caffeine is rapidly absorbed, and significant blood levels of caffeine are reached in about 30 minutes. Complete absorption occurs over the next 90 minutes. Although CNS effects

TABLE 7.1

Caffeine content in beverages, foods, and medicines.

Item	Caffeine content	
	Average (milligrams)	Range
Coffee (5-ounce cup)	100	50–150
Tea (5-ounce cup)	50	25–90
Cocoa (5-ounce cup)	5	2–20
Chocolate (semisweet, baking) (1 ounce)	25	15–30
Chocolate (milk) (1 ounce)	5	1–10
Soft drinks (12 ounces)	40	36–50
OTC* stimulants (No Doz, Vivarin)	100+	
OTC* analgesics (Excedrin)	65	
(Anacin, Midol, Vanquish)	33	
OTC* cold remedies (Coryban-D, Triaminicin)	30	
OTC* diuretics (Aqua-ban)	100	

*OTC, over the counter.

are appreciated in about 30 minutes, they take about 2 hours to reach maximum levels.

Caffeine is freely and equally distributed throughout the total amount of water in the body and, like all psychoactive drugs, it freely crosses the placenta to the fetus. Thus, caffeine is found in almost equal concentrations in all parts of the body, including the brain. Most of the caffeine is metabolized by the liver before it is excreted by the kidneys. Only about 10 percent of the drug is excreted unchanged (that is, without being metabolized). The half-life of caffeine is about 3 to 5 hours in most adults; it is longer in infants, pregnant women, and the elderly; and it is shorter in smokers. Concentrations of caffeine in breast milk may exceed the level that exists in the mother's plasma.

Pharmacological Effects

Caffeine is a powerful CNS stimulant. The cortex, being the most sensitive, is affected first, followed next by the brain stem and finally (if toxic doses of caffeine are taken) by the spinal cord. As a result of cerebral cortical stimulation, the earliest behavioral effects of caffeine include increased mental alertness, a faster and clearer flow of thought, wakefulness, and restlessness. Fatigue is reduced and the need for sleep is delayed. This increased mental awareness may result in sustained intellectual effort for prolonged periods of time without the disruption of coordinated intellectual or motor activity that usually follows an alteration in the function of the medulla (such as occurs with amphetamines or cocaine). However, tasks that involve delicate muscular coordination and accurate timing or arithmetic skills may be adversely affected.[3] The effects on the cerebral cortex occur after oral doses that are as small as 100 or 200 milligrams are consumed, that is, one to two cups of coffee. Heavy consumption (12 or more cups a day, or 1.5 grams of caffeine) can cause more intense effects, which are marked by agitation, anxiety, tremors, rapid breathing, and insomnia.

Only after massive doses (probably 2 to 5 grams) does the spinal cord become stimulated. Toxic stimulation of the spinal cord results in increased irritability of spinal reflexes, convulsions, coma and death. The lethal dose of caffeine is about 10 grams, which is equivalent to 100 cups of coffee. Thus, death from caffeine is highly unlikely.

Caffeine has a slight stimulant action on the heart, resulting in increased cardiac contractility and cardiac output, which is accompanied by dialation of the coronary arteries. (This action increases the supply of oxygen in the blood to meet the increased oxygen demand of the harder-working heart muscle.) It should be noted, however, that caffeine exerts an opposite effect on the cerebral blood vessels; it decreases blood flow to the brain secondary to cerebral vasoconstriction. Such action affords striking relief from headaches that are associated with increased blood pressure (hypertensive headaches) as well as relief from certain types of migraine headaches—conditions for which caffeine is used clinically.

Another action of caffeine is to relax the musculature of the bronchi of the lungs, although a closely related compound, theophylline, is more potent and more effective.

Mechanism of Action

For many years, the mechanism of action of caffeine was unclear; most of its described biochemical actions occur at blood levels that are higher than those usually encountered in persons who drink caffeine-containing beverages. As proposed in the early 1980s[4,5] and recently reviewed by Rall,[3] the leading concept today is that caffeine blocks the action

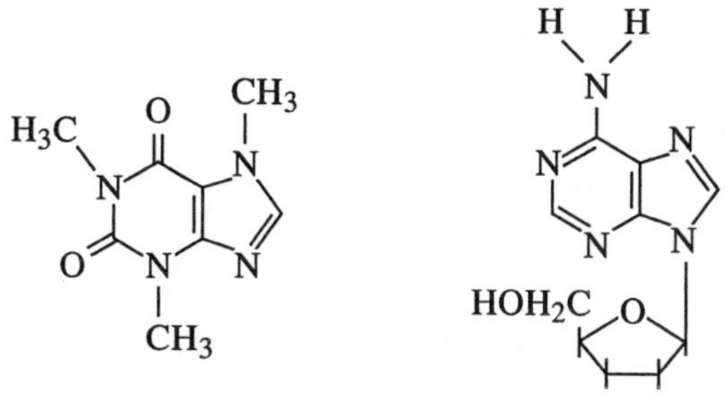

FIGURE 7.1

Structures of caffeine and adenosine.

(competitive antagonism) of adenosine receptors, which are located on cell membranes both in the CNS and in the peripheral nervous system. Adenosine is proposed to be an *autocoid** that acts on specific receptors on the surface of cells to produce behavioral sedation, to regulate oxygen delivery to cells, to dilate cerebral and coronary blood vessels, to produce bronchospasm (asthma), and to regulate other metabolic processes. Blockade of adenosine receptors by caffeine (note their structural similarity, shown in Figure 7.1) would thus account for its stimulant, anti–migraine headache, and antiasthma effects. Indeed, at levels that are comparable to those seen after a person drinks a few cups of coffee, caffeine occupies 50 percent of adenosine receptors, antagonizing the neuronal inhibition that is induced by adenosine.[6]

Side Effects

CAFFEINISM.   High doses of caffeine (higher than about 1000 mg) can cause a syndrome of unpleasant effects that are collectively referred to as *caffeinism*.[6] Nervousness, irritability, tremulousness, muscle hyperac-

---

*The term *autocoid*, derived from the Greek *autos* ("self") and *akos* ("medicine," or "remedy"), refers to a variety of locally acting, hormone-like or neurotransmitter-like substances that exert localized cellular regulatory functions. Studies involving adenosine and caffeine suggest a neuromodulatory role for adenosine and indicate that adenosine-releasing neurons constitute an important CNS depressant system that is blocked by caffeine.[7]

tivity and twitching, insomnia, elevated body temperature, rapid breathing, heart palpitations and arrhythmias, gastrointestinal upset, and diarrhea can all occur. Cessation of caffeine ingestion leads to a resolution of these symptoms.

PANIC ATTACKS   Patients who have a history of panic disorders may be particularly sensitive to the effects of caffeine.[3] Indeed, in one study[8] of such patients, moderate doses of caffeine (about 4 to 5 cups of coffee) precipitated panic attacks in about half of them. Here the implications are twofold: (1) in a person who experiences a panic attack, caffeine should not be overlooked as a possible treatable cause, and (2) any person who has a history of panic attacks should be counseled to avoid all caffeine-containing products or, at least, to use them in moderation and to be alert for signs of drug-induced precipitation of an attack.

CARDIOVASCULAR EFFECTS   Cardiovascular side effects of caffeine have been controversial, especially in terms of possible links between caffeine intake and cardiac irritability, cardiac arrhythmias, plasma catecholamine (adrenaline) levels, blood cholesterol, and heart attacks. Although many investigators have associated caffeine intake with increases in heart rate (tachycardia) and rhythm disturbances (arrhythmias), a recent study[9] reported that 275 milligrams (about three cups of coffee) neither induced nor increased the severity of cardiac arrhythmias. The authors, however, were careful to note that occasional patients did exhibit caffeine sensitization and may represent a subpopulation of heart patients for whom caffeine might be detrimental. Plasma catecholamine levels were unchanged in this study.

More disturbing were two studies[10,11] that reported a 2.5-fold increase in coronary artery disease and a twofold increase in heart attacks in middle-aged men who drank five or more cups of coffee daily. A recent study of 45,000 males failed to confirm this increased risk and concluded that

> the use of caffeinated coffee and the total intake of caffeine does not appreciably increase the risk of coronary artery disease or stroke.[12]

Thus, it is still controversial whether caffeine increases the risk of heart attacks. A conservative view is that caffeine should be used in moderation in patients who are at risk (that is, males, smokers, and those who have a positive family history of heart disease, obesity, hypertension, or elevated blood cholesterol levels). Interestingly, higher consumption of decaffeinated coffee is associated with a "marginally significant" increase in the risk of coronary artery disease:

> There seems to be little merit in switching from caffeinated coffee to decaffeinated coffee as a means of reducing the risk of cardiovascular disease.[12]

CANCER   Despite some early reports, there is now little evidence that caffeine plays a role in the cause of cancer in humans.[13,14]

BREAST DISEASE   Early reports indicated that caffeine use by women might be associated with the formation or enlargement of benign (noncancerous) lumps (fibrocystic lesions) in the breasts. Current thought is that no causative relationship exists.[15] However, it seems prudent to advise a patient who has known fibrocystic lesions to attempt a trial of a caffeine-free diet to determine whether the lesions reduce in size or become less painful.[16]

POSTSTIMULATION DEPRESSION   Although caffeine-induced cortical stimulation is much less pronounced than that induced by amphetamines, it must be remembered that once *any* stimulant agent is metabolized, a period of behavioral and mental depression will follow. This occurrence may be expressed as hypersomnia, emotional depression, or reduced physical and mental activity. Such should be considered when any stimulant (such as amphetamine, cocaine, or caffeine) is ingested to maintain wakefulness or performance for prolonged periods of time.

Tolerance and Dependence

Previously it was thought that, with the usually administered doses of caffeine, little tolerance of the CNS stimulant action develops. It was known that some slight tolerance might occur after prolonged ingestion of larger doses. It has recently been suggested, however, that caffeine does induce physiological dependence, even at low doses (one to two cups per day). Withdrawal symptoms include headache, irritability, fatigue, dysphoric mood changes, muscle pain and stiffness, flu-like feelings, nausea, and craving for coffee.[17] Snyder and Sklar[6] postulate that chronic caffeine ingestion increases the number of adenosine receptors (thus causing drug tolerance to develop), so that abrupt withdrawal of caffeine will expose a large number of receptors to adenosine. This occurrence would account for the withdrawal symptoms that occur.

Reproductive Effects

Certain drugs endanger the fetus when they are ingested by the mother during pregnancy. Such toxicities are usually manifested as either *mutagenesis* (changes in the genes) or *teratogenesis* (abnormal development). Indeed, caffeine may induce chromosomal breakage in a variety of nonmammalian species.[18] The doses that are required to induce such breakage, however, are massive in comparison with those that are usually consumed by humans.

It does not appear at this time that ingestion of tea or coffee increases mutation rates in humans, and most researchers have concluded, therefore, that caffeine does not constitute a *significant* toxic hazard to the fetus. One note of caution, however, was expressed by Goldstein et al.:

> Caffeine should be regarded as possibly hazardous to the fetus during the first three months of pregnancy.[19]

Such caution is warranted whenever any drug is ingested—especially a widely used drug that is freely distributed throughout the body and easily crosses the placenta. Modest reductions in birth weight have been reported in the offspring of mothers who ingest caffeine during pregnancy.[20]

NICOTINE

Together with caffeine and ethyl alcohol, nicotine is one of the three most widely used psychoactive drugs in our society. Despite the fact that nicotine currently has little therapeutic application in medicine, its extreme potency and widespread use give it considerable importance. Recent evidence indicates that nicotine and the other ingredients of tobacco are responsible for a wide variety of toxicities.

From the end of World War II to the mid-1960s, cigarette smoking was considered to be chic. Today, after 25 years of government reports on the increasing knowledge about the adverse health consequences of cigarettes, cigarette smoking is being increasingly shunned.[21] While 30 years ago, celebrities and athletes appeared in cigarette commercials, today they are rarely seen smoking. The impression that cigarette smoking is healthful, youthful, and adventurous is conveyed only by unknown actors in commercials that are accompanied by mandated health warnings. On the positive side, half of all persons who have ever smoked cigarettes have quit, and the prevalence of smoking has fallen from 50 percent in 1965 to 29 percent in 1989. About 1 million potential deaths have been averted or postponed by persons who have quit smoking. Millions more deaths will be avoided or postponed during the 1990s.[21] On the negative side, individual cigarette consumption has risen substantially (from 14 to 22 cigarettes per day among male smokers and from 7 to 17 cigarettes per day among female smokers during the period from 1949 to 1978). This occurrence may be related partially to a reduction in nicotine content, which has caused addicted smokers to smoke more heavily.[22] Also, during the late 1970s, about 30 percent of high-school students smoked cigarettes, and in 1990, only 20 percent smoked; that 20 percent figure has remained steady throughout the last decade (1980 to 1990). These numbers do not include high-school dropouts, 75 percent of whom are smokers. Those young smokers create a huge population who will eventually suffer significant toxicity and mortality as a direct consequence of their "habit," or "addiction."

As stated by the Surgeon General:

Smoking will continue as the leading cause of preventable, premature death for many years to come.[21]

In this discussion, it is important to note that nicotine, the primary active ingredient in tobacco, is only one of about 4000 compounds that are made available by the burning of cigarette tobacco. Thus, although the pharmacology of nicotine will be presented, it only accounts for the acute pharmacological effects and for the dependence on cigarettes. Long-term toxicities of cigarettes are related to multiple compounds that are contained in the product.

Pharmacokinetics

Nicotine is suspended in cigarette smoke in the form of minute particles ("tars"), and it is quickly absorbed into the bloodstream from the lungs when the smoke is inhaled. Most cigarettes contain between 0.5 and 2.0

milligrams of nicotine, depending on the brand. Approximately 20 percent (between 0.1 and 0.4 milligrams) of the nicotine in a cigarette is actually inhaled and absorbed into the smoker's bloodstream. Indeed, the physiological effects of smoking a single cigarette can be closely duplicated by the intravenous injection of these amounts of nicotine. This amount of nicotine is well below the lethal dose of the drug, which is considered to be approximately 60 milligrams.

When nicotine is administered orally in the form of snuff, chewing tobacco, or gum, absorption through the mucosal membranes of the mouth is quite efficient. Blood levels of nicotine that are reached through these routes of administration are comparable to those achieved as a result of smoking (Figure 7.2).

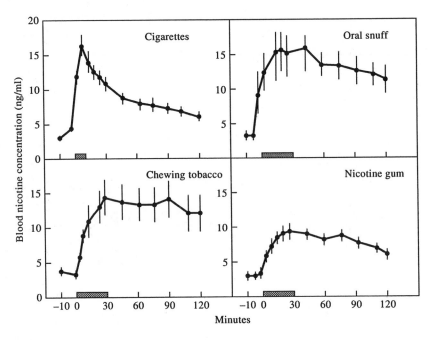

FIGURE 7.2

Blood nicotine concentrations during and after the use of cigarettes, oral snuff, chewing tobacco, and nicotine gum (two 2-mg pieces). Data represent average values for 10 subjects; vertical bars indicate SE. Shaded bars above the time axis indicate the period of tobacco or nicotine gum exposure. [From N. L. Benowitz, H. Porchet, L. Skeiner, and P. Jacob III, "Nicotine Absorption and Cardiovascular Effects with Smokeless Tobacco Use: Comparison with Cigarettes and Nicotine Gum," *Clinical Pharmacology and Therapeutics* 44 (1988): 24.]

Like most psychoactive drugs, nicotine is quickly and ubiquitously distributed, rapidly penetrating the brain, crossing the placental barrier, and appearing in all body fluids, including breast milk. Indeed, the breast-fed infant may have a blood level of nicotine that is as high as that of the mother. Approximately 80 to 90 percent of the nicotine that is administered to a person either orally or by smoking is metabolized by the liver before being excreted by the kidneys. The elimination half-life of nicotine in a chronic smoker is about 2 hours.

Pharmacological Effects

Nicotine appears to be the only pharmacologically active drug in tobacco smoke apart from carcinogenic tars.[22] It exerts powerful effects on the brain, the spinal cord, the peripheral nervous system, the heart, and various other body structures. Pharmacologically, nicotine appears to exert these actions at least partly by directly stimulating certain receptors that are sensitive to the transmitter acetylcholine. Mechanistically,

> the major action of nicotine consists initially in transient stimulation and subsequently in a more persistent depression of all autonomic ganglia.[23]

Acetylcholine is the neurotransmitter at the autonomic ganglia. The stimulation of acetylcholine receptors is manifested as CNS stimulation, increased blood pressure, increased heart rate, release of epinephrine (adrenaline) from the adrenal glands (producing symptoms that are characteristic of the fight/flight/fright response), and increased tone and activity of the gastrointestinal tract.

Nicotine stimulates the CNS at all levels, including the cerebral cortex, producing increased levels of behavioral activity. The drug is capable of inducing tremors and, in large doses, convulsions. As with all stimulant drugs, a period of depression follows. Nicotine causes nausea and vomiting by stimulating both the vomiting center in the brain stem and the sensory receptors in the stomach. Tolerance to this effect develops rapidly. Nicotine stimulates the hypothalamus to release a hormone, called *ADH* (antidiuretic hormone), that causes fluid retention. Nicotine reduces the activity of afferent nerve fibers coming from the muscles, leading to a reduction in muscle tone. This action may be involved (at least partially) in the relaxation that a person may experience as a result of smoking. Some facilitation of learning, memory, and alertness appears to occur and likely contributes to a reinforcing action of the drug. Nicotine also reduces weight gain. As summarized by Jaffe:

> Smokers weigh an average of 5–10 pounds less than nonsmokers. The nicotine in tobacco appears to suppress appetite for sweeter tasting food and to increase energy expenditure both at rest and during exercise.[24]

In addition to its effects on the CNS, normal doses of nicotine can increase heart rate, blood pressure, and cardiac contractility. In non-atherosclerotic coronary arteries, nicotine initiates vasodilation, increasing blood flow to meet the increased oxygen demand of the heart muscle. In atherosclerotic coronary arteries (which cannot dilate), however, cardiac ischemia can result when the oxygen supply fails to meet the oxygen demand that occurs as a result of the cardiac stimulation by the drug. This occurrence can precipitate angina or myocardial infarction (a heart attack).

Dependence

Nicotine induces both physiological and psychological dependence. It is, in fact, the most widespread example of drug dependence in the country. Indeed, the 1988 report of the Surgeon General contains the following conclusions:

> Cigarettes and other forms of tobacco are addicting.

> Nicotine is the drug in tobacco that causes addiction.

> The pharmacologic and behavioral processes that determine tobacco addiction are similar to those that determine addiction to drugs such as heroin and cocaine.

> More than 300,000 cigarette-addicted Americans die yearly as a consequence of their addiction.[25]

Nicotine is a behavioral reinforcer, though somewhat less powerful than amphetamines or cocaine,[24] which limits the ability of smokers to stop smoking. Continuation of smoking is not just a "choice" (as fostered by the tobacco industry) or a "habit." It is a true addiction, which is usually met with adverse health consequences.

Withdrawal from cigarettes is characterized by craving for nicotine, irritability, anxiety, anger, difficulty concentrating, restlessness, hunger, impatience, increased appetite, and insomnia.[26] The period of withdrawal appears to be about one month, as evidenced by persons who relapse after successfully completing the early stages of withdrawal.[26] Smoking cigarettes with less nicotine content usually fails to help persons cut down, because they merely smoke more cigarettes each day. Attempts to free persons from nicotine dependence by substituting nicotine-free cigarettes also fail. The newest treatment is the prescription chewing gum (Nicorette), each piece of which contains 2 milligrams of nicotine in a slow-release resin complex.[27] The idea is to substitute the gum for cigarettes in the hope that the person will tackle the psychological dependence and social components of smoking by first satisfying his or her physiological dependence on nicotine. Later, gum consumption can be slowly reduced and the individual withdrawn from the physiological dependence. Full withdrawal from cigarettes can take 6 months or longer. Nicotine-containing gum is not intended for nonsmokers because it may induce a physiological dependence on nicotine (thus, it is restricted by laws governing prescription drugs). Because it contains a fairly large dose of nicotine, it is not indicated in patients who have heart disease, in pregnant women, or in breast-feeding mothers.

The number of cigarettes one must smoke every day to be considered addicted is unclear, but those who smoke 15 or more cigarettes daily are very likely cigarette-dependent. Indeed, this may constitute the majority of the 50 million American smokers, who exhibit a mean smoking pattern of 18 cigarettes (female smokers) to 22 cigarettes (male smokers) every day.[28]

Side Effects and Toxicity

The acute side effects of nicotine usually consist of cortical stimulation, irritability, tremors, intestinal cramps, diarrhea, increased heart rate and blood pressure, nausea, vomiting, and water retention.

The serious side effects of nicotine (chronic cigarette toxicity) are many and alarming. Serious toxicity occurs secondary to the nicotine, carbon monoxide, and tars that are found in cigarette smoke.[29] It is estimated that more than 434,000 persons in the United States die annually from tobacco use. Of these, 82,000 deaths are caused by noncancerous lung diseases; 110,000 deaths are caused by lung cancer; 30,000 deaths are caused by cancers of other body organs; and more than 200,000 deaths result from heart and vascular diseases. A person's life is shortened 14 minutes for every cigarette smoked. In other words, a 30- to 40-year-old person who smokes two packs of cigarettes every day loses an estimated 8 years of his or her life. More than 50 million people (one out of every six Americans alive today) will die from the effects of smoking cigarettes years before they otherwise would. Cigarette smoking, the nation's greatest public health hazard, is, ironically, the nation's most preventable cause of premature death, illness, and disability.[30] Internationally, similar statistics are appearing, with a current estimate that global tobacco use is responsible for nearly 2.5 million deaths per year.[31]

In 1964, the Surgeon General released the first Surgeon General's Report on the health consequences of smoking, recognizing that cigarette smoking is a cause of cancer and other serious diseases. The major conclusions from the more than 20 Surgeon General's Reports are summarized in Tables 7.2 and 7.3 and culminate in the following five conclusions from the 1989 report:

1. The prevalence of smoking among adults decreased from 40 percent in 1965 to 29 percent in 1987. Nearly half of all living adults who ever smoked have quit.
2. Between 1964 and 1985, approximately three-quarters of a million smoking-related deaths were avoided or postponed as a result of decisions to quit smoking or not to start. Each of these avoided or postponed deaths represented an average gain in life expectancy of two decades.
3. The prevalence of smoking remains higher among blacks, blue-collar workers, and less educated persons than in the overall population. The decline in smoking has been substantially slower among women than among men.
4. Smoking begins primarily during childhood and adolescence. The age of initiation has fallen over time, particularly among females. Smoking among high school seniors leveled off from 1980 through 1987 after previous years of decline.
5. Smoking is responsible for more than one of every six deaths in the United States. Smoking remains the single most important preventable cause of death in our society.[32,33]

The effects on the heart as a result of the combined action of carbon monoxide and nicotine in cigarette smoke are as follows: carbon monoxide decreases the amount of oxygen that is delivered to heart muscle, while nicotine increases the amount of work that is required by the heart (by increasing heart rate and blood pressure). Both carbon

TABLE 7.2

Surgeon General's Reports on smoking and health, 1964–1988.

Year	Subject/Highlights
1964	First official report of the Federal Government on smoking and health. Concluded that "Cigarette smoking is a health hazard of sufficient importance in the United States to warrant appropriate remedial action." Concluded that cigarette smoking is a cause of lung cancer in men and a suspected cause of lung cancer in women. Identified many other causal relationships and smoking-disease associations.
1967	Confirmed and strengthened conclusions of 1964 Report. Stated that "The case for cigarette smoking as the principal cause of lung cancer is overwhelming." Found that evidence "strongly suggests that cigarette smoking can cause death from coronary heart disease." 1964 Report had described this relationship as an "association." Also concluded that "Cigarette smoking is the most important of the causes of chronic non-neoplastic bronchiopulmonary diseases in the United States." Identified measures of morbidity associated with smoking.
1968	Updated information presented in 1967 Report. Estimated smoking-related loss of life expectancy among young men as 8 years for "heavy smokers" (over 2 packs per day) and 4 years for "light smokers" (less than 1/2 pack per day) (US PHS 1968b).
1969	Also supplemented 1967 Report. Confirmed association between maternal smoking and infant low birthweight. Identified evidence of increased incidence of prematurity, spontaneous abortion, stillbirth, and neonatal death.
1971	Reviewed entire field of smoking and health, with emphasis on most recent literature. Discussed new data indicating associations between smoking and peripheral vascular disease, atherosclerosis of the aorta and coronary arteries, increased incidence and severity of respiratory infections, and increased mortality from cerebrovascular disease and nonsyphilitic aortic aneurysm. Concluded that smoking is associated with cancers of the oral cavity and esophagus. Found that "Maternal smoking during pregnancy exerts a retarding influence on fetal growth."
1972	Examined evidence on immunological effects of tobacco and tobacco smoke, harmful constituents of tobacco smoke, and "public exposure to air pollution from tobacco smoke." Found tobacco and tobacco smoke antigenic in humans and animals; tobacco may impair protective mechanisms of immune system; nonsmokers' exposure to tobacco smoke may exacerbate allergic symptoms; carbon monoxide in smoke-filled rooms may harm health of persons with chronic lung or heart disease; tobacco smoke contains hundreds of compounds, several of which have been shown to act as carcinogens, tumor initiators, and tumor promoters. Identified carbon monoxide, nicotine, and tar as smoke constituents most likely to produce health hazards of smoking.
1973	Presented evidence on health effects of smoking pipes, cigars, and "little cigars." Found mortality rates of pipe and cigar smokers higher than those of nonsmokers but lower than those of cigarette smokers. Found that cigarette smoking impairs exercise performance in healthy young men. Presented additional evidence on smoking as risk factor in peripheral vascular disease and problems of pregnancy.
1974	Tenth Anniversary Report. Reviewed and strengthened evidence on major hazards of smoking. Reviewed evidence on association between smoking and atherosclerotic brain infarction and on synergistic effect of smoking and asbestos exposure in causing lung cancer.
1975	Updated information on health effects of involuntary (passive) smoking. Noted evidence linking parental smoking to bronchitis and pneumonia in children during the first year of life (US DHEW 1975).
1976	Compiled selected chapters from 1971-75 Reports.

TABLE 7.2 (continued)

Surgeon General's Reports on smoking and health, 1964–1988.

Year	Subject/Highlights
1977-78	Combined 2-year Report focused on smoking-related health problems unique to women. Cited studies showing that use of oral contraceptives potentiates harmful effects of smoking on the cardiovascular system.
1979	Fifteenth Anniversary Report. Presented most comprehensive review of health effects of smoking ever published, and first Surgeon General's Report to carefully examine behavioral, pharmacologic, and social factors influencing smoking. Also first Report to consider role of adult and youth education in promoting nonsmoking. First Report to review health consequences of smokeless tobacco. Many new sections, including one identifying smoking as "one of the primary causes of drug interactions in humans."
1980	Devoted to health consequences of smoking for women. Reviewed evidence that strengthened previous findings and permitted new ones. Noted projections that lung cancer would surpass breast cancer as leading cause of cancer mortality in women. Identified trend toward increased smoking by adolescent females.
1981	Examined health consequences of "the changing cigarette," i.e., lower tar and nicotine cigarettes. Concluded that lower yield cigarettes reduced risk of lung cancer but found no conclusive evidence that they reduced risk of cardiovascular disease, chronic obstructive pulmonary disease, and fetal damage. Noted possible risks from additives and their products of combustion. Discussed compensatory smoking behaviors that might reduce potential risk reductions of lower yield cigarettes. Emphasized that there is no safe cigarette and that any risk reduction associated with lower yield cigarettes would be small compared with benefits of quitting smoking.
1982	Reviewed and extended understanding of the health consequences of smoking as a cause or contributory factor of numerous cancers. Included first Surgeon General's Report consideration of emerging epidemiologic evidence of increased lung cancer risk in nonsmoking wives of smoking husbands. Did not find evidence at that time sufficient to conclude that relationship was causal, but labeled it "a possible serious public health problem." Discussed potential for low-cost smoking cessation interventions.
1983	Examined health consequences of smoking for cardiovascular disease. Concluded that cigarette smoking is one of three major independent causes of coronary heart disease (CHD) and, given its prevalence, "should be considered the most important of the known modifiable risk factors for CHD." Discussed relationships between smoking and other forms of cardiovascular disease.
1984	Reviewed evidence on smoking and chronic obstructive lung disease (COLD). Concluded that smoking is the major cause of COLD, accounting for 80 to 90 percent of COLD deaths in the United States. Noted that COLD morbidity has greater social impact than COLD mortality because of extended disability periods of COLD victims.
1985	Examined relationship between smoking and hazardous substances in the workplace. Found that for the majority of smokers, smoking is a greater cause of death and disability than their workplace environment. Risk of lung cancer from asbestos exposure characterized as multiplicative with smoking exposure. Observed special importance of smoking prevention among blue-collar workers because of their greater exposure to workplace hazards and their higher prevalence of smoking.
1986	Focused on involuntary smoking, concluding that "Involuntary smoking is a cause of disease, including lung cancer, in healthy nonsmokers." Also found that, compared with the children of nonsmokers, children of smokers have higher incidence of

TABLE 7.2 (concluded)

Surgeon General's Reports on smoking and health, 1964–1988.

Year	Subject/Highlights
	respiratory infections and symptoms and reduced rates of increase in lung function. Presented detailed examination of growth in restrictions on smoking in public places and workplaces. Concluded that simple separation of smokers and non-smokers within same airspace reduces but does not eliminate exposure to environmental tobacco smoke.
1986	Special Report of advisory committee appointed by the Surgeon General to study the health consequences of smokeless tobacco. Concluded that use of smokeless tobacco can cause cancer in humans and can lead to nicotine addiction.
1988	Established nicotine as a highly addictive substance, comparable in its physiological and psychological properties to other addictive substances of abuse.

From reference 28.

monoxide and nicotine serve to increase the incidence of atherosclerosis[*] (narrowing) and thrombosis (clotting) in the coronary arteries. These three actions (and others as well) seem to underlie the fivefold to nineteenfold increase in the risk of death from coronary heart disease in smokers as compared to nonsmokers. If a smoker also has preexisting hypertension or diabetes, the risk is even greater.

In the lungs, chronic smoking results in a smoker's syndrome, which is characterized by difficulty in breathing, wheezing, chest pain, lung congestion, and increased susceptibility to infections of the respiratory tract. Cigarette smoking impairs ventilation and greatly increases the risk of emphysema (a form of irreversible lung damage).

---

[*]Atherosclerosis first appears as fatty deposits inside large arteries and progresses, over years, to occlusion of the arteries throughout the body; the result is clinically manifested as strokes or peripheral vascular ischemic disease. In a large study of arteries collected from young men who had died of violent causes, a history of cigarette smoking was associated with a threefold to fourfold increase in atherosclerosis of the coronary arteries and abdominal aorta.[34] This was the first report of cigarette-induced, severe atherosclerosis in persons under 25 years of age. It emphasizes that in males, cigarette-induced atherosclerosis begins at a young age, and it reinforces the fact that smoking must be controlled for the long-range prevention of adult vascular disease.

TABLE 7.3

Summary of the principal effects of cigarette smoking.

Effect first discussed in Surgeon General's Reports	Year first discussed in a Surgeon General's Report	Current knowledge in 1989
MORTALITY AND MORBIDITY		
Overall mortality, increased in men	1964	Overall mortality increased in men and women
Overall morbidity, increased	1967	Overall morbidity increased
CARDIOVASCULAR		
CHD* mortality increased in men	1964	A major cause of coronary heart disease in men and women
Cerebrovascular disease (stroke), mortality increased	1964	A cause of cerebrovascular disease (stroke)
Atherosclerotic aortic aneurysm, mortality increased	1967	Increased mortality from atherosclerotic aortic aneurysm
Atherosclerotic peripheral vascular disease, risk factor	1971	A cause and most important risk factor for atherosclerotic peripheral vascular disease
CANCER		
Lung cancer, the major cause in men	1964	The major cause of lung cancer in men and women
Laryngeal cancer, a cause in men	1964	The major cause of laryngeal cancer in men and women
Oral cancer (lip), a cause (pipe smoking)	1964	A major cause of cancer of the oral cavity (lip, tongue, mouth, pharynx)
Esophageal cancer, associated with	1964	A major cause of esophageal cancer
Bladder cancer, associated with	1964	A contributory factor for bladder cancer
Pancreatic cancer, increased mortality	1967	A contributory factor for pancreatic cancer
Renal cancer, increased mortality	1968	A contributory factor for renal cancer
Gastric cancer, associated with	1982	An association with gastric cancer
Cervical cancer, possible association with	1982	An association with cervical cancer

PULMONARY

Chronic bronchitis, the major cause	1964	The major cause of chronic bronchitis
Emphysema, increased mortality	1964	The major cause of emphysema

WOMEN

Low-birth-weight babies, associated with	1964	A cause of intrauterine growth retardation
Unsuccessful pregnancy, associated with	1980	A probable cause of unsuccessful pregnancies

OTHER EFFECTS

Tobacco habit, related to psychological and social drives	1964	Cigarette smoking and other forms of tobacco use are addicting
Involuntary smoking, irritant effect	1972	A cause of disease, including lung cancer, in healthy nonsmokers
Peptic ulcer disease, associated with	1964	A probable cause of peptic ulcer disease
Occupational interactions, adverse	1971	Adverse occupational interactions that increase the risk of cancer
Alcohol interactions, adverse	1971	Adverse interactions with alcohol that increase the risk of cancer
Drug interactions, adverse	1979	Adverse drug interactions
Nonmalignant oral disease, associated with	1969	An association with nonmalignant oral disease
Smokeless tobacco, associated with oral cancer	1979	Smokeless tobacco is a cause of oral cancer

From the U.S. Department of Health and Human Services.[33]
*CHD, coronary heart disease.

About nine million Americans suffer from cigarette-induced chronic bronchitis and emphysema.

The relation between smoking and cancer is now beyond question. Cigarette smoking is the major cause of lung cancer in both men and women, causing approximately 112,000 deaths in the United States every year. High incidences of cigarette-induced cancers of the mouth, voice box, and throat are also noted. Concomitant alcohol ingestion greatly increases the incidence of these problems. Finally, cigarette smoking is a primary cause of many, if not most, of the nearly 10,000 deaths every year that result from bladder cancer. Similar statistics apply to cancer of the pancreas. Newly recognized in the 1989 Surgeon General's Report is that cigarette smoking is associated with cancer of the uterine cervix. How cancer is caused by the compounds in cigarette smoke is unclear, but at least 23 of the more than 2000 compounds identified in cigarette "tar" have been determined to be carcinogenic.

Historically, society has focused on the adverse effects of smoking in men, but some reports also focus on women.[35] More women now die from cigarette-induced lung cancer than from breast cancer, and cigarettes are now the leading cause of cancer-related deaths in women. Women who smoke also suffer higher incidences of coronary heart disease and heart attacks than do women who do not smoke. In addition to the direct effects of cigarettes on smokers, data indicate that adverse consequences can be imposed on nonsmokers by the environmental pollution that is caused by smokers.[36,37] Indeed, in 1988 more than 3825 Americans died from lung cancer that was caused by other persons' smoking, or passive smoke. Over and above this figure, an additional 37,000 deaths every year have been estimated to follow from heart disease that was contracted as an effect of passive smoke inhalation.

Effects in Pregnancy

There is now irrefutable evidence that cigarette smoking adversely affects the developing fetus.[38] Cigarettes increase the rates of spontaneous abortion, stillbirth, and early postpartum death. Indeed, in 1988, 2552 deaths of infants were attributed to the mothers' smoking. Pregnant women who smoke have approximately twice the number of stillborn infants as do nonsmoking mothers, with a relation existing between the number of cigarettes smoked every day and the percentage of stillbirths. There is evidence that infants born of nonsmoking mothers may be heavier than those born of smoking mothers. Cigarette smoking reduces oxygen delivery to the developing fetus, causing fetal hypoxia, which can result in long-term, irreversible intellectual and physical deficiencies.

As has been so often stressed throughout this book, psychoactive drugs are readily distributed through the placenta and exert potent effects on the developing fetus. Because nicotine is among the most commonly used psychoactive drugs in our society, the situation is even more serious. Nicotine is deleterious to the fetus and, therefore, is contraindicated during pregnancy. Because a woman often does not realize that she is pregnant until 6 to 8 weeks or longer after conception, cigarettes are contraindicated for all women who might become pregnant. The evidence is conclusive: if we are interested in the effects of drugs on the fetus, on fetal development, and on the health of the newborn infant, nicotine should be contraindicated throughout the entire 9 months of pregnancy and during breast-feeding thereafter.

As a response to these toxicities, the warning placed on cigarette packs and advertisements in 1970 ("Warning: The Surgeon General has determined that cigarette smoking is dangerous to your health") has been replaced by four new statements that are used on a rotating basis. These warnings read as follows:

Surgeon General's Warning: Smoking causes lung cancer, heart disease, and emphysema.

Surgeon General's Warning: Quitting smoking now greatly reduces serious risks to your health.

Surgeon General's Warning: Smoking by pregnant women may result in fetal injury and premature birth.

Surgeon General's Warning: Cigarette smoke contains carbon monoxide.

Although these statements are an improvement on the old warning, they greatly understate the toxicities of cigarettes and the health consequences of continued cigarette smoking. On an encouraging note, a progression toward intolerance of smoking has occurred during recent years, with government and private agencies establishing work spaces that are smoke-free. Factors that continue to be a source of discouragement are (1) the continued denial of cigarette-induced toxicity by cigarette manufacturers, (2) the continued smoking by impressionable youth, and (3) the continued political contradictions. Those contradictions lead (on the one hand) to receipt of income from taxes on cigarettes but (on the other hand) to the subsidization of tobacco growing and the production of cigarettes, as well as to the tax-draining payment of billions of dollars for the social and health consequences that result from long-term cigarette-induced toxicity. It is to be hoped that the Surgeon General's dream of a smokeless society[21] may be realized, but this can only be achieved through governmental actions that are consistent with the data and warnings of its own expert advisors.

STUDY QUESTIONS

1. Differentiate the CNS stimulant actions of caffeine from those of amphetamines or cocaine.
2. Describe the mechanism of action of caffeine. How does this mechanism explain the clinical effects of the drug?
3. What is the relation between panic attacks and caffeine?
4. Discuss the effects of caffeine on the cardiovascular system.
5. What evidence is there for and against the use of caffeine by women who are pregnant or breast-feeding?
6. Discuss the political, health, and economic dichotomies that are related to tobacco.
7. List some of the statistics that are relevant to the health effects of cigarettes.
8. Separate the acute effects of nicotine from the long-term effects of smoking. Organize and discuss the long-term problems that occur in persons who smoke cigarettes.
9. Are cigarettes addicting or are they merely habit forming? Defend your position.
10. Discuss Nicorette gum. Describe its clinical uses and limitations.

NOTES

1. D. Grady, "Don't Get Jittery over Caffeine," *Discover* 7(7) (1986): 73–79.

2. G. L. Clementz and J. W. Dailey, "Psychotropic Effects of Caffeine," *American Family Physician* 37 (1988): 167–172.

3. T. W. Rall, "Drugs Used in the Treatment of Asthma," in A. G. Gilman, T. W. Rall, A. S. Nies, and P. Taylor, eds., *Goodman and Gilman's The Pharmacological Basis of Therapeutics*, 8th ed. (New York: Pergamon, 1990), pp. 618–637.

4. T. W. Rall, "Evolution of the Mechanism of Action of Methylxanthines: From Calcium Mobilizers to Antagonists of Adenosine Receptors," *Pharmacologist* 24 (1982): 277–287.

5. T. V. Dunwiddie, "The Physiological Role of Adenosine in the Central Nervous System," *International Review of Neurobiology* 27 (1985): 63–139.

6. S. H. Snyder and P. Sklar, "Behavioral and Molecular Actions of Caffeine: Focus on Adenosine," *Journal of Psychiatric Research* 18 (1984): 91–106.

7. P. J. Marangos and J. P. Boulenger, "Basic and Clinical Aspects of Adenosinergic Neuromodulation," *Neuroscience and Biobehavioral Reviews* 9 (1988): 421–430.

8. D. S. Charney, G. R. Heniger, and P. L. Jatlow, "Increased Anxiogenic Effects of Caffeine in Panic Disorders," *Archives of General Psychiatry* 42 (1985): 233–243.

9. L. B. Chelsky, J. E. Cutler, K. Griffith, J. Krow, J. H. McClelland, and J. H. McAnulty, "Caffeine and Ventricular Arrhythmias: An Electrophysiological Approach," *Journal of the American Medical Association* 264 (1990): 2236–2240.

10. A. Z. LaCroix, L. A. Mead, K.-Y. Liang, C. B. Thomas, and T. A. Pearson, "Coffee Consumption and the Incidence of Coronary Heart Disease," *The New England Journal of Medicine* 315 (1986): 977-982.

11. L. Rosenberg, J. R. Palmer, J. P. Kelly, D. W. Kaufman and S. Shapiro, "Coffee Drinking and Nonfatal Myocardial Infarction in Men Under 55 Years of Age," *American Journal of Epidemiology* 128 (1988): 570–578.

12. D. E. Grobbee, E. B. Rimm, E. Giovannucci, G. Colditz, M. Stampfer, and W. Willett, "Coffee, Caffeine, and Cardiovascular Disease in Men," *New England Journal of Medicine* 323 (1990): 1026–1032.

13. H. M. Phelps and C. E. Phelps, "Caffeine Ingestion and Breast Cancer. A Negative Correlation," *Cancer* 61 (1988): 1051–1054.

14. P. C. Pozniak, "The Carcinogenicity of Caffeine and Coffee: A Review," *Journal of the American Dietetic Association* 85 (1985): 1127–1133.

15. W. Levinson and P. M. Dunn, "Nonassociation of Caffeine and Fibrocystic Breast Disease," *Archives of Internal Medicine* 146 (1986): 1773–1775.

16. L. C. Russell, "Caffeine Restriction as Initial Treatment for Breast Pain," *Nurse Practitioner* 14 (1989): 36–37.

17. R. R. Griffiths, S. M. Evans, S. J. Heishman, K. L. Preston, C. A. Sannerud, B. Wolf, and P. P. Woodson, "Low-Dose Caffeine Physical Dependence in Humans," *Journal of Pharmacology and Experimental Therapeutics* 255 (1990): 1123–1132.

18. A. Goldstein, L. Aronow, and S. M. Kalman, *Principles of Drug Action* (New York: Harper & Row, 1968), pp. 647–653, 663–668.

19. A. Goldstein, L. Aronow, and S. M. Kalman, *Principles of Drug Action* (New York: Harper & Row, 1968), p. 733.

20. T. R. Martin and M. B. Bracken, "The Association Between Low Birth Weight and Caffeine Consumption During Pregnancy," *American Journal of Epidemiology* 126 (1987): 813–820.

21. U.S. Department of Health and Human Services, *Reducing the Health Consequences of Smoking: 25 Years of Progress. A Report of the Surgeon General*, (Rockville, Md.: U.S. Department of Health and Human Services, 1989), pp. *iii–viii.*

22. H. P. Rang and M. M. Dale, "Non-Therapeutic Drugs: Nicotine, Alcohol and Cannabis," in H. P. Rang and M. M. Dale, eds., *Pharmacology* (Edinburgh: Churchill Livingstone, 1987), p. 679.

23. P. Taylor, "Agents Acting at the Neuromuscular Junction and Autonomic Ganglia," in A. G. Gilman, T. W. Rall, A. S. Nies, and P. Taylor, eds., *Goodman and Gilman's The Pharmacological Basis of Therapeutics*, 8th ed. (New York: Pergamon, 1990), pp. 180–181.

24. J. H. Jaffe, "Drug Addiction and Drug Abuse," in A. G. Gilman, T. W. Rall, A. S. Nies, and P. Taylor, eds., *Goodman and Gilman's The Pharmacological Basis of Therapeutics*, 8th ed. (New York: Pergamon, 1990), pp. 545–549.

25. U. S. Department of Health and Human Services, *The Health Consequences of Smoking: Nicotine Addiction. A Report of the Surgeon General* (Rockville, Md.: U.S. Department of Health and Human Services, 1988), pp. *i–vii.*

26. J. R. Hughes, S. W. Gust, K. Skoog, R. M. Keenan, and J. W. Fenwick,

"Symptoms of Tobacco Withdrawal: A Replication and Extension," *Archives of General Psychiatry* 48 (1991): 52–59.

27. J. Grabowski and S. M. Hall, eds., *Pharmacological Adjuncts in Smoking Cessation*, National Institute on Drug Abuse, Research Monograph No. 53, Department of Health and Human Services Publication No. (ADH) 85-1333 (Washington, D.C.: U.S. Government Printing Office, 1985).

28. U.S. Department of Health and Human Services, *Reducing the Health Consequences of Smoking: Nicotine Addiction. A Report of the Surgeon General* (Rockville, Md.: U.S. Department of Health and Human Services, 1988), pp. 16–17.

29. M. E. Jarvik, "Biological Factors Underlying the Smoking Habit," in M. E. Jarvik, J. W. Cullen, E. R. Gritz, T. M. Vogt, and L. J. West, eds., *Research on Smoking Behavior*, National Institute on Drug Abuse Research Monograph 17 (Washington, D.C.: U.S. Government Printing Office, 1977), pp. 122–146.

30. W. Pollin, in M. E. Jarvik, J. W. Cullen, E. R. Gritz, T. M. Vogt, and L. J. West, eds., *Research on Smoking Behavior*, National Institute on Drug Abuse Research Monograph 17 (Washington, D.C.: U. S. Government Printing Office, 1977), pp. *v–vi*.

31. M. Barry, "The Influence of the U.S. Tobacco Industry on the Health, Economy, and Environment of Developing Countries," *New England Journal of Medicine* 324 (1991): 917–920.

32. U.S. Department of Health and Human Services, *Reducing the Health Consequences of Smoking: 25 Years of Progress. A Report of the Surgeon General* (Rockville, Md.: U.S. Department of Health and Human Services, 1989), pp. 8–10.

33. U.S. Department of Health and Human Services, *Reducing the Health Consequences of Smoking: 25 Years of Progress. A Report of the Surgeon General* (Rockville, Md.: U.S. Department of Health and Human Services, 1989), pp. 98–99.

34. Pathobiological Determinants of Atherosclerosis in Youth (PDAY) Research Group, "Relationship of Atherosclerosis in Young Men to Serum Lipoprotein Cholesterol Concentrations and Smoking," *Journal of the American Medical Association* 264 (1990): 3018–3024.

35. U.S. Department of Health, Education and Welfare, *The Health Consequences of Smoking for Women: A Report of the Surgeon General* (Washington, D.C.: U.S. Government Printing Office, 1980).

36. J. R. White and H. F. Froeb, "Small-Airways Dysfunction in Non-Smokers Chronically Exposed to Tobacco Smoke," *New England Journal of Medicine* (27 March 1980): 720–723.

37. U.S. Department of Health and Human Services, *The Health Consequences of Involuntary Smoking. A Report of the Surgeon General* (Washington, D. C.: U.S. Government Printing Office, 1986).

38. U.S. Department of Health and Human Services, *Reducing the Health Consequences of Smoking: 25 Years of Progress. A Report of the Surgeon General* (Rockville, Md.: U.S. Department of Health and Human Services, 1989), pp. 71–76.

Antidepressants and Lithium

Drugs Used in Affective Disorders

Depressive illness, manic illness, and manic-depressive illness are mood, or affect, disorders in contrast to schizophrenia, which is a thought disorder. A depressive episode is characterized by dysphoria, or loss of interest or pleasure in all (or almost all) of a person's usual activities or pastimes. Depression that is clinically significant is characterized by feelings of intense sadness and despair; inability to experience joy or pleasure in usual activities; decreased sexual drive; mental slowing and loss of concentration; pessimism; feelings of helplessness, worthlessness, or self-reproach; inappropriate guilt; recurrent thoughts of death and hopelessness; blunted affect; anorexia; fatigue; insomnia; and so on. Anxiety almost invariably occurs in persons who are depressed, which can lead to a misdiagnosis and inappropriate or improper treatment. About 10 to 15 percent of depressed persons may display suicidal thoughts or acts at some point during their lives.[1]

Mania is, in most respects, the opposite of depression. Manic patients exhibit excessive enthusiasm, emotional euphoria, elation, extreme self-confidence, flight of ideas, excessive speech, excessive sociability, and impaired judgement, which is often accompanied by delusions of grandeur, irritability, insomnia, and hyperactivity, all of which are inappropriate to the surroundings or the circumstances.

A patient who suffers from *bipolar depression* oscillates between depression and mania. There is strong evidence that this condition may be hereditary, which would suggest that a biochemical abnormality may exist in persons who suffer from this disorder.[2] Patients who suffer from unipolar depression do not swing into bouts of mania, and little evidence exists to suggest a genetic cause for that condition. As stated:

> There is disagreement about whether these two clinical categories represent fundamentally different disorders. One view is that unipolar depression may be either "reactive" in origin or "endogenous," the former being a non-psychotic reaction to distressing circumstances, such as bereavement or poverty, while the latter is, like bipolar depression, the result of a biochemical abnormality within the brain. There is some evidence that these two types of depressive illness respond differently to antidepressant drugs. Some patients suffering from bipolar depression also show symptoms associated with schizophrenia, whereas patients with unipolar depression often show symptoms of anxiety neurosis, so the depressive illnesses appear as a broad continuum stretching from what is probably a fundamental biochemical disturbance to psychological disturbances that are initiated by external events.[2]

Thus, patients who experience bipolar depression or endogenous unipolar depression resemble patients who are psychotic, and their disorders appear to have both a hereditary link and a biochemical origin.

Patients who experience these major depressions respond to tricyclic antidepressants or other antidepressant drugs, to monoamine oxidase inhibitors, and, in severe or drug-resistant cases, to electroconvulsive shock therapy (ECT) in addition to psychotherapy.

Patients who experience reactive, or exogenous unipolar, depression seldom display evidence of a psychosis, do not exhibit bouts of mania, and do not appear to possess a genetic or biochemical origin for their depression. Anxiety and agitation are often present in these patients. The antidepressant drugs are rarely appropriate in the treatment of such persons, and they certainly should not be a treatment of first and only choice. Professional counseling may often resolve the problems that are associated with reactive depression, often without drug therapy.

Attempts to identify the underlying causes of major depressive disorders have led to inconclusive results.[2,3] Most investigators agree that a neurochemical imbalance is probably involved and, in some cases, is genetically determined. Pharmacological evidence points to an involvement of at least two, and perhaps three, biological amines (norepinephrine, serotonin, and, perhaps, but less likely, dopamine) in the brain.

Indeed, if one attempts to reconcile 40 years of pharmacological research that correlates the clinical or behavioral effects of antidepressants with their biochemical actions, one can postulate an (admittedly simplistic) biological amine deficiency theory of depression and, conversely, a biological amine excess theory of mania. We will refer to this combination of actions as the *biological amine theory of mania and depression*.

The Biological Amine Theory of Mania and Depression

In 1965, it was first postulated that depression might be caused by a functional deficit of specific transmitters at certain sites in the brain, while mania might result from a functional excess of the same transmitters. Some of the evidence in support of this claim follows.

First, reserpine has been shown both to induce severe depression and, concomitantly, to deplete norepinephrine and serotonin from the neurons that release them. Second, the antidepressant drugs exert important actions on both of these transmitters to potentiate their neurotransmitter action. Third, strong evidence for genetic predisposition has led to speculation that the underlying biological ideology of major depressive episodes may include an abnormal, hypoactive function of the neurotransmission of norepinephrine and serotonin or of the receptors for these transmitters. Antidepressant drugs do not appear to potentiate the neurotransmission of dopamine very effectively, in contrast to the behavioral stimulants, cocaine and the amphetamines, which potentiate transmission primarily at dopamine synapses. Indeed, cocaine and the amphetamines are poor antidepressants, despite the fact that they are behavioral stimulants and euphoriants. Thus, although the stimulant action of such drugs as cocaine and the amphetamines may be caused by the increased neurotransmission of dopamine, relief of major depression appears to result from the increased neurotransmission of norepinephrine and serotonin.

Although reasonable correlations are observed between drug-induced increases in the levels of norepinephrine and serotonin and positive, mood-elevating effects in persons who are depressed, several limitations and inconsistencies in this pattern are also seen. One major difficulty is that the time course of action is vastly different for the biochemical effect than it is for the clinical response. Although neurotransmission of norepinephrine and serotonin is augmented soon after the drug is taken, the clinical antidepressant effect may not appear for two weeks or longer. Thus, altering the rate of neurotransmission may be only an initial step. A more complex series of events may then occur that eventually result in secondary, adaptive changes that are the consequence of a potentially complex cascade of cellular events.[3] Second, cocaine and amphetamines augment biological amine neurotransmission (Chapter 6), but they are not effective as antidepressants, even though they can induce a manic paranoia or psychosis. Perhaps the preference of amphetamines and cocaine for dopamine neurons (rather than for norepinephrine and serotonin neurons) might at least partially account for this discrepancy. As stated by Baldessarini:

> A few tentative generalizations may be made from these observations, together with the clinical and behavioral effects of antidepressant drugs. First, blockade of *dopamine* transport seems to be associated with *stimulant* rather than antidepressant activity. Second, inhibition of serotonin uptake may well contribute to antidepressant activity. Finally, inhibitory actions on the uptake of norepinephrine seem to correspond with antidepressant activity. However, there is increasing doubt that inhibition of the uptake of norepinephrine or serotonin *per se* is a sufficient explanation for the antidepressant action of these drugs.[3]

Investigations into the delay of the therapeutic effect of antidepressants have given rise to a *biological amine receptor hypothesis*. This hypothesis postulates that the receptors for norepinephrine and serotonin mediate the clinical effects of antidepressant drugs. Thus, either blocking the active reuptake of transmitter or inhibiting the action of monoamine oxidase (see the following discussion) produces longer-term biochemical, cellular adaptive changes such as reductions in the number of biological amine receptors or in the activity of a "second messenger" enzyme (adenylate cyclase). Conversely, depression might be caused by an abnormality (genetically or otherwise induced) in the regulation of these receptors, which may be corrected by the administration of an antidepressant drug (that "down-regulates" the receptors).[4] The factors that are involved in the pathology of bipolar or endogenous unipolar depression are currently the focus of intense research. The lack of adequate animal models for the study of depression is a major limitation.

Mania and the bipolar manic-depressive affective disorder are less common than major unipolar depressions. Patients who experience mania (and its milder form, hypomania) are treated with lithium. Short-term treatment is sometimes all that a patient may need, whereas long-term treatment may be needed to prevent the recurrence of manic episodes.

Lithium, at therapeutic blood levels (see the following discussion), may inhibit the release of norepinephrine from nerve terminals. This finding is consistent with our monoamine hypothesis. In addition, lithium inhibits the breakdown of certain chemical intermediates that serve to modulate the action of several CNS transmitters. This occurrence may lead to a decreased neuronal responsiveness, especially in hyperactive neurons, thus modulating the function of those neurons that might contribute to states of mania. Again, much remains to be learned about the biological and neurochemical basis of mania and the pharmacological action of lithium in helping people who suffer from this disorder.

Therapy for Major Depressive Illness

Therapy for the pharmacological treatment of major depression includes the use of (1) the tricyclic antidepressants, (2) the newer "second-generation" antidepressants, (3) serotonin uptake inhibitors, (4) monoamine oxidase (MAO) inhibitors, and (5) electroconvulsive therapy.

Other agents have been tried and, generally, have been rejected. One such agent is L-tryptophan, the amino acid precursor of serotonin. The claimed effectiveness of large doses of L-tryptophan is inconsistent, short-lived, and less than that achieved as a result of other therapies. In 1990, L-tryptophan was linked to a rare blood disorder, called *eosinophilia-myalgia syndrome*,[5] and was removed from the market by the Food and Drug Administration. Another drug (gamma-hydroxybutyric acid, GHB), which has also been sold through health-food outlets as an L-tryptophan replacement, is causing severe gastrointestinal, respiratory, and CNS problems, and it should also be avoided because it is ineffective and dangerous.

Tricyclic Antidepressants

The term *tricyclic antidepressant* is derived from the fact that these drugs all have a three-ring molecular core (Figure 8.1), and all produce relief from depression in persons who experience major depressive illness.[3] In general, these drugs also share the ability to inhibit, or block, the active

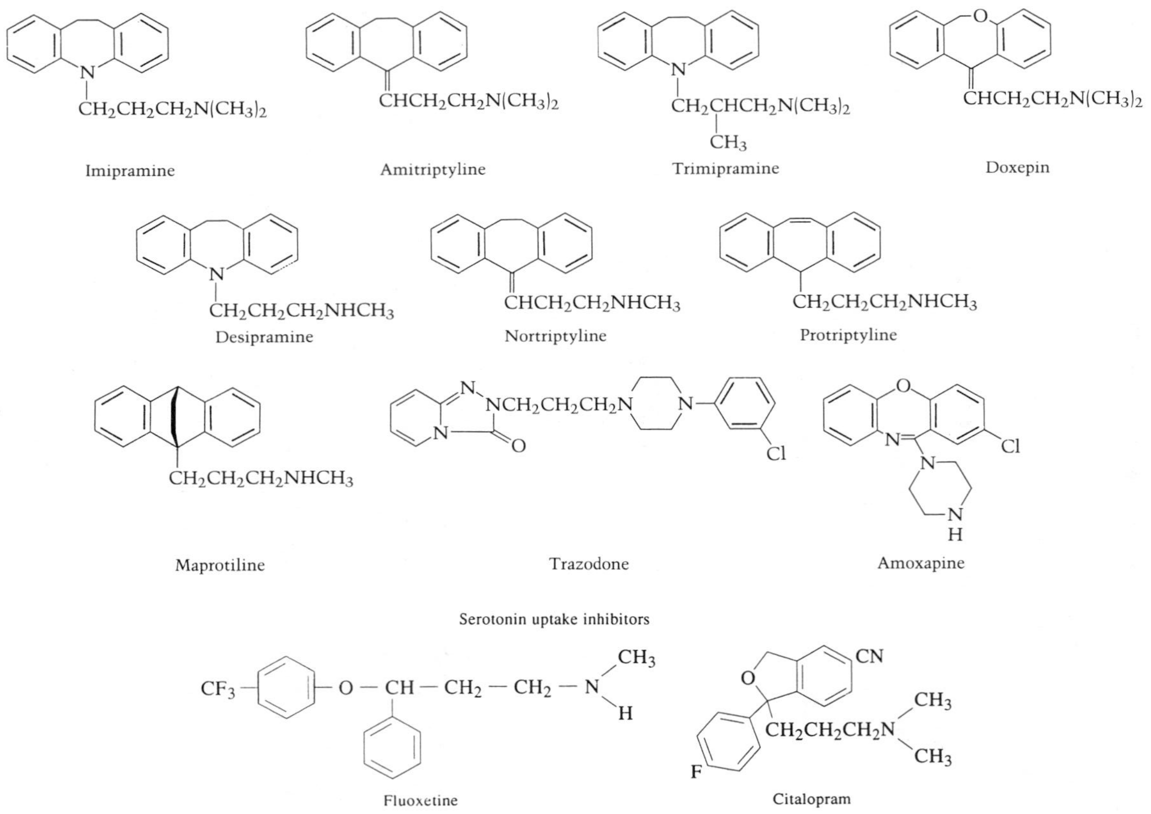

FIGURE 8.1

Tricyclic and second-generation antidepressants.

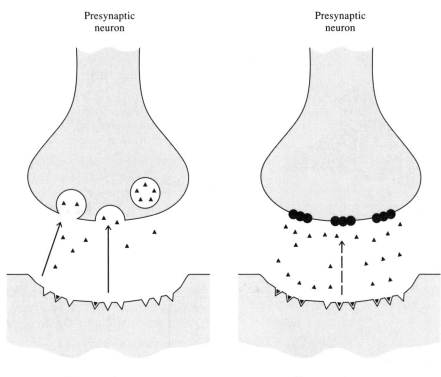

Presynaptic neuron   Presynaptic neuron

Postsynaptic neuron   Postsynaptic neuron

▲ Norepinephrine or serotonin

● Tricyclic antidepressant drug

FIGURE 8.2

Normal mechanism of inactivation of norepinephrine or serotonin by presynaptic uptake (*left*) and its inhibition by tricyclic antidepressant drugs (*right*). [From S. H. Snyder, *Drugs and the Brain* (New York: Scientific American Library, 1986), p.106.]

neuronal uptake of both norepinephrine and serotonin into the presynaptic nerve terminals from which they were originally released (Figure 8.2). None of these agents, however, is ideal for clinical use

TABLE 8.1

Drugs used in affective disorders: Antidepressants.

Drug name Generic (trade)	Sedative activity	Anticholinergic* activity	Elimination half-life (hours)	Reuptake inhibition[†]		
				NE	5-HT	DA
TRICYCLIC COMPOUNDS						
Imipramine (Tofranil)	Moderate	Moderate	5–20	++	+	0
Desipramine (Norpramin)	Low	Low	12–75	+++	0	0
Trimipramine (Surmontil)	High	High	8–10	+	0	0
Protriptyline (Vivactil)	Low	Moderate	55–125	++	+/–	0
Nortriptyline (Pamelor, Aventil)	Moderate	Low	15–35	++	+	0
Amitriptyline (Elavil)	High	High	20–35	+	++	0
Doxepin (Adapin, Sinequan)	High	High	8–24	++	+	0
SECOND-GENERATION COMPOUNDS						
Amoxapine (Asendin)[††]	Low	Low	8–10	++	0	0
Maprotiline (Ludiomil)	Moderate	Moderate	27–58	++	0	0
Trazodone (Desyrel)	Moderate	Low	6–13	0	++	0
Fluoxetine (Prozac)	None	None	24–96	0	+++	0
Bupropion (Wellbutrin)	None	None	14	+/–	0	++
MAO INHIBITORS: IRREVERSIBLE						
Phenelzine (Nardil)	Low	None	2–4**	0	0	0
Isocarboxazid (Marplan)	None	None	1–3**	0	0	0
Tranylcypromine (Parnate)	None	None	1–3**	0	0	0
MAO INHIBITORS: REVERSIBLE						
Moclobemide (NA)[‡]	None	Low	1–3**	0	0	0
Brofaramine (NA)	None	Low	12–15**	0	0	0
Cimoxatone (NA)	None	Low	9–16**	0	0	0

*Anticholinergic side effects include dry mouth, blurred vision, tachycardia, urinary retention, and constipation. [†]NE, norepinephrine; 5-HT, serotonin; DA, dopamine [††]Also has antipsychotic effects due to dopamine receptor blockage (Chapter 7). **Half-life does not correlate with clinical effect (see text). [‡]Trade name not available; not available for use in the United States.

because they have a slow onset of action, their effectiveness is frequently unreliable or unpredictable, they all cause prominent and bothersome side effects, and their toxicity is difficult to manage if an overdose is taken.

These drugs do not produce euphoria or other pleasurable effects, and they have few discernible psychological effects in normal patients. Thus, they have no recreational or behavior-reinforcing value, so abuse and psychological dependence are not a concern. The choice of drug is determined by effectiveness, tolerance of side effects, and duration of action.

The tricyclic antidepressants are currently the drugs that are most widely used for the treatment of persons who experience major depression. This use is well established, and their therapeutic effectiveness is well delineated. Tricyclic antidepressants elevate mood, increase physical activity and activities of daily living, improve appetite and sleep patterns, and reduce morbid preoccupation in 60 to 70 percent of persons who suffer from major depression.[1] They are useful in treating patients who are experiencing acute episodes of depression as well as in preventing relapses, serving as maintenance therapy for persons who are prone to major depressive episodes.

Pharmacological Effects

CENTRAL NERVOUS SYSTEM   As stated previously, the tricyclic antidepressants do not have a stimulating or mood-elevating effect in *normal* persons. In such persons, drowsiness, confusion, motor incoordination, hypotension, dry mouth, and blurred vision commonly occur. These effects are often interpreted as unpleasant and may resemble those seen in persons who are using phenothiazines (Chapter 10).

In contrast to the effects in normal persons, when tricyclic antidepressants are administered over a 2- to 3-week period to *depressed* patients, an elevation of mood occurs. Like the result of receptor desensitization, the antidepressant effect may represent a dulling of depressive ideation rather than a stimulation of euphoria.[3] The tricyclic antidepressants markedly alter patients' sleep patterns; they suppress REM sleep, increase slow-wave sleep, and decrease the number of nocturnal awakenings. Sedation is a prominent feature of many of these drugs (Table 8.1), which can be a limiting factor in terms of patients' willingness to take the medication and, ultimately, in therapeutic success.

PERIPHERAL NERVOUS SYSTEM   The tricyclic antidepressants exert a variety of effects on the peripheral nervous system. These effects occur largely from the blockade of acetylcholine receptors (anticholinergic effects are listed in Table 8.1), which results in blurred vision, dry mouth, tachycardia, constipation, and urinary retention. In addition, these drugs also have an effect on the heart and blood vessels, which frequently is manifested as postural hypotension (that is, a drop in blood pressure when the patient rises from a recumbent position). A complex picture of cardiac depression, combined with increased electrical irritability of the heart (which is evidenced as cardiac arrhythmias), may also occur. Cardiac depression becomes life-threatening when an overdose of tricyclic antidepressant is taken for attempted suicide. In such a situation, the patient commonly exhibits excitement, delirium, and convulsions, followed by respiratory depression and coma, which can persist for several days. Cardiac arrhythmias can lead to ventricular fibrillation, cardiac arrest, and death. These arrhythmias are extremely difficult to treat. One must presume, therefore, that all these drugs (used to treat severe depression) are potentially lethal in doses that are commonly available to patients who have a preexisting risk of suicide. As a general rule, "It is unwise to dispense more than a week's supply of an antidepressant to an acutely depressed patient."[3]

Drug Administration

The tricyclic antidepressants are quite well absorbed when they are administered orally. Because most of them have relatively long half-lives (Table 8.1), they should only be taken once a day at bedtime to minimize their unwanted side effects, especially the persistent sedation.

The tricyclic antidepressants are metabolized in the liver, and some of these drugs (for example, imipramine, amitriptyline) are converted into pharmacologically active intermediates that are detoxified later (Figure 8.3). This combination of a pharmacologically active drug and its active metabolites yields a very long duration of clinical effect (up to 3 to 4 days), especially in elderly patients. Further, drug accumulation can occur and, therefore, an increased incidence of side effects and toxicity.

The initial treatment period is considered to be in a range of 4 to 8 weeks—a time period that is necessary to make a reasonable evaluation of the patient. Excessive sedation can occur during the first few weeks of therapy, and this occurrence can reduce patient compliance. This is a critical point at which patients should be evaluated to determine whether a drug failed because it was ineffective or because it was not

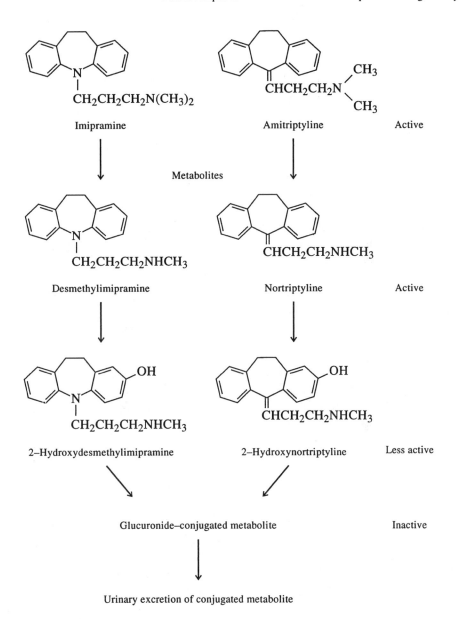

Parent compound .... Uptake blocking activity

$CH_2CH_2CH_2N(CH_3)_2$

Imipramine

$CHCH_2CH_2N\begin{smallmatrix}CH_3\\CH_3\end{smallmatrix}$

Amitriptyline ...... Active

Metabolites

$CH_2CH_2CH_2NHCH_3$

Desmethylimipramine

$CHCH_2CH_2NHCH_3$

Nortriptyline ...... Active

$CH_2CH_2CH_2NHCH_3$ OH

2–Hydroxydesmethylimipramine

$CHCH_2CH_2NHCH_3$ OH

2–Hydroxynortriptyline ...... Less active

Glucuronide–conjugated metabolite ...... Inactive

Urinary excretion of conjugated metabolite

FIGURE 8.3

Metabolism of imipramine and amitriptyline.

taken. For patients who are undergoing long-term therapy, continuous administration of lower doses is usually preferred. Therapy is usually continued long enough to ensure that any observed improvements in the patient are drug induced and not merely the natural waxing and waning of depressive states. Following the initial phase of therapy, dosage can be reduced gradually. However, if signs of relapse are observed, the initial dosage can be reinstituted. In elderly patients, drugs with short half-lives and inactive metabolites should be used (Table 8.1). In addition, dosages should be markedly reduced for elderly patients, and close medical supervision should be maintained. Elderly patients who have cardiac disease are especially susceptible to serious side effects.

Drug interactions that involve the tricyclic antidepressants are commonplace and potentially serious. These drugs markedly potentiate the effects of alcohol, and deaths have occurred as a result—severe respiratory depression has followed the drinking of a normally harmless amount of alcohol.[2] Other drug–drug interactions involve the combination of tricyclic antidepressants and drugs that are used to treat high blood pressure, arthritis, epilepsy, and parkinsonism. Conscious awareness of these problems and close monitoring of the patient are essential.

Therapeutically, major depression is a primary indication for prescribing these drugs. Tricyclic antidepressants are also effective in treating children who experience enuresis (bed-wetting); and they have been tried in patients who have other problems, including anorexia nervosa, bulimia, obsessive-compulsive disorders, panic disorder, chronic pain, migraine headaches, posttraumatic stress disorder, and peptic ulcer disease.[6,7]

Second-Generation (Atypical) Antidepressants

The slow onset of action and the relative severity of the side effects of the tricyclic antidepressants have led to a search for more effective, less toxic, and more rapid-onset antidepressant agents. Drugs that have a different chemical structure have been the goal of research in the hope that an alteration in structure will produce less toxic and more effective drugs. Early efforts (during the late 1970s and early to mid-1980s) were most often met with disappointment. Newer agents (for the 1990s) appear to be quite promising. These agents have been grouped under such terms as *second-generation, atypical,* or *new-generation antidepressants*

TABLE 8.2

Relative advantages and potential drawbacks of second-generation antidepressants compared to tricyclic antidepressants.

Drug	Advantages	Potential drawbacks
Maprotiline	Sedating and may be useful for agitation Does not antagonize antihypertensive effects of clonidine	Increased incidence of seizures Increased lethality in overdose Long half-life; therefore, accumulates Increased incidence of rashes
Amoxapine	Low sedation Low anticholinergic Possible role as monotherapy for psychotic depression ? Rapid onset	Marked potential for parkinsonian side effects and tardive dyskinesia Inability to separate antidepressant from "antipsychotic" effect Increased lethality in overdose
Trazodone	Relative safety in overdose Sedating; therefore, may be useful in controlling agitation and hostility in geriatric patients May be used as a hypnotic in conjunction with MAO inhibitors	Efficacy not clearly established May induce or exacerbate ventricular arrhythmia Potential for priapism
Fluoxetine	Low sedative, anticholinergic, hypotensive side effects No weight gain, maybe weight loss No prolongation of cardiac conduction Efficacy in obsessive-compulsive disorders	Anxiety, nausea, insomnia Long half-life; therefore, accumulates ? Efficacy in panic ? Indirect dopamine blocking effects Pharmacokinetic interactions with tricyclics and benzodiazepines
Bupropion	Low incidence of sedative, hypotensive, and anticholinergic side effects No weight gain Lack of ECG changes	Propensity for "overstimulation," with insomnia, tremor Low efficacy in panic, also ? obsessive-compulsive disorders Increased incidence of seizures in bulimia May induce perceptual abnormalities, psychosis Increases in prolactin

to distinguish them from the older tricyclic antidepressants. Their pharmacokinetic data, relative advantages, and potential disadvantages in comparison to the standard tricyclic antidepressants are listed in Tables 8.1 and 8.2.

Specific Agents

Maprotiline was one of the first clinically available drugs with modifications of the basic tricyclic structure. It has a long half-life, blocks norepinephrine uptake, and is comparable to imipramine (a "gold standard" of tricyclic antidepressants) in terms of efficacy. However, it offers few, if any, therapeutic advantages. A major limitation of maprotilene is that it tends to cause seizures, presumably because of the accumulation of active metabolites.

Amoxapine was another early drug with structural modification of the tricyclic structure. Its effectiveness is equivalent to that of imipramine, although amoxapine may be slightly more effective in relieving anxiety and agitation. Amoxapine exhibits a high incidence of serious neuroleptic side effects, and it is lethal when an overdose is taken. A recent report discusses the closely monitored use of amoxapine in patients who suffer from a panic disorder.[8]

Trazodone is a chemically unique antidepressant (Figure 8.2). It primarily blocks the reuptake of serotonin, having less of an effect on the reuptake of norepinephrine. Trazodone has a short onset of action (½ to 1 week), but 2 to 5 weeks are still required to produce an optimal effect. Some studies question its overall efficacy.[9] Few fatalities have occurred in patients who have taken an overdose of trazodone. Drowsiness is its most common side effect, occurring in about 20 percent of patients. Uncommonly, priapism (prolonged and painful penile erections) limits its use in males.

Fluoxetine, which was released during the late 1980s as the first *selective serotonin reuptake inhibitor*, has now become the most widely prescribed antidepressant. Fluoxetine is the first of the second-generation antidepressants to be considered a first-to-be-prescribed antidepressant (not just for patients who have failed other drug therapy), particularly for patients who are at the less severe end of the depressive spectrum.[9,10] Its efficacy has been established primarily in outpatients, and its role in patients who experience severe endogenous depression remains to be documented.

Fluoxetine has a long half-life (1 to 4 days) and its active metabolite (norfluoxetine) has a half-life of about 1 to 2 weeks. The antidepressant action thus tends to build with time and repeated doses, presumably as the blood levels of both the parent compound and its active metabolite build. With time, therefore, daily doses stabilize at a low daily level. The relation between the clinical effects, blood levels, and daily doses of fluoxetine is still unclear. As a result of the long half-lives of fluoxetine and norfluoxetine, a 5-week drug-free interval is recommended between the cessation of fluoxetine administration and the initiation of alternative drug therapy.

Fluoxetine is also used to treat persons who suffer from obsessive-compulsive disorder. Although we are still uncertain about the neurochemistry of depression,[11] obsessive-compulsive disorder appears to involve a dysfunction of the neurotransmission of serotonin.[8,12–14] Indeed, the mainstay of pharmacological treatment of persons who suffer from obsessive-compulsive disorder continues to be the antidepressant drugs whose prominent action is to block serotonin reuptake. Fluoxetine and clomipramine (long used in Europe and Canada for obsessive-compulsive disorder and introduced into the United States in 1990 under the trade name Anafranil) are both clinically effective. They are both being studied for use in patients who have this disorder. Other drugs that potentiate the action of serotonin are being developed. These drugs include derivatives of fluoxetine (for example, *fluvoxamine*) as well as structurally novel compounds (for example, *citalopram* and *sertraline*).

Fluoxetine has been used effectively in the treatment of patients who experience *panic and anxiety disorders,* either alone or in combination with the benzodiazapine derivative alprazolam (Xanax).[15] The long-term pharmacological treatment of *obesity* has, until now, been disappointing. A consistent effect of fluoxetine and other serotonin-potentiating drugs, however, has been anorexia secondary to the enhancement of satiety feelings and reduced carbohydrate intake.[16,17] Finally, fluoxetine and other serotonin-potentiating antidepressants appear to be effective in reducing *alcohol consumption* in heavy drinkers, which suggests an innovative approach to moderating the alcohol intake of problem drinkers.[18–21]

Side effects that are associated with fluoxetine include nervousness, anxiety, sexual dysfunction, motor restlessness, and muscle rigidity. The limitations to drug treatment that are caused by these side effects are still being evaluated.

Bupropion was withheld from distribution for several years because it causes serious toxicities. It is now available as a newly marketed antidepressant. It differs from the other antidepressants in that it selectively inhibits dopamine reuptake (a cocaine-like action). Bupropion is effective in the treatment of depression, but it is not effective in the treatment of panic disorders. Because of its dopamine potentiation, it has been successfully tried in the treatment of children who have attention-deficit disorders.[22] Side effects of bupropion include behavioral stimulation, anxiety, restlessness, tremor, and insomnia. Its potential for abuse is unclear because the drug may resemble the behavioral stimulants more than it resembles the antidepressants. More serious toxicities include the induction of psychosis *de novo* and generalized seizures.

Sertraline (Zoloft) is a new antidepressant compound that possesses potent serotonin reuptake inhibitor activity. It is currently awaiting release for clinical use in the United States. As with fluoxetine and trazodone, the inhibition of serotonin reuptake leads to enhanced serotonin neurotransmission and indirectly results in the "down-regulation" of norepinephrine receptors. Sertraline is as effective as the tricyclic antidepressants in treating major depression. It may also be useful in treating obsessive-compulsive disorder. Comparisons with fluoxetine are unavailable.

Monoamine Oxidase Inhibitors

The traditional monoamine oxidase (MAO) inhibitors are a small group of older drugs that have long been considered alternative drugs for the treatment of patients who experience major depressive illnesses; their limitations include side effects, possibly serious toxicities, and limited efficacy.[23] They were introduced during the late 1950s, and they have a checkered and controversial history. They disappeared from use during the late 1960s (because of serious and even fatal reactions with certain cheeses and other foods), reappeared during the early 1980s, when their usefulness was reaffirmed, and now their use is decreasing again as the second-generation antidepressants gain in popularity.

Currently, however, a new class of MAO inhibitors is being developed, which is reviving interest in MAO inhibition as a mechanism of action for antidepressant drugs. These new drugs are *short-acting, reversible, selective* inhibitors of a recognized subtype of MAO enzyme. This discussion, therefore, will focus on these two classes of MAO inhibitors—one older and of limited use and one newer and more promising.

Irreversible MAO Inhibitors

Three MAO inhibitors are currently available (phenelzine, tranyl-cypromine, and isocarboxazid). All three share the ability to produce an irreversible block of the enzyme monoamine oxidase—an enzyme that is located within the nerve terminals of norepinephrine, dopamine, and serotonin neurons. Blockade of this enzyme (which normally modu-lates the amount of transmitter that is present) allows large amounts of transmitters to accumulate in the nerve terminals. As a result, more transmitter is released when neuronal stimulation occurs. In addition, these drugs also block the action of several other enzymes nonselectively, and they cause numerous interactions with other drugs by interfering with their metabolism in the liver.

Recently, two subtypes of MAO have been identified. MAO-A is found in norepinephrine and serotonin nerve terminals of the brain (locus caeruleus), in human placenta, in the intestine, and in peripheral norepinephrine-secreting nerve terminals. MAO-B is found in neurons (usually dopamine-secreting) in the brain (dorsal raphe nucleus) and in blood platelets (a component of blood that is responsible for the initiation of clotting). The older, irreversible MAO inhibitors are nonselective and inhibit both forms of the enzyme; the inhibition of MAO-A is presumably responsible for the antidepressant activity, and the inhibition of MAO-B is responsible for side effects, including serious drug interactions that occur when the patient eats cheeses and other foods (see the next section).

PHARMACOKINETICS AND MECHANISM OF ACTION   As shown in Table 8.1, the elimination half-life of tranylcypromine is about 2 hours. This rapid rate of elimination results in a rapid decline in plasma levels of the drug (Figure 8.4a), but it does not correlate with its degree of MAO inhibition (Figure 8.4b). The reason for this discrepancy is that after tranylcypromine is absorbed, it is metabolized to a reactive intermediate compound, which then binds irreversibly with MAO-A and MAO-B by forming a tight covalent bond between the intermediate compound and the enzyme. The remaining amount of drug that is not converted to the intermediate compound is metabolized rapidly and then excreted.[24] This course of events is illustrated in Figure 8.4b. Here, the upper sinusoidal tracing reflects the rapid rise and fall in the blood (plasma) levels of tranylcypromine that is given orally three times a day for 7 days. Plasma levels rise rapidly, fall rapidly, and do not tend to exhibit drug accumulation (because of rapid metabolism of the drug by the liver). The irreversible inhibition of MAO occurs slowly; a level of 70 percent inhibition is reached by day 7. After the patient stops taking the drug, MAO activity returns very slowly, which reflects the irreversible inhibition of any enzyme that was present initially and the synthesis of new enzyme, which is biologically active and can be detected.

Thus, the limitations of irreversible enzyme inhibition include a slow onset of maximum effects, little predictability of the amount or quality of therapeutic effect, difficulty in controlling the effects by alterations of dosage, and long duration of the effects. It is not surprising, therefore, that the irreversible MAO inhibitors are used only when other types of therapy have proved to be inadequate or incomplete.

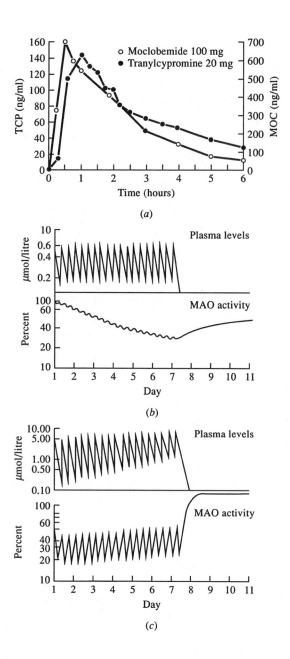

FIGURE 8.4

(a) Concentration profiles of moclobemide and tranylcypromine after an oral dose. TCP, tranylcypromine; MOC, moclobemide. (b) Tranylcypromine (10 mg, three times a day) plasma levels and MAO activity. (c) Moclobemide (150 mg, three times a day) plamsa levels and MAO activity. [From R. Amrien et al.[24]]

Severe and often unpredictable side effects also limit the widespread use of MAO inhibitors. The most severe problems with these drugs involve interactions between MAO inhibitors and (1) other drugs that the patient might be taking or (2) numerous foods that patients might occasionally eat (see the following discussion). Use of these agents, therefore, is potentially hazardous, and extensive patient education, combined with close supervision by a physician, is necessary. In addition, REM sleep is abolished by these three drugs and intense REM rebound occurs when their use is discontinued.[25]

MAO is not only responsible for the regulation of intracellular levels of norepinephrine, serotonin, and dopamine, but also for the hepatic (liver) metabolism of transmitter-like substances, such as *tyramine* (metabolized by MAO-B). Tyramine is a substance that is widely found in foods, such as aged cheese, red wine, kippered and pickled herring, chicken livers, figs, yeast, and so on. The presence of tyramine in the body from such sources, which potentially can occur when MAO is inhibited, can precipitate a hypertensive crisis that is characterized by severe increases in blood pressure, intense headache, increased heart rate, palpitations, and other effects that can be very severe or even fatal. Thus, serious food limitations are required of patients who take nonspecific MAO inhibitors.

Reversible MAO-A Inhibitors

As stated previously, several *short-acting, selective, reversible* MAO inhibitors are being investigated. The one that is currently of most interest is *moclobemide;* two others (brofaramine and cimoxatone) are also being studied. All three drugs are highly selective in their ability to inhibit MAO-A, and all are reversible in action. Thus, they have a much improved safety profile.[26] These drugs block MAO-A, which is responsible for their antidepressant effects, but do not block MAO-B, which leaves tyramine metabolism unaffected (thus, the "cheese syndrome" is less of a concern).[27] In addition, unlike the effects of the older compounds, REM sleep is relatively unaffected by these drugs.[25]

Figure 8.4 demonstrates that the half-lives and plasma decay curves of moclobemide and tranylcypromine are virtually identical. With moclobemide, however, the inhibition of MAO tends to parallel the plasma concentration of drug (Figure 8.4c). This figure shows a profile of a patient in whom moclobemide was administered orally three times a day for seven days. With each dose, MAO activity fell and then returned as the drug was metabolized and its plasma level fell. At the cessation of therapy, MAO activity rapidly returned to normal. These kinetics are similar to the kinetics of most drugs, but they differ from those of tranylcypromine because an irreversible, covalent bond is not formed. From Figure 8.4, it is apparent that MAO inhibition achieves a maximum level after even the first dose of moclobemide. Drug effects can be controlled easily, plasma concentration parallels pharmacological effects, and the effect has a short duration with no aftereffects. Because of the specificity of enzyme blockade (MAO-A), side effects are minimal.

In conclusion, these newer, selective, reversible MAO-A inhibitors offer distinct advantages over the older agents. Presumably, clinical usefulness and tolerability will be increased. Indeed, one author[26] has referred to these agents as the "gentle MAO inhibitors".

Electroconvulsive Therapy

Electroconvulsive therapy (ECT) is a safe, rapidly acting, and very effective form of treatment for persons who are suffering from major depression.[28,29]

ECT has been used for longer than 50 years, and its rate of effectiveness is between 80 and 90 percent. Indeed, no comparative study has shown that other types of intervention (even drugs) are superior to ECT.[30] Many depressed elderly patients, especially those with psychotic symptoms, do not respond to drugs, but they do improve with ECT.[31] Despite its efficacy, however, there is a decline in the use of ECT, especially in the United States, where about 100,000 treatments are administered each year. In Great Britain, which has a much smaller population, about twice as many treatments are performed annually. Social-political considerations appear to be involved in the generation of public attitudes about ECT.

The history of inducing seizures to treat depressive illness dates back to 1934, and it has included the use of insulin overdoses, chemically induced seizures, and electrically induced seizures. Currently, electroconvulsive therapy is the only modality that is used. The safety of ECT has been greatly increased by modern anesthesia techniques, which include administration of low doses of barbiturates to produce unconsciousness and muscle relaxants to prevent injuries to the patient's body.[32] Indeed, ECT, combined with short-acting intravenous anesthetics and muscle relaxants, results in a technically simple, safe regimen to produce brain seizures that can ameliorate depression effectively.

Persons who exhibit endogenous depression are helped the most by ECT; elderly patients and those who have a history of failed drug therapy, recurrent bouts of depression, or suicidal tendencies are prime candidates.

Physiological effects are characterized by increases in heart rate and blood pressure and, occasionally, by cardiac arrhythmias. Cardiac arrhythmias usually resolve spontaneously or can be treated relatively easily by the attending physician. CNS effects include seizures (which are not usually accompanied by muscle contractions, because the patient is medicated for the procedure) and a resulting increase in oxygen consumption, and the release of multiple transmitters.

Memory loss is the most troublesome side effect to patients who undergo ECT; however, only a small fraction of patients claim or exhibit long-term major impairments of memory. Following the induction of seizures, alterations occur in multiple aspects of brain activity. Thus, it is very difficult to determine which of the alterations that occur in transmitter function are responsible for the mood-elevating effect. However, it is known that ECT activates norepinephrine transmission, reduces serotonin reuptake, and increases the sensitivity of dopamine receptors. Thus, improved transmitter function may correlate with its clinical effectiveness. Some postulate that ECT is

> essentially nonspecific; nonphysiological depolarizations are distinctly important for the restoration of aberrant intravesicular transmitter ratios with resultant therapeusis.[33]

According to current estimates, complications occur in about 1 in 1700 treatments, and the risk is generally attributed to the anesthetic. Memory losses in patients are difficult to substantiate, and most arguments concerning ECT are now being focused on that unknown factor.

Lithium

Lithium (Li$^+$) is the lightest of the alkali metals, and it shares some of the same characteristics as sodium and potassium. Lithium is currently the most widely used drug for the management of patients who have bipolar depressive disorder. It is used to treat patients who experience acute mania and those who require maintenance therapy. Emerging data suggest that it is effective in the treatment of other disorders as well, especially in augmenting antidepressant drug therapy for patients who experience resistant depression, converting nonresponders to responders.[34,35] Other uses of lithium include (1) treatment of obsessive-compulsive syndrome, (2) antiviral therapy in persons with herpes simplex infections, (3) additional therapy along with antipsychotic medications in certain schizophrenic patients, and (4) a possible treatment for certain types of alcoholics.[36]

History

Lithium was used during the 1920s as a sedative-hypnotic compound and as an anticonvulsant drug. During the late 1940s, lithium chloride was employed as a salt substitute for patients with heart disease. This use resulted in cases of severe toxicity and death. At about the same time, however, an Australian scientist noted that when lithium was administered to guinea pigs, these animals became lethargic. When lithium was administered to manic patients, somewhat spectacular effects occurred. However, because of the notorious reputation of lithium, it took longer than 20 years for this agent to be accepted by the medical community as an effective treatment for mania. Today, its further uses are being explored actively.

Pharmacokinetics

Lithium is absorbed rapidly and completely when it is administered orally. Peak blood levels are reached within one to three hours, and correlations exist between the levels of lithium in the blood and its therapeutic efficacy. Because lithium closely resembles normal salt (sodium chloride), when a patient lowers his or her salt intake or loses excessive amounts of salt (such as through sweating), lithium blood levels will rise and intoxication may follow (see the following discussion).

Lithium crosses the blood-brain barrier slowly and incompletely; concentrations in cerebral spinal fluid (CSF) only reach about 50 percent of those in plasma. Lithium is excreted by the kidneys in two phases: about half of an oral dose is excreted within 12 hours, and the rest (which represents the amount of lithium that is taken up by cells) is excreted over the next one to two weeks. Thus, when therapy is initiated, lithium will accumulate slowly over about two weeks, until a steady state (or plateau) is reached.

The therapeutic dose of lithium is determined by close monitoring of blood levels of the drug. Indeed, lithium has a very narrow "therapeutic window," below which drug failure will occur and above which side effects and toxicity will dominate. Older reports and even modern textbooks[2,3] claim that an approximate therapeutic value is

1 mEq per liter (one milliequivalent of lithium per liter of blood), with serum toxicity occurring at levels that are higher than 2 mEq per liter. A recent review, however, notes that blood levels that are between 0.6 and 0.8 mEq per liter may be satisfactory for many patients:

> Patients who are doing well at levels of 0.8 to 1.0 mEq/L can probably stay at these levels, but if side effects are troublesome, the levels should be reduced to 0.6 to 0.8 mEq/L. Ideally, all patients should be maintained at the lowest effective blood level. Unfortunately, it is not possible to predict this level in advance. In view of these recent findings, it may make more sense to err in the direction of too high a level rather than too low.[36]

Pharmacodynamics

In therapeutic concentrations, lithium has almost no discernible psychotropic effect in normal persons.[3] It does not induce sedation, depression, or euphoria, which differentiates it from other psychoactive drugs. Indeed, it exhibits few effects on the brain aside from its specific action on mania.

The mechanism through which lithium exerts its antimanic effect is a matter of speculation. It does seem to decrease the release of both norepinephrine and serotonin, and it may slightly alter their reuptake into nerve terminals—actions in directions that are consistent with the biological amine hypothesis. Although its effects on biological amines occur very rapidly, the antimanic effect often takes 1 to 2 weeks to develop (which is indicative of either receptor adaptation or slow accumulation of the drug to therapeutic levels). Antimanic effects may involve a "second messenger" system[*] in the postsynaptic neuron,

---

[*]Most models of psychoactive drug action focus on a drug's effects on the presynaptic release or the active reuptake of the chemical neurotransmitter as well as the interactions of the neurotransmitter with its receptor. Activation of a postsynaptic receptor (by either an excitatory neurotransmitter or an agonist drug) will trigger (within the postsynaptic neuron) a complex cascade of electrical and biochemical responses that result in activation of the postsynaptic neuron. This postsynaptic, intraneuronal process is called the *second messenger system*, which translates postsynaptic receptor activation into neuronal activity. Increasingly, the enzymes that are involved in the chemical reactions within this second messenger system are recognized as a site of psychoactive drug action. Here, lithium may not work within the synaptic cleft, but it inhibits specific enzyme systems (phosphoinositide and/or adenyl cyclase enzymes) so that the postsynaptic neuron is "down-regulated" or stabilized, reducing its response to norepinephrine or serotonin.[37,38,39]

which alters the postsynaptic response to norepinephrine and serotonin.

The mechanism by which an antimanic drug produces a useful effect in the treatment of patients who are experiencing severe resistant depression is also unclear. Some investigators[40] claim that it exerts a net enhancing effect on serotonin neurons, both presynaptic and postsynaptic.

Side Effects and Toxicity

The occurrence and intensity of side effects are, in most cases, directly related to plasma concentrations of lithium. As levels fall below about 0.6 mEq per liter, side effects become much less bothersome than when the blood levels are 1.0 mEq per liter or higher. These effects consist of nausea, vomiting, diarrhea, tremor, and polyuria (increased volume of urine). As plasma levels increase, toxicity also increases, which includes fatigue, muscle weakness, slurred speech, and worsening tremors. Thyroid gland function becomes depressed, and the thyroid gland may enlarge (resulting in goiter). At high concentrations, more serious toxic effects occur, which include muscle rigidity, coma, and death.

Despite this potential toxicity and narrow "therapeutic window," lithium can be well tolerated by patients as long as they are monitored appropriately. Its use in patients who suffer from mania and resistant depression is well established, and its potential use in patients who have other kinds of problems should become more clearly delineated in coming years.

Many patients who do not respond to lithium or who cannot tolerate its side effects have been treated with one of the two newer antiepileptic drugs (Chapter 13): carbamazepine (Tegretol) or valproic acid (Depakene). Experience with (and efficacy of) these alternatives is quite limited.[1,41]

STUDY QUESTIONS

1. Differentiate among exogenous depression, endogenous depression, and bipolar depression.
2. What is the correlation between depression and the biological amine transmitters in the brain?
3. Differentiate cocaine and the amphetamines from clinical antidepressants.
4. What might account for the 2- to 3-week therapeutic delay that occurs when a patient takes a tricyclic antidepressant?
5. Compare and contrast imipramine and fluoxetine.
6. Discuss the results that occur when an overdosage of a tricyclic antidepressant is taken by a patient. Identify the patients who are at risk, the dose of the drug, the side effects, and the treatment.
7. How does MAO inhibition result in antidepressant activity?
8. Compare and contrast tranylcypromine and moclobemide.
9. What are your feelings about the use of ECT? State your reasons.
10. To what endpoint is lithium administered? What are the reasons for this procedure? Describe the "therapeutic window" for lithium.

NOTES

1. American Medical Association, "Drugs Used in Mood Disorders," in *Drug Evaluations, Annual 1991* (Milwaukee, Wis.: American Medical Association, 1990), pp. 257–283.
2. H. P. Rang and M. M. Dale, "Drugs Used in Affective Disorders," in H. P. Rang and M. M. Dale, *Pharmacology* (Edinburgh: Churchill Livingstone, 1987), pp. 513–529.
3. R. J. Baldessarini, "Drugs and the Treatment of Psychiatric Disorders," in A. G. Gilman, T. W. Rall, A. S. Nies, and P. Taylor, eds., *Goodman and Gilman's The Pharmacological Basis of Therapeutics,* 8th ed. (New York: Pergamon, 1990), pp. 404–423.
4. S. M. Stahl and L. Palazidou, "The Pharmacology of Depression," *Trends in Pharmacological Sciences* 7 (1986): 349–354.

5. E. A. Belongia, C. W. Hedberg, G. J. Gleich, K. E. White, A. N. Mayeno, D. A. Loegering, S. L. Dunnette, P. L. Pirie, K. L. MacDonald, and M. T. Osterholm, "An Investigation of the Cause of the Eosinophilia Myalgia Syndrome Associated with Tryptophan Use," *New England Journal of Medicine* 323 (1990): 357–365.

6. W. K. Goodman and D. S. Charney, "Therapeutic Applications and Mechanism of Action of Monoamine Oxidase Inhibitors and Hetero-cyclic Antidepressant Drugs," *Journal of Clinical Psychiatry* 46 (1985): 6–24.

7. P. J. Orsulak and D. Waller, "Antidepressant Drugs: Additional Clinical Uses," *Journal of Family Practice* 28 (1989): 209–216.

8. D. D. Gold, "Management of Panic Disorder: Case Reports Support a Potential Role for Amoxapine," *Hospital Formulary* 25 (1990): 1178–1184.

9. H. K. Manji, M. V. Rudorfer, and W. Z. Potter, "The New Antidepressants," *Hospital Therapy* (May–July 1990): 683–700, 767–790, 911–929.

10. H. Freeman, ed., "Progress in Antidepressant Therapy," *British Journal of Psychiatry* 153, Supplement 3 (1988): 7–115.

11. H. Meltzer, "Serotonergic Dysfunction in Depression," *British Journal of Psychiatry* 155, Supplement 8 (1989): 25–31.

12. D. L. Murphy, J. Zohar, C. Benkelfat, M. T. Pato, T. A. Pigott, and T. R. Insel, "Obsessive-Compulsive Disorder as a 5-HT Subsystem-Related Behavioral Disorder," *British Journal of Psychiatry* 155, Supplement 8 (1989): 15–24.

13. M. A. Jenike, "Drug Treatment of Obsessive-Compulsive Disorder," in M. A. Jenike, L. Baer, and W. E. Minichiello, eds., *Obsessive-Compulsive Disorders: Theory and Management*, 2d ed. (Chicago: Year Book Medical Publishers, 1990), pp. 249–265.

14. M. A. Jenike, I. Baer, and J. H. Greist, "Clomipramine versus Fluoxetine in Obsessive-Compulsive Disorder: A Retrospective Comparison of Side Effects and Efficacy," *Journal of Clinical Psychopharmacology* 10 (1990): 122–124.

15. J. C. Ballenger, G. Burrows, R. DuPont, I. M. Lesser, R. Noyes, J. Pecknold, A. Rifkin, and R. Swinson, "Alprazolam in Panic Disorder and Agoraphobia: Results from a Multicenter Trial. I: Efficacy in Short-Term Treatment," in J. C. Ballenger, ed., *Clinical Aspects of Panic Disorder, Frontiers in Clinical Neuroscience*, vol. 9 (New York: Wiley, 1990), pp. 219–237.

16. J. McGuirk and T. Silverstone, "The Effect of the 5-HT Re-uptake In-

hibitor Fluoxetine on Food Intake and Body Weight in Healthy Male Subjects," *International Journal of Obesity* 14 (1990): 361–372.

17. M. D. Marcus, R. R. Wing, L. Ewing, E. Kern, M. McDermott, and W. Gooding, "A Double-Blind, Placebo-Controlled Trial of Fluoxetine plus Behavior Modification in the Treatment of Obese Binge-Eaters and Non-Binge Eaters," *American Journal of Psychiatry* 147 (1990): 876–881.

18. C. A. Naranjo and E. M. Sellers, "Serotonin Uptake Inhibitors Attenuate Ethanol Intake in Problem Drinkers," *Recent Developments in Alcoholism* 7 (1989): 255–266.

19. K. Gill and Z. Amit, "Serotonin Uptake Blockers and Voluntary Alcohol Consumption. A Review of Recent Studies," *Recent Developments in Alcoholism* 7 (1989): 225–248.

20. C. A. Naranjo, K. E. Kadlec, P. Sanhueza, R. D. Woodley, and E. M. Sellers, "Fluoxetine Differentially Alters Alcohol Intake and Other Consummatory Behaviors in Problem Drinkers," *Clinical Pharmacology and Therapeutics* 47 (1990): 490–498.

21. D. A. Gorelick, "Serotonin Uptake Blockers and the Treatment of Alcoholism," *Recent Developments in Alcoholism* 7 (1989): 267–281.

22. C. D. Casat, D. Z. Pleasants, D. H. Schroeder, and D. W. Parler, "Bupropion in Children with Attention-Deficit Disorder," *Psychopharmacology Bulletin* 25 (1989): 198–201.

23. G. D. Tollefson, "Monoamine Oxidase Inhibitors: Review," *Journal of Clinical Psychiatry* 44 (1983): 280-288.

24. R. Amrien, S. R. Allen, T. W. Guentert, D. Hartmann, T. Lorscheid, M.-P. Schoerlin and D. Vranesic, "The Pharmacology of Reversible Monoamine Oxidase Inhibitors," *British Journal of Psychiatry* 155, Supplement 6 (1989): 66–71.

25. J. M. Monti, "Effect of a Reversible Monoamine Oxidase-A Inhibitor (Moclobemide) on Sleep of Depressed Patients," *British Journal of Psychiatry* 155, Supplement 6 (1989): 61–65.

26. R. G. Priest, "Antidepressants of the Future," *British Journal of Psychiatry* 155, Supplement 6 (1989): 7–8.

27. E. S. Paykel and J. L. White, "European Study of Views on the Use of Monoamine Oxidase Inhibitors," *British Journal of Psychiatry* 155, Supplement 6 (1989): 9–17.

28. R. R. Crowe, "Electroconvulsive Therapy: Current Perspectives," *New England Journal of Medicine* 311 (1984): 163–166.

29. C. E. Coffey and R. D. Weiner, "Electroconvulsive Therapy: An Update," *Hospital and Community Psychiatry* 41 (1990): 515–521.

30. E. Persad, "Electroconvulsive Therapy in Depression," *Canadian Journal of Psychiatry* 35 (1990): 175–182.

31. M. A. Jenike, "Treatment of Affective Illness in the Elderly with Drugs and Electroconvulsive Therapy," *Journal of Geriatric Psychiatry* 22 (1989): 77–122.

32. B. L. Selvin, "Electroconvulsive Therapy—1987," *Anesthesiology* 67 (1987): 367–385.

33. B. H. King and E. H. Liston, "Proposals for the Mechanism of Action of Convulsive Therapy: A Synthesis," *Biological Psychiatry* 27 (1990): 76–94.

34. J. B. Murray, "New Applications of Lithium Therapy," *Journal of Psychology* 124 (1990): 55–73.

35. H. R. Kim, N. J. Delva, and J. S. Lawson, "Prophylactic Medication for Unipolar Depressive Illness: The Place of Lithium Carbonate in Combination with Antidepressant Medication," *Canadian Journal of Psychiatry* 35 (1990): 107–114.

36. J. W. Jefferson, "Lithium: The Present and the Future," *Journal of Clinical Psychiatry* 51, Supplement (1990): 4–8.

37. J. M. Baraban, P. F. Worley, and S. H. Snyder, "Second Messenger Systems and Psychoactive Drug Action: Focus on the Phosphoinositide System and Lithium," *American Journal of Psychiatry* 146 (1989): 1251–1260.

38. R. H. Belmaker, A. Livne, G. Agam, D. G. Moscovich, N. Grisaru, G. Schreiber, S. Avissar, A. Danon, and O. Kofman, "Role of Inositol-1-Phosphate Inhibition in the Mechanism of Action of Lithium," *Pharmacology and Toxicology* 66, Supplement 3 (1990): 76–83.

39. P. C. Waldmeier, "Mechanism of Action of Lithium in Affective Disorders: A Status Report," *Pharmacology and Toxicology* 66, Supplement 3 (1990): 121–132.

40. L. H. Price, D. S. Charney, P. L. Delgado, and G. R. Heninger, "Lithium and Serotonin Function: Implications for the Serotonin Hypothesis of Depression," *Psychopharmacology* 100 (1990): 3–12.

41. H. G. Pope, Jr., S. L. McElroy, P. E. Keck, and J. L. Hudson, "Valproate in the Treatment of Acute Mania," *Archives of General Psychiatry* 48 (1991): 62–68.

The Opioid Analgesics
Morphine and Other Narcotics

In this chapter, we discuss the pharmacological, physiological, psychological, and behavioral effects of a group of compounds that are referred to as *opioids, opiates, narcotic analgesics,* and *strongly addictive analgesics.* The term *opioid* refers to any natural or synthetic drug that exerts actions on the body that are similar to those induced by morphine (the major pain-relieving agent that is obtained from the opium poppy), the actions of which are antagonized by naloxone (discussed later). Opioids include the opiate narcotics (pain-relieving agents that are extracted from the opium poppy), substances that are structurally related to morphine, synthetic drugs with structures that may be quite different from that of morphine, and various endogenous (that is, naturally occurring in the body) neuroactive peptides that exert analgesic actions. *Opium* is an extract of the exudate of the incised capsule of the poppy, *Papaver somniferum,* which has been used for social and medicinal purposes for thousands of years to produce euphoria, analgesia, sleep, and relief from diarrhea.[1] The term *narcotic* has numerous connotations. In this text, the term *opioid* is used to refer to all substances, natural and synthetic, that possess morphine-like actions.

Historical Background

Morphine occurs naturally and is obtained from the opium poppy. The earliest descriptions of the psychological and physiological effects of opium were written in about 300 B.C., although references to opiates have been found dating to about 3000 B.C. Opium appears to have been used in early Egyptian, Greek, and Arabic cultures primarily for its constipating effect in the treatment of diarrhea. Later, opium's sleep-inducing properties were noted by Greek and Roman writers, such as Homer, Virgil, and Ovid. Opium was frequently used by the ancient Greeks to treat a variety of medical problems, including snake bite, asthma, cough, epilepsy, colic, urinary complaints, headache, and deafness. Opium was also used recreationally and was readily available during that time. Addiction to opium was common, even among the high-standing military and political figures of Rome.

From the early Greek and Roman days through the sixteenth and seventeenth centuries, the medicinal and recreational uses of opium were well established throughout Europe. Because much of the opium came from the Near East and the Orient, a bustling trade in opium existed between the East and the West. Indeed, control of opium was a central issue during the opium wars in China in 1839.

Throughout the centuries (from 3000 B.C. to A.D. 1800), the opiates that were used medicinally and recreationally consisted of crude opium, which was obtained from the opium poppy. Opium, however, is a resinous material that contains at least 20 different substances. It was not until the early 1800s that morphine was isolated from opium. The purification of morphine revolutionized the use of opiates, and since then, morphine (rather than crude opium) has been used throughout the world for the medical treatment of pain and diarrhea.

In the United States, morphine and opium were widely used during the nineteenth century. Opium and morphine were freely available from physicians, drugstores, and general stores; by mail order; and in patent medicines that were sold through a variety of channels. It was not until after the Civil War (when opiate addiction was referred to as the "soldier's disease") and the invention of the hypodermic needle (in 1856) that a new type of drug user appeared in the United States—one who administered opiates to himself by injection.

By the early part of the twentieth century, the use of opium was widespread, and concern began to mount about the possible dangers of opiates and the dependence that they might induce. By 1914, the Harrison Narcotic Act was passed, and the use of most opiate products was placed under strict controls. Nonmedical uses of opiates were banned.

The use of opiates is deeply entrenched in society; it is widespread, attractive, difficult to treat, and impossible to stop. The pharmacology of the opiates should be discussed in the same manner as that of any other class of psychoactive drugs that has effects that can be pleasurable to the user, affect behavior, produce a pattern of tolerance and physiological dependence, and have a potential for compulsive misuse. Emotional reactions and extensive legal efforts will probably fail to eradicate the recreational use of these drugs. The opiates will continue to be used in medicine because they are irreplaceable as pain-relieving agents. In addition, the profound effects of opiates on the CNS induce an enormous liability for compulsive abuse—a liability that is likely to resist any efforts at total control.

Pain and Its Perception

Pain is associated with the activation of electrical activity in small-diameter sensory (afferent) fibers of peripheral nerves. These sensory nerves originate in peripheral tissues (such as skin, muscle, and abdominal viscera) and are activated by various mechanical, thermal, chemical, or injury stimuli. Because these nerves are activated by noxious (painful) stimuli, their receptors are called *nociceptors* (Figure 9.1). The electrical discharge in these nerves is conducted to their synaptic terminals, which are located in the dorsal horn of the spinal cord, where a chemical transmitter, called *substance P,* is released.

Substance P, a peptide that is 11 amino acids in length, is a neurotransmitter. When it is released, it activates (excites) other neurons that transmit information about noxious stimuli to the brain by means of two specialized afferent pathways: the spinothalamic tract and the spinoreticular tract (Figure 9.2). Thus, pain is first "perceived" in the spinal cord; and this perception is relayed to the brain stem and the thalamus and, eventually, to higher centers in the brain (such as the limbic system and the somatosensory cortex) for interpretation. The dorsal horn of the spinal cord, the thalamus, the brain stem, and the limbic system are all rich in both opioid peptides (*enkephalins, endorphins,* and *dynorphins*) and opioid receptors (discussed in the following text). These centers in the brain are important as sites of action for morphine-like drugs as well as for pain sensation.

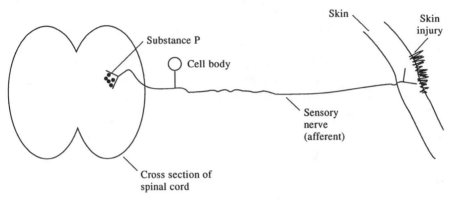

FIGURE 9.1

Activation of peripheral nociceptive (pain) fibers results in the release of substance P from nerve terminals in the dorsal horn of the spinal cord. The cell body for the nerve is located in the dorsal root ganglion.

Thus, pain is transmitted from the peripheral nociceptors to the brain after passing through the spinal cord. As Figure 9.3 illustrates, at least two descending pathways in the spinal cord modulate (or "gate") the transmission of pain impulses. One pathway originates in the locus caeruleus of the medulla and sends descending axons to the dorsal horn, where the neurotransmitter norepinephrine is released. There, norepinephrine *inhibits* the release of substance P and thus reduces nociception (that is, it is analgesic). This path is important in the mechanism for pain relief, because an injection of norepinephrine-like agonists (adrenaline or clonidine) into the spinal fluid will cause analgesia.[2,3]

The second descending analgesic pathway originates in the midbrain (in the periaquaductal gray matter) and in the medulla (the nucleus raphe magnus) and sends axons down the spinal cord. These axons also synapse on the terminals of nociceptive neurons that are located (once again) in the dorsal horn of the spinal cord. Here, the neurotransmitter serotonin is released.[4] This pathway is an important

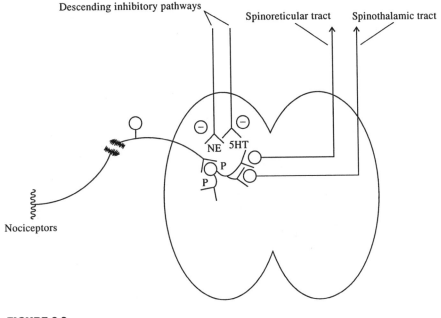

FIGURE 9.2

Release of substance P in the dorsal horn of the spinal cord with transmission of secondary relay pathways to higher centers. Descending inhibitory pathways (−) are also shown (expanded in Figure 9.3). NE, norepinephrine; 5HT, serotonin.

site of action for opioid analgesics, because (1) these areas of the midbrain and medulla are rich in both opioid peptides and opioid receptors, (2) electrical stimulation of these areas in the brain stem causes intense analgesia that is blocked by the narcotic antagonist naloxone,[5,6] and (3) serotonin induces the release of opioid peptides in the dorsal horn and the latter substances inhibit substance P release.

Thus, descending norepinephrine and serotonin pathways modulate noxious stimuli by directly or indirectly reducing the release of substance P in the spinal cord. The process by which the release of substance P is reduced is not clear, but it seems to involve the activation of opioid neurons, which release opioid peptides (mainly metenkephalin and beta-endorphin), which, in turn, strongly inhibit the release of substance P. This inhibition would cause a strong analgesic action.

Using this model, we can visualize several sites of action for analgesic drugs. Drugs that potentiate serotonin might cause analgesia by activating descending inhibitory pathways. Such might be the case with

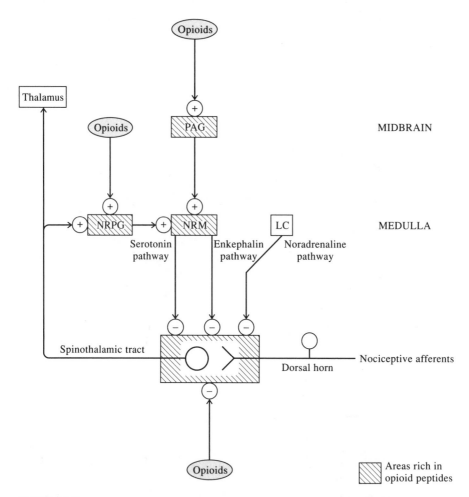

FIGURE 9.3

Sites of action of opioids on pain transmission. Opioids excite neurons in the periaqueductal gray matter (PAG) and in the nucleus reticularis paragigantocellularis (NRPG), which in turn project to the nucleus raphe magnus (NRM). From there, NRM serotoninergic and enkephalinergic neurons run to the substantia gelatinosa of the dorsal horn and exert an inhibitory influence on transmission. Opioids also act directly on the dorsal horn. The locus caeruleus (LC) sends noradrenergic neurons to the dorsal horn, which also inhibits transmission. The pathways shown in this diagram represent a considerable oversimplification, but they depict the general organization of the supraspinal control mechanisms. [From H. P. Rang and M. M. Dale,[1] p. 550.]

tricyclic antidepressants, because they are effective clinically in the treatment of persons who suffer from chronic pain syndromes. Drugs that potentiate norepinephrine may cause analgesia in a similar way. Indeed, two such drugs (adrenaline and clonidine) have analgesic properties. In addition, clonidine is useful in ameliorating the symptoms of opioid withdrawal in persons who are addicted to narcotics (see the following discussion). Whether these effects follow from a spinal cord action is not yet clear. Finally, the substantia gelatinosa of the dorsal horn of the spinal cord and the midline structures of the medulla, midbrain, and medial thalamus are rich in opioid peptides and receptors. Morphine-like drugs exert their analgesic action by stimulating the opioid receptors in those areas.

So far, we have discussed the afferent transmission of nociceptive impulses and its modulation, which is caused by descending inhibitory influences (serotonin and norepinephrine) as well as local opioid influences. We have not addressed the *affective* component of pain—the component that determines our emotional response by reducing the distress that is associated with the pain. The affective component of pain may be the underlying factor in the mechanism of chronic pain states for which often no objective cause can be identified.[7] Chronic pain states may arise from deficits in the central (CNS) processing of nociceptive afferent actions, whereby input that might be innocuous in some persons may debilitate others. In such persons, treatment with opioids is not effective (and sometimes harmful because dependence can develop). Thus, for these persons, treatment is focused on behavior modification, cognitive-behavioral therapy, or self-management approaches that include biopsychosocial models of therapy.

Opioid Receptors and Drug Classification

From the previous discussion, it is apparent that opioid receptors are located in specific areas of the brain and spinal cord. Opioid receptors are not all identical; several distinct types exist, and each one has a different affinity for binding with various opioid analgesics.[8,9] The major categories of receptors have been identified; they have been designated as *mu, kappa, delta,* and *sigma* receptors. At least two subtypes of some of these receptors have also been identified (for example, mu-1 and mu-2).

Different opioid analgesics interact with different receptors and this factor, together with the location of those receptors, can provide a profile of pharmacological activity. Thus, before discussing specific drugs, each receptor for the opioids will be examined briefly.

Mu receptors are located mostly at supraspinal sites, which are responsible for morphine-induced analgesia. Such areas include the medial thalamus and brain-stem areas (locus caeruleus, periaquaductal gray matter of the midbrain, and the nucleus raphe magnus of the medulla). Activation of mu receptors in these areas seems to underlie the analgesic, respiratory depressant, miotic (pin-point pupils), euphoric, and physical dependence properties of morphine and its related drugs. It is thought that the mu-1 subtype modulates analgesia and euphoria primarily, while the mu-2 subtype modulates respiratory depression. As yet, no specific mu-1 analgesics are clinically available and, thus, analgesia cannot be separated from respiratory depression in patients who are taking opioids. In addition, the intense analgesia that is caused by opioids has not been separated from the euphoria that is induced. All analgesics that stimulate mu receptors induce euphoria, have potent behavioral reinforcing properties, and thus are capable of causing drug dependence. Some mu receptors are also located in the spinal cord, and these receptors may modulate at least part of the spinal analgesia that is induced by morphine.

Kappa receptors are located principally within the dorsal horn of the spinal cord. Thus, they are responsible for inducing analgesia by depressing the initial relay site of pain transmission. The analgesia that is produced by the opioid peptides appears to be exerted through these spinal kappa receptors. However, other kappa receptors are located in the brain stem (medullary reticular formation), because kappa-specific drugs produce miosis and sedation. Euphoria, physical dependence, and respiratory depression are not mediated by kappa receptors.

Delta receptors are poorly delineated as yet, but they may be involved at brain-stem and spinal levels in the production of certain aspects of analgesia and in some of the positive reinforcing properties of morphine.

Sigma receptors appear to be located primarily in the limbic system of the brain (amygdala and hippocampus). Activation of these receptors results in psychotomimetic, hallucinogenic, and dysphoric responses to certain opioids. Sigma receptors might also interact with other non-opioid drugs. The psychedelic properties of the dissociative anesthetics ketamine and phencyclidine (PCP; see Chapter 11) may be exerted through PCP- or ketamine-induced stimulation of sigma receptors.

Using this knowledge of opioid receptors, we can develop a classification scheme for opioid analgesics. First, we can tabulate the ac-

TABLE 9.1

Classification of opioid analgesics by their ability to produce analgesia (agonists) or block the actions of morphine (antagonists).

Pure agonists	Mixed agonist–antagonists	Pure antagonists
Morphine	Nalbuphine (Nubain)	Naloxone (Narcan)
Codeine	Butorphanol (Stadol)	Naltrexone (Trexan)
Heroin	Pentazocine (Talwin)	
Meperidine (Demerol)	Buprenorphine (Buprenex)	
Methadone (Dolophine)	Dezocine (Dalgan)	
Oxymorphone (Numorphan)		
Hydromorphone (Dilaudid)		
Fentanyl (Sublimaze)		

tivity of each drug at each type of receptor and indicate whether it activates (agonistic action) or inhibits (antagonistic action) receptor function. We can thus categorize each drug as a pure agonist, a pure antagonist, or a mixed agonist–antagonist (Table 9.1). Pure agonists include most of the morphine-like drugs. All these drugs exhibit a high binding affinity (and exert high activity) with mu receptors but have low affinity for kappa or sigma receptors (morphine: Table 9.2). Pure antagonists (naloxone: Table 9.2) bind to opioid receptors (with varying affinity), but they do not exert agonist activity at any receptor. Finally, the mixed agonist–antagonists (pentazocine, butorphanol, nalbuphine, and dezocine: Table 9.2) exhibit modest morphine-like activity at some receptors, but they can also antagonize the effects of morphine at some, or all, of the receptors. Several such agents are available clinically, and most of them show some affinity for sigma receptors, which results in the production of unpredictable dysphoric or psychedelic effects.

Morphine

Opium (the crude resinous exudate obtained from the opium poppy) contains two pharmacologically active analgesic drugs: *morphine* and *codeine*. Morphine is the more effective pain-relieving drug; it represents approximately 10 percent of the crude exudate. Codeine is closely related to morphine structurally, but it is much less potent and constitutes only 0.5 percent of the crude exudate.

TABLE 9.2

Classification of opioid agonists and antagonists by actions at opioid receptors.

| Compound | Receptor types* | | | |
	Mu	Kappa	Sigma	Delta
Morphine	+++	+	0	+
Naloxone	– –	–	–	–
Pentazocine	+/0	+	+	NA
Butorphanol	+/0	+	+	NA
Nalbuphine	–	+	+/0	NA
Buprenorphine	+	–	0	NA
Fentanyl	+++	+	0	+
Dezocine	+	+	NA	+

*The mu receptor is thought to mediate supraspinal analgesia, respiratory depression, euphoria, and physical dependence; the kappa receptor, spinal analgesia, miosis, and sedation; the sigma receptor, dysphoria, hallucinations, and respiratory and vasomotor stimulation. Categorizations are based on best inferences about actions in humans. See text for further explanation. Agonists are indicated by one or more plus signs, antagonists by one or more minus signs, and agents which have no significant action at the receptor by zero. NA, data not available.

The primary medical uses of morphine include the relief of pain, the treatment of diarrhea, and the relief of cough—all disorders for which opium has been used since well before the sixteenth century. Despite intensive research, few other drugs have come close to morphine in terms of its effectiveness as an analgesic. Although morphine and codeine are extremely effective for the relief of cough, they have largely been replaced by newer nonnarcotic drugs that have a very low potential for compulsive abuse. Nevertheless, morphine and codeine retain vital roles in the armamentarium of the physician as essential agents in the struggle against pain.

Pharmacokinetics

Morphine may be administered orally, rectally, or by injection. In general, absorption of morphine from the gastrointestinal tract (oral or rectal) is slow and incomplete compared to that which follows injection: blood levels reach only about half of that achieved when the drug is injected. Absorption through the rectum is adequate, and several opioids (morphine, hydromorphone, oxymorphone) are available in suppository form. The use of such preparations might be indicated in patients who suffer from muscle-wasting diseases (such as in patients with terminal cancer), who cannot tolerate other routes of administration. Highly fat-soluble opioids (such as fentanyl, discussed later) are absorbed readily from the oral mucosa, and this route of administration is being investigated as a possible way to treat patients with narcotics.

Morphine is most often administered by intramuscular, subcutaneous, or intravenous injection. The problems and limitations of the injection of drugs (delineated in Chapter 1) include accidental overdose, rapid onset of adverse drug reactions, the necessity of using sterile techniques, and the inability to retrieve the drug if too much is administered. Drug "antagonism" may sometimes be accomplished by administering the specific pharmacological antagonist, naloxone (Narcan), which is discussed later in this chapter.

As is well known from the history of opium smoking among people of Eastern cultures, the opiates (including morphine) may be administered by inhalation and absorbed through the lungs, either by sniffing the powdered drug or, more commonly, by inhaling the smoke from burning crude opium. In either case, the opiates are rapidly and completely absorbed. In fact, the rapidity of onset of drug action that occurs when opium is smoked rivals that following intravenous injection.

Opioids achieve significant levels in the brain within seconds to minutes after an intravenous injection. The more water-soluble (lipid-insoluble) opioids, such as morphine, penetrate the blood-brain barrier somewhat more slowly than do the more lipid-soluble opioids. Thus, morphine exists in the bloodstream in a relatively lipid-insoluble form, which does not cross the blood-brain barrier easily (it is fairly impermeable to such compounds). Only small amounts of morphine (20 percent) ever penetrate the brain. In contrast, heroin crosses the blood-brain barrier easily. This difference may explain why the "flash" or "rush" following intravenous injection of heroin is so much more intense than that perceived after injection of morphine. The opiates also reach all body tissues, including the fetus; infants born of addicted mothers are physically dependent on opiates and exhibit withdrawal symptoms that require intensive therapy.[10]

Morphine is metabolized by the liver, and its metabolites are excreted by the kidneys. The metabolism of morphine is rapid, and its duration of action is about 4 to 5 hours. This factor is critically important to drug-dependent persons, because they must continually seek and administer the drug at intervals that are as short as 3 to 5 hours. The half-life of morphine is about 2 hours.

Urine screening tests to determine whether a person has used narcotics will detect codeine and morphine as well as their metabolites.

Because heroin (discussed later) is metabolized to morphine and because street heroin also contains acetylcodeine (which is metabolized to codeine), heroin use is suspected when both morphine and codeine are present in a patient's urine. Thus, assays cannot be used to determine which drug (heroin, codeine, or morphine) has been used. Furthermore, codeine is widely available in cough syrups and analgesic preparations, and even poppy seeds contain small amounts of morphine. Thus, depending on the drug that was taken originally, morphine and codeine may be detected in a patient's urine for 2 to 4 days after he or she has taken an opioid.

Pharmacological Effects

Morphine exerts its major effects primarily by stimulating opioid receptors that are located in the centers of the brain (within the CNS) that have just been described. Morphine is the prototype of a pure narcotic agonist (Table 9.1). It produces a syndrome that consists of analgesia, euphoria, sedation, respiratory depression, and pupillary constriction.

ANALGESIA   Morphine produces intense analgesia, reducing the intensity of pain by blocking the release of substance P in the spinal cord and, at the same time, reducing the distress that is associated with pain by altering its central processing (at the level of the thalamus, limbic system, and cerebral cortex). Thus, morphine is analgesic because it stimulates opioid receptors in the brain stem, in the spinal cord, and in the brain. Experimentally, analgesia can be produced in animals by injecting morphine directly into the periaquaductal gray matter, the nucleus raphe magnus, or the dorsal horn of the spinal cord. An injection of naloxone (Narcan) (discussed later) or the surgical interruption of the descending inhibitory opioid pathways will block the analgesia that is induced by morphine.

EUPHORIA   Morphine produces a pleasant euphoric state, which includes a strong feeling of contentment, well-being, and lack of concern. Indeed, this is part of the affective, or reinforcing, response of the drug.

Regular users and those who are psychologically attracted to morphine describe the effects of intravenous injection in ecstatic and, often, in sexual terms. However, the euphoric effect becomes progressively less intense after a while. Then, users will inject the drug for one or more of several possible reasons: as an attempt to reexperience the extreme euphoria that occurred after the first few injections, to maintain a state of pleasure and well-being, to prevent mental discomfort that may be associated with reality, or to prevent the occurrence of withdrawal symptoms.

Perhaps part of the psychological attraction to morphine is related to its ability to alter a person's perception of pain by inducing a lack of concern for (or indifference to) it. Medical practitioners and researchers often tend to describe pain in physical terms (for example, in terms of a person who has cancer or breaks a leg). However, pain also occurs that is emotional or psychological in origin, for which no organic cause may be ascribed. Thus, some persons who are attracted to the opiates may be attempting to dull psychological pain, which may partly account for the profound psychological effects and the feeling of well-being that have been reported following the use of these drugs.

Because morphine exerts these powerful effects on pain and emotion by stimulating receptors that bind with naturally occurring opioid peptides, we might ask what role these peptides play in our bodies. Are they "natural analgesics" or "natural euphoriants"? The answer to this question is not clear, especially since the pure narcotic antagonist naloxone, when it is injected intravenously into a normal person, does not induce pain or dysphoria. In marathon runners, however, endorphin levels in plasma increase fourfold;[11,12] these natural analgesics reduce depression and provide an overall feeling of well-being (a "runner's high"). Endorphins may, therefore, be part of a natural euphoric reward system. However, naloxone (even in very large doses) does not either antagonize this natural "high" or reduce the levels of endorphin in plasma.

SEDATION   Morphine produces sedation and drowsiness, but the level of sedation is not as deep as that produced by the general CNS depressants. Although persons who are taking morphine will doze, they can usually be awakened readily. During this state, "mental clouding" is prominent, which is accompanied by a lack of concentration and by apathy, complacency, lethargy, and reduced mentation.

DEPRESSION OF RESPIRATION   Morphine causes a profound depression of respiration secondary to stimulating brain-stem mu receptors. A great reduction in the respiratory rate occurs even at therapeutic doses and, when the dose is increased, the rate slows even further, respiratory volume decreases, breathing patterns become shallow and irregular, and, finally, breathing ceases. The mechanism for this occurrence is a drug-induced decrease in the respiratory center's sensitivity to higher levels of carbon dioxide in the blood. Depression of respiration is the major acute side effect of morphine, and it is the cause of death when a person takes an acute drug overdose.

SUPPRESSION OF COUGH   Opiates suppress the "cough center," which is also located in the brain stem. Thus, opiate narcotics are frequently used as cough suppressants. Codeine appears to be particularly effective in suppressing cough, and it is widely used for that purpose.

PUPILLARY CONSTRICTION   Morphine (as well as other mu and kappa agonists) causes pupillary constriction (miosis), which is precipitated by a stimulant action on an ophthalmic control center in the brain stem (the oculomotor nucleus). Pupillary constriction in the presence of analgesia is characteristic of narcotic ingestion.

NAUSEA AND VOMITING   Morphine stimulates receptors in an area of the medulla that is called the *chemoreceptor trigger zone*. Such stimulation of the chemoreceptor trigger zone produces nausea and vomiting, which are the most characteristic and unpleasant side effects of morphine and other narcotics.

GASTROINTESTINAL SYMPTOMS   Morphine and the other opioids have been used for centuries to relieve diarrhea and to treat dysentery—uses that were prevalent long before these agents were used as analgesics or euphoriants. They cause intestinal tone to increase, motility to decrease, feces to dehydrate, and intestinal spasm (and cramping) to occur. This combination of a decreased propulsion, an increased intestinal tone, a decrease in the rate of movement of food, and dehydration hardens the stool and further retards the advance of fecal material. All these effects contribute to the constipating properties of opiates. Indeed, nothing more effective has been developed yet for treating severe diarrhea.

OTHER EFFECTS   Morphine (but not the other opioids) releases histamine, which causes localized itching or more severe allergic reactions, including bronchoconstriction (an asthma-like constriction of the bronchi of the lungs).

Tolerance and Dependence

Tolerance to morphine and to the other opiate narcotics varies according to the patient's physiological response, the dose, and the frequency of administration. Tolerance to the respiratory depressant, analgesic, euphoric, and sedative effects will develop as a result of using any opiate, but tolerance to both the pupil-constricting and constipating effects does not usually develop to the same extent.

The rate at which tolerance develops varies widely. When there is only intermittent use of morphine and other opiate narcotics, little, if any, tolerance will develop. Thus, when a person's "sprees" of drug use are separated by prolonged periods of time without using drugs, the opiates will retain their initial efficacy. For example, if a person uses morphine or other opioids for recreational purposes only occasionally, low doses may continue to be effective and may not have to be increased markedly (unless, of course, a greater or more intense effect is desired). As drug use is increased, greater dependence and greater tolerance occur. As soon as a pattern of repeated administration appears, tolerance may become so marked that phenomenal doses have to be administered to either maintain a degree of euphoria or prevent withdrawal discomfort (avoidance of discomfort is the more usual case). Tolerance appears to be less a result of the induction of drug-metabolizing enzymes in the liver than it is of the adaptation of CNS neurons to the presence of the drug.

In addition to the development of tolerance to one opiate, *cross-tolerance* also develops, so that a person who becomes tolerant to one opiate will also exhibit a tolerance to all other natural or synthetic opiates, even if they are chemically dissimilar. Cross-tolerance, however, does not develop between the opiate narcotics and the sedative-hypnotics. Thus, a person who has developed a tolerance for morphine will also have a tolerance for heroin but not for alcohol or barbiturates. This point is extremely important, because accidental death may result from the additive effects of using a sedative and an opiate together. For example, if a person takes moderate doses of opiates and then drinks alcohol or takes a sedative, an additive depression of respiration will occur and, ultimately, could lead to coma and death. Deaths from the combined effects of opiates and general depressants are common.

In Chapter 1, we described *physical dependence* as a state in which a person does not function properly without taking a particular drug. Physical dependence is characterized by a withdrawal (or abstinence) syndrome when that drug is not administered.

Symptoms of withdrawal from the opiate narcotics are characterized by restlessness and craving for the drug, sweating, extreme anxiety, fever, chills, violent retching and vomiting, increased respiratory rate (panting), cramping, insomnia, explosive diarrhea, and intense aches and pains. The magnitude of these withdrawal symptoms depends on the dose, the frequency of drug administration, and the duration of drug dependence.

Withdrawal is seldom life-threatening, although it is uncomfortable and seemingly unbearable. Too often, extremely vivid accounts of the withdrawal symptoms are presented as part of an attempt to discourage the recreational use of heroin, opium, morphine, or other opiate narcotics. However, the dependence and withdrawal syndrome are not the only reasons that these drugs should not be used for casual or recreational purposes. Exposure to an opiate narcotic may lead to a powerful compulsion for misuse and dependence. Such an outcome is particularly likely if the opiate narcotic is used by intravenous injection. Finally, the development of tolerance leads to a need for large doses of drugs to prevent withdrawal, alleviate pain (physical or psychological), and attempt to maintain a state of euphoria. Drugs are extremely expensive when they are purchased illegally, even though they may be inexpensive when they are available legitimately (for example, by prescription). Further, tolerance and dependence on opiates are harmful to an addict, but the lengths to which he or she must go to procure an adequate supply of drugs may be even worse. A person who has access to inexpensive, medical-quality narcotics and sterile needles and syringes that are supplied through legitimate sources may be capable of leading a fairly normal life despite his or her tolerance to, and physical dependence on, an opiate. The same may be said for patients who are receiving treatment with chronic methadone maintenance (see the following discussion).

Other Pure Agonist Opioids

As discussed previously, pure opioid agonists are potent mu-receptor stimulants; they produce less activity at other opioid receptors. Morphine is the prototype of an agonist opioid, but several others are also available. Comments on several of these opioids follow.

Heroin (diacetylmorphine) is produced from morphine by a chemical alteration that slightly modifies the structure (Figure 9.4). Heroin is

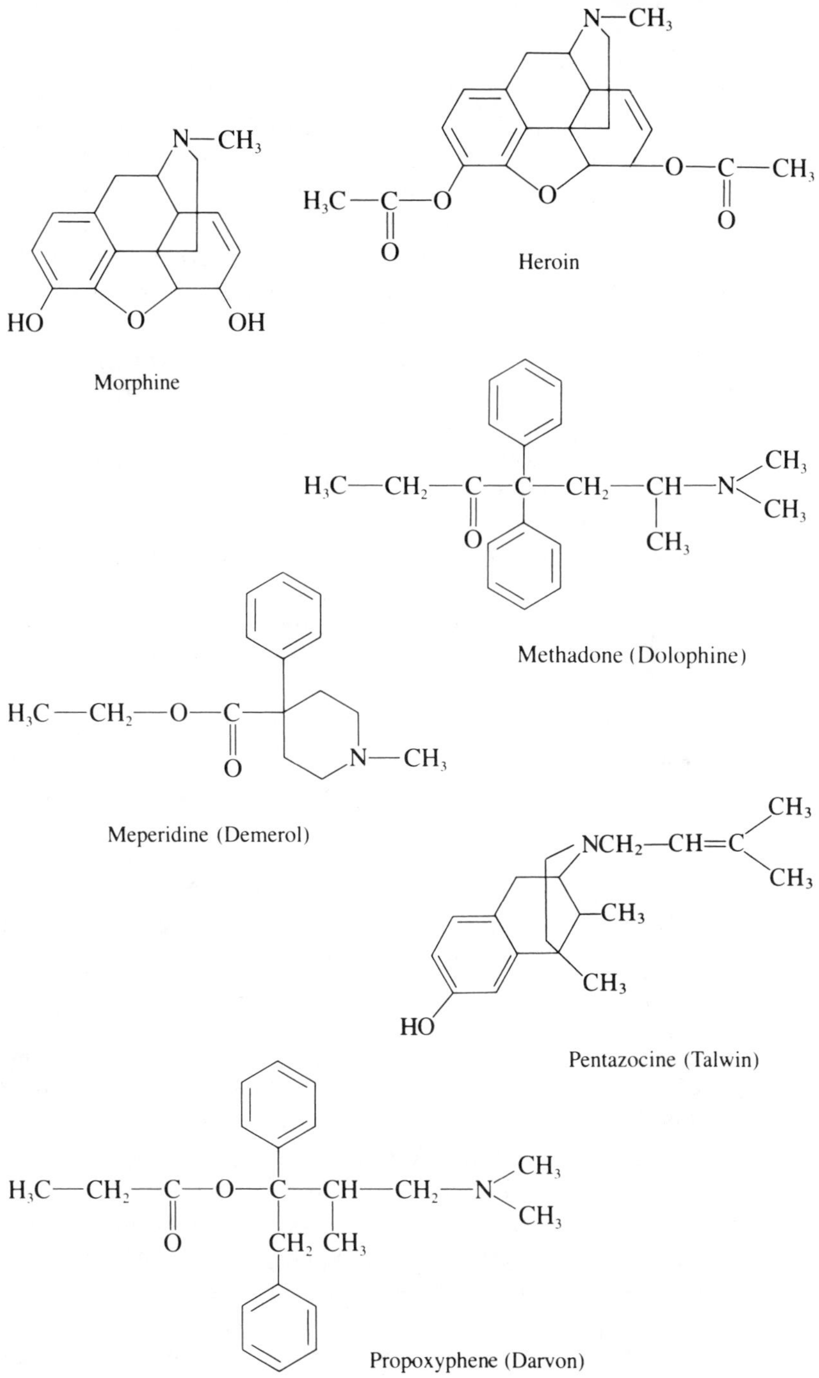

FIGURE 9.4

Structural formulas of morphine, heroin, and four synthetic narcotic analgesics.

about three times more potent than morphine (thus, one-third as much is used). Its increased solubility in lipids leads to faster penetration through the blood-brain barrier, producing an intense "rush" when it is injected intravenously. Heroin is metabolized to morphine, which is eventually metabolized and excreted. Heroin (also called "horse") is still legally available in Great Britain and is used clinically in that country. The drug is not legally available in the United States, but illicit use of heroin is increasing. In addition to its use by injection, smoking of heroin is increasing in popularity. This trend toward smoking of the drug tends to "legitimize" the illicit use of the drug because needles and the risk of hepatitis and AIDS are avoided. When heroin is smoked with crack cocaine, euphoria is intensified, the anxiety and paranoia that are associated with cocaine are tempered, and the depression that follows after the effects of cocaine wear off is reduced. Unfortunately, this combination creates a polydrug addiction that is extremely difficult to treat.

Codeine, with morphine, occurs naturally in opium. It is only about one-tenth as potent as morphine, but it is absorbed better than morphine when it is taken orally. Codeine is often combined with aspirin or acetaminophen (Tylenol) in oral tablets for use as a moderately effective analgesic drug. Codeine causes constipation and reduces cough, which explains its former use as an antidiarrheal and anticough compound. However, nonaddicting compounds are currently available for these purposes.

Hydromorphone (Dilaudid) and *oxymorphone* (Numorphan) are both structurally related to morphine. Both of these drugs are effective mu-receptor stimulants that are about six to ten times more potent than morphine.

Meperidine (Demerol) is a synthetic opioid whose structure is dissimilar to that of morphine (Figure 9.4). Originally, meperidine was thought to be free of many of the undesirable properties that are associated with the use of opioids that are structurally related to morphine. It is now recognized that meperidine is addictive and can be substituted for morphine or heroin in addicts. Meperidine is widely prescribed medically. It is one-tenth as potent as morphine, it produces a similar type of euphoria, and it is equally liable to cause dependence. Unlike morphine, meperidine toxicity is associated with tremors, delirium, hyperreflexia, and convulsions. These effects seem to be produced by a metabolite of meperidine (normeperidine) that has a long half-life (about 18 hours) and causes CNS excitation.

Methadone (Dolophine) is a synthetic opiate whose pharmacological activity is very similar to that of morphine. As stated:

The outstanding properties of methadone are its effective analgesic activity, its efficacy by the oral route, its extended duration of action in suppressing withdrawal symptoms in physically dependent individuals, and its tendency to show persistent effects with repeated administration.[13]

One of the most important reasons for using methadone today is to control the withdrawal symptoms of opiate addicts who are attempting to recover. In this situation, orally administered methadone is substituted for the injected opiate to which the patient is addicted, and the patient is later withdrawn slowly from the methadone. A second important reason for using methadone is to provide maintenance programs for persons who are dependent on opiates. Methadone is an effective agent when it is administered orally, and it has an extended duration of action. Thus, it is used as a substitute for other opiate narcotics. These uses of methadone are discussed further in the following text.

Propoxyphene (Darvon) is an analgesic compound that is structurally very similar to methadone (Figure 9.4). As an analgesic, its potency is less than that of codeine (about one-half) but greater than that of therapeutic doses of aspirin. When propoxyphene is taken in large doses, opiate-like effects are seen; and when it is used intravenously, it is recognized by addicts as a narcotic. When it is taken orally, it does not have much potential for abuse. Some cases of drug dependence have been reported, but to date they have not been of major concern. Because commercial intravenous preparations of propoxyphene are not available, intravenous abuse is encountered only when persons attempt to inject solutions of the powder that is contained in capsules, which are intended for oral use.

Fentanyl (Sublimaze) and two related compounds, *sufentanil* (Sufenta) and *alfentanil* (Alfenta), are short-acting, intravenously administered, agonist opioids that are structurally related to meperidine. These compounds are intended to be used primarily as general anesthetics. Both of these compounds are 80 to 500 times more potent than morphine as analgesics, and both have short durations of action. They can have a profound effect on breathing, both by depressing respiration and by inducing spastic paralysis of the chest-wall muscles. Death from these agents is invariably caused by respiratory failure. In illicit use, fentanyl is known as "China White." Numerous derivatives (such as methylfentanyl) can be manufactured illegally; they emerge periodically and usually cause multiple fatalities.

In attempts to control the manufacture and distribution of illicit derivatives of fentanyl ("designer drugs"), the Federal Drug Enforcement Agency (DEA) added an emergency provision to the Comprehensive Crime Control Act of 1984. This provision authorized the DEA temporarily to declare any drug a Schedule I narcotic substance if it poses an immediate public health hazard. Since 1985, dozens of analogue drugs have been placed under Schedule I control, including the fairly widespread hallucinogenic amphetamine MMDA (methoxy-methylene-dioxyamphetamine), which is popularly known as "ecstasy," certain meperidine (Demerol) derivatives, especially MPPP (1-methyl-4-phenyl-4-propionoxypiperidine), and MPTP (1-methyl-4-phenyl-1,2,5,6-tetrahydropyridine). Both MPPP and MPTP are neurotoxic byproducts of meperidine, and both induce a severe, irreversible, and progressive parkinsonian disease state.

The Emergency Scheduling Provision of the Comprehensive Crime Control Act was first invoked for the fentanyl analogue 3-methylfentanyl in 1985. Since then, many other fentanyl analogues have also been placed under control. Newer legislation makes it illegal to engage in any drug activities using these illicit analogues, regardless of whether the "designer drug" in question has been duly scheduled under the DEA's Controlled Substance Act. Thus, it is unlawful to manufacture, distribute, or possess, with the intent to distribute, a controlled substance analogue intended for human consumption unless the action is in conformance with the Federal Food, Drug, and Cosmetic Act.

Buprenorphine (Buprenex) is a newer agent whose action is characterized by a limited stimulation (partial agonist action) of mu receptors. This action is responsible for its analgesic effectiveness. It has a very long duration of action, presumably because of its strong binding to mu receptors. Such binding, however, occasionally limits its reversibility by naloxone when a reversal is considered to be necessary.

Opioids with Mixed Actions

Four drugs that all bind in varying degrees to three types of opioid receptors (mu, kappa, and sigma) are pentazocine (Talwin), butorphanol (Stadol), dezocine (Dalgan), and nalbuphine (Nubain). These drugs are either unable to exert any actions at all on these receptors (and thus act as competitive *antagonists* of more potent opiates) or their actions are limited (whereupon they are termed *partial antagonists* at their receptors). The characterization of the action of these drugs (as far as it is known for each agent) is presented in Table 9.2.

Pentazocine and butorphanol are very weak mu agonists and have somewhat stronger sigma and kappa effects. Their actions are characterized by moderate analgesia with prominent behavioral alterations, including, at high doses, psychotomimetic effects. Because of their minimal mu effects, neither of these drugs has much potential for producing respiratory depression or physical dependence. Obviously, this characteristic also limits their analgesic effectiveness. When these drugs are administered to morphine- or heroin-dependent persons, they usually precipitate a withdrawal syndrome, because they displace the more potent opioids from the mu receptors. (Hence, they are called *mixed agonist–antagonist opioids*.)

In recent years, abuse of pentazocine has been increasing, and the combination of pentazocine with tripelennamine, an antihistamine, has been especially popular. This combination of drugs is called "T's and blues," and it has caused serious medical complications, including seizures, psychotic episodes, skin ulcerations, abscesses, and muscle-wasting. (The latter three effects are caused by the repeated injections, rather than by the drugs themselves.)

Nalbuphine is primarily a kappa agonist, which accounts for its limited analgesic effects. Because it is also a mu antagonist, it is not likely to produce profound analgesia, respiratory depression, or patterns of abuse. It is relatively devoid of sigma effects, and psychotomimetic effects are rarely observed. Structurally (Figure 9.5), nalbuphine is closely related to naloxone (Narcan), which is a pure narcotic antagonist (discussed in the following section).

Dezocine was introduced in 1990 as the newest of the mixed agonist–antagonist opioids. It is a moderate mu agonist and a weak delta and kappa agonist. Dezocine has few psychotomimetic effects. However, this drug can substitute for morphine. Its clinical efficacy and potential for abuse have not yet been determined.

Opioid Antagonists

In the previous discussion, we noted that when opioids that have mixed agonist–antagonist actions were administered to persons who were not addicts, a morphine-like action was observed, but when they were administered to persons who were morphine or heroin dependent, they would not substitute for the original drug and a withdrawal syndrome would occur. This apparent contradiction in action can be explained in the following manner. When the drugs are administered to nonaddicted

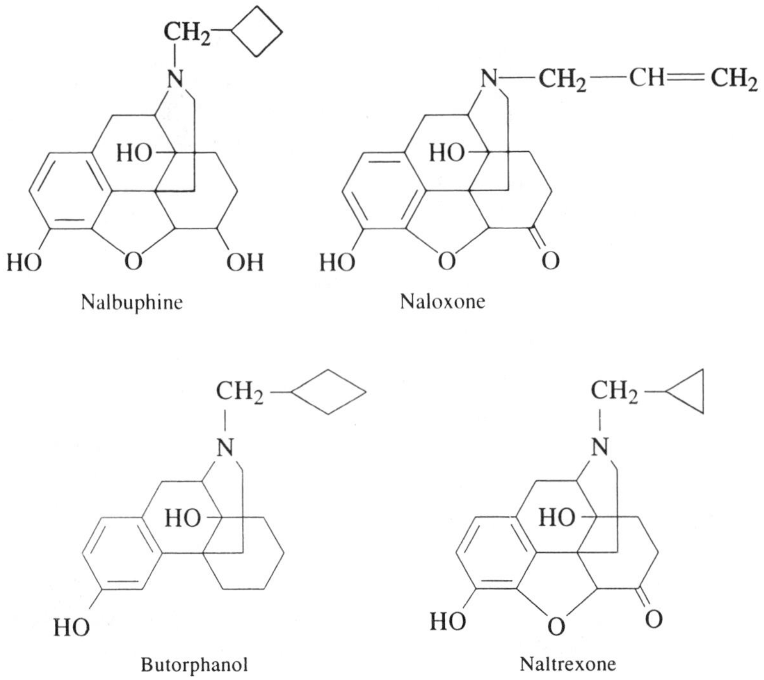

FIGURE 9.5

Structural formulas of four morphine analogues. Naloxone and naltrexone (*right*) are *pure* antagonists, while nalbuphine and butorphanol (*left*) have *mixed* agonistic-antagonistic properties.

persons, they attach to kappa or mu receptors and produce the characteristic (although mild) narcotic actions of analgesia, sedation, euphoria, and respiratory depression. However, when they are administered to a person who is already physically dependent on morphine, heroin, or another narcotic analgesic, they occupy the receptors and thus physically impede the access of the more potent drug to the mu receptor.

In contrast, two drugs (naloxone and naltrexone) have *no* agonist effects of their own, but they antagonize the effects of opiates at all their receptors. These two drugs are called *pure narcotic antagonists.* In essence, they have *affinity* for all opioid receptors, but after binding, they exert no intrinsic activity (that is, after attachment, no receptor stimulation or activation occurs).

Naloxone (Narcan) produces very few pharmacological effects when it is administered to normal persons. However, it rapidly precipitates withdrawal when it is given to narcotic-dependent persons. Naloxone is devoid of agonist (morphine-like) effects and, therefore, is not subject to abuse. It antagonizes the actions of morphine at all its receptors (mu receptors are ten times more sensitive to naloxone than are kappa receptors). Naloxone also antagonizes the actions of endogenous opioid peptides as well as those of morphine-like drugs. It is being used extensively to explore the physiological role of these peptides in persons who are in pain or in other stressful situations.

Naloxone is used to reverse the respiratory depression that follows acute narcotic intoxication (overdoses) and to reverse narcotic-induced respiratory depression in newborns of mothers who have received narcotics. The limitations of naloxone include its short duration of action and the necessity of using a parenteral route of administration (because the drug is poorly absorbed orally).

Naltrexone (Trexan) became clinically available in 1985 as a new narcotic antagonist that is administered orally. Its actions resemble those of naloxone, but naltrexone is well absorbed orally and has a long duration of action, necessitating only a single daily dose of 50 to 100 milligrams. It is useful in narcotic treatment programs when it is desirable to maintain a person on chronic therapy with a narcotic antagonist. In persons who take naltrexone, subsequent injections of an opiate will produce little or no effect. Naltrexone appears to be particularly effective for the treatment of narcotic addicts who realize that they have more to gain by being drug-free than by being drug-dependent.

Opioid Narcotics and Crime

The relation between the use of opioids and the occurrence of crime is complex. Blum and his associates state:

> No known drug, by itself, can be shown to "cause" crime, although when the use of a drug is illegal, the "crime" clearly rests upon the person's decision to acquire, possess, or use the drug illicitly.[14]

If the use of a drug is defined as a crime, drug use *must* lead to crime. Laws have been passed to control the manufacture, distribution, and sale of opioids and many other psychoactive drugs so that the mere illegal possession, use, or sale of any of these drugs is necessarily a crime.

Other factors in the relation between opioids and crime are perhaps more serious. For example, the illegal procurement of opioids is extremely expensive. A well-developed heroin habit may cost an addict hundreds of dollars every day. Obviously, there are very few legitimate ways that most people can earn this amount of extra money. By making these drugs illegal, by making addicts criminals, and by restricting trade by incarcerating small-volume dealers (which forces prices upward), the laws encourage addicts to commit crimes to maintain their drug supply.

There is little evidence to indicate that crimes of violence are a direct consequence of the use of opioid narcotics. Persons who are addicted to opioids are usually quiet, passive, and seldom prone to violence. However, there is little doubt that among those addicts who have a background of delinquency, the use of opioids is part of their total social activity, which includes crime. The use of opioids by these persons may encourage or perpetuate their associations in social or antisocial groups that may pose problems for the community as well as for society.

Within the last few years, a significant change has occurred in the pattern of illicit drug use in our society. Whereas most opiate users were formerly antisocial persons in our society, the current widespread use of opiates and other psychoactive drugs has involved all kinds of persons and has permeated all facets of community life. This factor tends to weaken even further the causal relation between drugs and crime. Persons in this new generation who use drugs often do not use them continuously, and thus they may not develop tolerance or physical dependence. They use opioids, at least initially, only on "sprees" and do not need to buy large quantities. Further, an addict is not necessarily a degenerate criminal, and he or she is not necessarily shabby, ill-shod, or malnourished. A person who is tolerant to, and dependent on, an opiate and who is socially or financially capable of obtaining an adequate supply of good-quality drugs and sterile syringes and needles may maintain his or her proper social and occupational functions, remain in fairly good health, and suffer little serious incapacitation as a result of the dependence.

Treatment of the Opioid User

The precise motivations for a person to become dependent on opiate narcotics are far from clear. In the United States, three basic patterns of opiate use and dependence can be seen:

One involves individuals whose drug use begins in the context of medical treatment and who obtain the initial supplies through medical channels. This group constitutes a very small percentage of the addicted population. Another pattern begins with experimental or recreational drug use, and progresses to more intensive use; this pattern involves primarily adolescents and young adults, with males outnumbering females. Most of these individuals are introduced to the drug by other users. Thus, drug use spreads from one friend to another in epidemic fashion. A third pattern involves users who begin in one or another of the preceding ways but later switch to oral opioids [methadone] obtained from organized treatment programs.[15]

The analgesia and euphoria that are induced by opioid narcotics are attractions for persons who use them. However, additional contributions to the incidence of opiate dependence appear to be sociological or psychological rather than the result of a physiological or organic deficit in the addict. For example, in 1971, when opium and heroin were widely available in the Far East, about 45 percent of U.S. Army enlisted men in Vietnam used opioids at least once.[16] About half of these users reported that at some time during their tour of duty in Vietnam, they were physically dependent on drugs. It is unlikely that this large number of young men had a consistent organic deficit. Rather, the ready availability of opioids and the traumatic situation in which the soldiers were involved predisposed them to the use of these agents. Therefore, it can be seen that before any attempt is made to withdraw an addict permanently from opioid use, his or her underlying motivation for seeking the drug's positive reinforcement, or reward (the euphoria, sedation, and analgesia), must be determined. In recent years, it has become clear that treatment and rehabilitation of opioid users cannot reside solely in attempts to withdraw them from the drug; the positive reinforcements or life situations that are associated with opioid use must also be changed. As Jaffe states:

> The indications for treatment vary with the drugs being used as well as with the social and cultural factors determining the particular pattern of drug use. Some patterns of drug use, such as weekly use of marijuana, do not require treatment any more than does the occasional smoking of tobacco or the social use of alcohol. Such casual use is not without hazard, and it may jeopardize vocational status, especially as programs for testing the presence

of drugs in body fluids expand. However, such patterns of use do not necessarily constitute a treatable disorder. It is likely that changing views about drug use will continue to create grey areas where the indications for treatment are unclear. However, there is general agreement that treatment is appropriate for the adverse consequences of drug use and for the compulsive drug user who voluntarily seeks help.[17]

Until recently, few thought that a heroin addict could ever be satisfactorily rehabilitated and maintained in a functional, drug-free state, and addicts were routinely sentenced to imprisonment. Statistics indicate that such periods of imprisonment were neither an effective treatment nor sufficient rehabilitation for the addict. At least 90 percent of those persons who were incarcerated for opioid use relapsed within 6 months of their release.

We have now entered a more enlightened time and recognize that an addict is ill and not necessarily a criminal (recall the discussion of alcoholism). We handle the treatment and rehabilitation of the narcotic addict with a more positive, medically oriented approach. No longer do all physicians adhere to the concept that drug withdrawal must be the first step in treatment or that effective rehabilitation requires a carefully controlled, drug-free environment. The latter concept of rehabilitation started with the development of residential communities such as the Synanon Foundation in California, which are comprised of social programs of group living and community involvement to assist former addicts. Although these programs are effective, they are not capable of handling large numbers of drug-dependent persons.

Such considerations have led to the development of new programs that have been designed to allow withdrawal of addicts from illicit drugs while they remain functioning members of their own communities, by providing oral doses of narcotics so that they do not need to purchase drugs on the street. In this manner, the addict's dependence on the needle, the subcultural involvement, and the criminal orientation are decreased. It would be possible, of course, to continue to give these patients the intravenous drugs that they had been using (heroin, morphine, and so on) and either maintain them on a particular dose (provided by a legitimate source) or else reduce the dose over a period of several days. However, as mentioned previously, we can improve on this method by substituting methadone, which can be administered orally and can be substituted for any other opioid analgesic.

With *methadone substitution,* the opioid that was originally used (usually injected) is replaced by an orally administered agent. The dose of methadone is then reduced slowly over a period of 10 to 14 days. The withdrawal symptoms are rarely worse than those of a moderate "flu-like" syndrome. The dose of methadone that is employed varies with the patient's health and the amount of drug that was formerly used. Unfortunately, the relapse rate following methadone substitution is high—approaching 60 to 70 percent.

With *methadone maintenance,* addicts are stabilized on methadone and, it is postulated, remain productive members of their communities, so that it may not be necessary to withdraw the methadone. More recently, however, it has been found that after 1 to 2 years, many former heroin addicts who have been maintained on methadone can be gradually withdrawn from this drug successfully over a period of several weeks. The withdrawal discomforts are relatively minor, and some patients are able to complete the withdrawal process and not relapse to the use of heroin, morphine, or other opioid. Others have completed the withdrawal process but have later returned to using heroin. Still others have discontinued the withdrawal process and have remained on methadone maintenance.

Methadone-substitution and methadone-maintenance programs have been in operation for several years, and studies conclude that methadone is an effective aid in the treatment of heroin addiction. It is also clear that methadone must be combined with intensive psychological counseling and the adoption of a productive lifestyle. It is not enough merely to switch addicts from heroin to methadone and then return them to the street. This has happened in some programs and, in many cases, the addict has responded by either compulsively abusing the methadone or returning to the use of heroin. Alternatives must be provided to help addicts find a new lifestyle and positive reinforcements to replace the motivation to use opioids, so that they can become adjusted successfully. Once these rein-forcements are found, consideration can be given to the possibility of discontinuing the methadone. Too-rapid removal of methadone should be avoided, however, because it may be more socially acceptable to maintain an opioid addict on methadone than to return him or her to the street and to former habits of drug acquisition and use.

Several nonnarcotic drugs have been tried to aid in opioid with-drawal, and one agent has been found to be quite useful. Clonidine (Catapres) is an antihypertensive drug that is used clinically to lower blood pressure in patients who have hypertension. Pharmacologically, it stimulates certain specialized catecholamine receptors in the spinal cord (alpha-2 receptors, which ultimately modulate the release of substance P in the spinal cord: Figure 9.4). Clonidine effectively suppresses withdrawal symptoms in addicts who are withdrawing from low-to-moderate doses of methadone.[18,19]

In treatment, methadone is discontinued abruptly, and clonidine is administered for 7 to 10 days to suppress symptoms. The clonidine is then withdrawn gradually over 3 to 4 days. The drug is more effective in suppressing the physical signs and symptoms of withdrawal (nausea, vomiting, and diarrhea) than it is in treating the psychological discomforts and drug craving.

In addicts who desire more rapid withdrawal, methadone doses can be lowered gradually until the patient becomes uncomfortable, at which time either naloxone or naltrexone can be administered to precipitate complete withdrawal. Clonidine is then administered to ameliorate the symptoms of the precipitated withdrawal. Such therapy, however, is seldom used.

At present, the pharmacologically optimal method of withdrawal for an addict is to place him or her on oral methadone and, after prolonged methadone maintenance and gradual dosage reduction, the patient is withdrawn with the assistance of clonidine. This procedure is followed by long-term maintenance with the antagonist naltrexone. Such a scheme appears to provide the safest and the most effective method of withdrawal in those patients who desire to remain drug-free.

STUDY QUESTIONS

1. Describe the location of opioid receptors in the brain and the spinal cord.
2. How are pain impulses modulated as they enter the spinal cord?
3. What is substance P and how is it influenced by narcotic analgesics?
4. (a) What is an opioid agonist? (b) What is an opioid antagonist? (c) What is a mixed agonist–antagonist? (d) Give an example of each.
5. What might lead a person to misuse or abuse opioid narcotics?
6. Differentiate between naloxone and naltrexone. How might each of these drugs be used?
7. Describe the various ways that opioid dependence might be handled or treated.

8. Why are tricyclic antidepressants analgesic? (Answer from your knowledge of descending spinal-cord analgesic pathways.)

9. Differentiate between the opioid modulation of afferent pain impulses and the affective component of pain.

10. Give evidence for and against the existence of endogenous opioid peptides (e.g., endorphins) that serve as "natural opioids."

NOTES

1. H. P. Rang and M. M. Dale, *Pharmacology* (Edinburgh: Churchill Livingstone, 1987), pp. 553–554.

2. Y. Kuraishi, N. Hirota, Y. Sato, et al., "Noradrenergic Inhibition of the Release of Substance P from the Primary Afferents in the Rabbit Spinal Dorsal Horn," *Brain Research* 359 (1985): 177–182.

3. J. C. Eisenach, D. M. Dewan, J. C. Ruse, and J. M. Angelo, "Epidural Clonidine Produces Antinociception, but Not Hypotension, in Sheep," *Anesthesiology* 66 (1987): 496–501.

4. T. L. Yaksh and P. R. Wilson, "Spinal Serotonin Terminal System Mediates Antinociception," *Journal of Pharmacology and Experimental Therapeutics* 208 (1979): 446–453.

5. C. A. DiFazio, "Pharmacology of Narcotic Analgesics," *The Clinical Journal of Pain* 5, Supplement 1 (1989): S5–S7.

6. K. H. Gwirtz, "Intraspinal Narcotics in the Management of Postoperative Pain," *Anesthesiology Review* 17 (1990): 16–28.

7. R. W. Hansen and K. E. Gerber, *Coping with Chronic Pain: A Guide to Patient Management* (New York: Guilford, 1990).

8. J. H. Jaffe and W. R. Martin, "Opioid Analgesics and Antagonists," in A. G. Gilman, T. W. Rall, A. S. Nies, and P. Taylor, eds., *Goodman and Gilman's The Pharmacological Basis of Therapeutics*, 8th ed. (New York: Pergamon, 1990), pp. 485–489.

9. R. M. Brown, D. H. Clouet, and D. Friedman, eds., *Opiate Receptor Subtypes and Brain Function*, National Institute on Drug Abuse, Monograph No. 71, Department of Health and Human Services Publication No. ADM. 86-1462 (Washington, D.C.: U.S. Government Printing Office, 1986).

10. L. P. Finnegan and S. M. Ehrlich, "Maternal Drug Abuse During Preg-

nancy: Evaluation and Pharmacotherapy for Neonatal Abstinence," in M. W. Adler and A. Cowan, eds., *Modern Methods in Pharmacology, Volume 6, Testing and Evaluation of Drugs of Abuse* (New York: Wiley-Liss, 1990), pp. 255–263.

11. D. A. Mahler, L. N. Cunningham, G. S. Skrinar, W. J. Kraemer, and G. L. Colice, "Beta-Endorphin Activity and Hypercapnic Ventilatory Responsiveness after Marathon Running," *Journal of Applied Physiology* 66 (1989): 2431–2436.

12. G. A. Sforzo, "Opioids and Exercise. An Update," *Sports Medicine 7* (1989): 109–124.

13. J. H. Jaffe and W. R. Martin, "Opioid Analgesics and Antagonists," in A. G. Gilman, T. W. Rall, A. S. Nies, and P. Taylor, eds., *Goodman and Gilman's The Pharmacological Basis of Therapeutics,* 8th ed. (New York: Pergamon, 1990), p. 508.

14. R. H. Blum et al., *Society and Drugs,* vol. 1 (San Francisco: Jossey-Bass, 1969), p. 290.

15. J. H. Jaffe, "Drug Addiction and Drug Abuse," in A. G. Gilman, T. W. Rall, A. S. Nies, and P. Taylor, eds., *Goodman and Gilman's The Pharmacological Basis of Therapeutics,* 8th ed. (New York: Pergamon, 1990), p. 531.

16. L. Robins, *The Vietnam Drug User Returns: Final Report, September 1973,* Special Action Office Monograph, Series A, No. 2 (Washington, D.C.: U. S. Government Printing Office, 1974).

17. J. H. Jaffe, "Drug Addiction and Drug Abuse," in A. G. Gilman, T. W. Rall, A. S. Nies, and P. Taylor, eds., *Goodman and Gilman's The Pharmacological Basis of Therapeutics,* 8th ed. (New York: Pergamon, 1990), p. 560.

18. J. H. Jaffe, "Drug Addiction and Drug Abuse," in A. G. Gilman, T. W. Rall, A. S. Nies, and P. Taylor, eds., *Goodman and Gilman's The Pharmacological Basis of Therapeutics,* 8th ed. (New York: Pergamon, 1990), pp. 565–567.

19. D. S. Charney et al., "Clonidine and Naltrexone," *Archives of General Psychiatry* 39 (1982): 1327–1332.

Antipsychotic (Neuroleptic) Drugs
Drugs for Treating Schizophrenia

The term *psychosis* refers to a group of mental disorders that are considered to be endogenous in origin. Persons who suffer from psychosis display an impaired capacity to recognize reality, communicate, or associate with others to such a degree that they cannot deal with even the ordinary demands of life. The psychoses are severe psychiatric disorders, and persons who suffer from them exhibit a marked impairment of behavior as well as a serious inability to think coherently, to comprehend reality, or to gain insight into their abnormality. These conditions often include delusions and hallucinations.

Psychoses are often divided into three major subclassifications, which are based on the origin of a person's disorder: (1) a "brain syndrome" (a loss of nerve-cell function) (for example, the type of disorder that would occur in drug intoxication or dementia; Chapter 3), (2) affective disorders (for example, depression and mania; Chapter 8), and (3) schizophrenia.

Schizophrenia literally means "splitting of the mind." It refers to a number of psychotic disorders with various cognitive emotional and behavioral manifestations including thought disturbances, delusions, hallucinations (usually auditory), disturbed sense of self and a loss of reality testing. Characteristics are distinctive changes in reasoning[1] and concept formation. Symptoms typically become evident in schizophrenics during adolescence or early adulthood and are highly disabling. The etiology of schizophrenia includes a strong hereditary factor, but the exact genetic alteration remains unknown. Exacerbations of symptoms are common in patients who have this disorder, which may signify a chronic state of schizophrenia. Patients who suffer from chronic schizophrenia often experience a progressive impairment of insight, judgment, and affect. Chronic schizophrenia is particularly important from a pharmacological point of view, because antipsychotic drugs are most effective in patients who are experiencing acute exacerbations of schizophrenia. They are less effective in those who suffer from sustained, or progressive, impairments. Indeed, the principal benefit of antipsychotic drugs may be the prevention of acute exacerbations; they can reduce the exacerbation rate in chronic schizophrenics by about one-half to two-thirds of that seen in nontreated patients.

Thought disturbances that are experienced by schizophrenic patients include a distortion of reality, delusions, and hallucinations (usually auditory). Mood and behavior disorders are characterized by ambivalence, apathy, withdrawal, and bizarre activity. The estimated incidence of schizophrenia is 0.5 to 1 percent of the general population.

Minor versus Major Tranquilizers

The benzodiazepine sedatives, or tranquilizers (discussed in Chapter 5), reduce anxiety states and neurotic behavior. They are not effective in the management of schizophrenic patients. In contrast, the neuroleptic tranquilizers discussed in this chapter are effective in the treatment of schizophrenic persons. They reduce the frequency of relapses and make such patients more manageable and functional.

The term *minor tranquilizer* refers to the benzodiazepine (or meprobamate) type of sedative. The terms *major tranquilizer, neuroleptic, antipsychotic,* or *antischizophrenic* refer to drugs that are capable of relieving the symptoms of schizophrenia. Major tranquilizers induce a behavioral state that is characterized by psychomotor slowing, emotional quieting, and an indifference to external stimuli. This triad of characteristics describes what is called a *neuroleptic state.*

Note that the word *tranquilizer*, by definition, implies the induction of a tranquil, calm, or pleasant state. This state may indeed be produced by minor tranquilizers, because sedative-hypnotic compounds can induce a state of disinhibition, euphoria, and relief from anxiety. However, the psychological effects that are induced by neuroleptic (or major) tranquilizers are seldom pleasant or euphoric; and they may be unpleasant or dysphoric when they are administered to persons who are not psychotic. Hence, these agents are seldom encountered as drugs of abuse. Their importance in medicine, however, is well established. In addition, laboratory studies of these agents have contributed to our knowledge about the physiological and biochemical bases of behavior and of mental disease.

Historical Background

Clinical descriptions of schizophrenic patients date back at least to 1400 B.C. Isolation of, and caring for, these patients was the only known therapy until the 1930s. Before that time, therapeutic attempts to treat schizophrenic patients included such activities as twirling them on a stool until they lost consciousness or dropping them through a trap door into an icy lake. The effectiveness of such treatments was very doubtful.

Alternatively, and more humanely, some were treated with more individualized care, which today would resemble group and social therapy. Such treatment was probably a moderately effective therapeutic approach. However, when huge mental hospitals were introduced during the twentieth century, the personal approach disappeared; moral treatment and the therapeutic gains that were made by such individualized attention were no longer seen.

In 1933, Sakel introduced insulin coma as a form of therapeutic treatment. This method involved the injection of insulin until the patient became hypoglycemic enough to lose consciousness and lapse into a coma. A series of several of these treatments was reported to be helpful for schizophrenic patients. Shortly thereafter, drug-induced convulsions and electroconvulsive therapy (ECT) were introduced. A series of those treatments frequently brought relief to patients who were experiencing acute psychotic episodes. Today, such therapies have been abandoned (except for ECT, which is effective in treating major depression; Chapter 8).

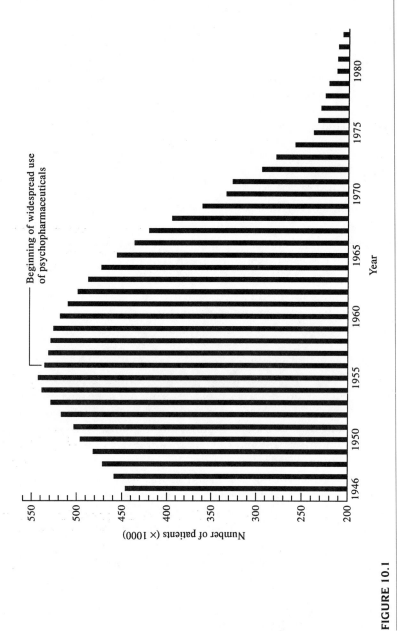

FIGURE 10.1

Numbers of resident patients in state and local government mental hospitals in the United States from 1946 through 1983. Note the dramatic change in the total population of mental hospitals that began in 1956 with the introduction of psychoactive drugs into therapy.

Thus, prior to 1950, effective drugs for the treatment of psychotic patients were virtually nonexistent; and such patients were usually permanently or semipermanently hospitalized. By 1955, more than half a million persons in the United States were residing in mental hospitals. However, in 1956, a dramatic and steady reversal in this trend occurred (see Figure 10.1). By 1983, fewer than 220,000 patients were institutionalized. This decline in the number of residents in mental hospitals has occurred despite a doubling in the numbers of *admissions* to state hospitals. We now stabilize patients on medication and discharge them from institutions quite rapidly.* What accounts for such a dramatic shift in the treatment of schizophrenic patients? The answer lies in the history of a class of drugs called *phenothiazines*.

In 1952, a French surgeon named Laborit introduced promethazine (the first of the phenothiazines) to deepen the anesthesia that was induced in patients to whom barbiturates were administered. Later that year, researchers in France developed a second phenothiazine—chlorpromazine (Thorazine). This drug was administered in a "cocktail" to patients the night before surgery to allay their fears and anxieties. Chlorpromazine was found to lower the amount of anesthetic drugs that were needed for a patient without inducing a loss of consciousness, because it appeared to cause a profound alteration of the patient's mental awareness. Patients who had received chlorpromazine were quiet, conscious, sedated, and quite uninterested in, or unconcerned about, what was going on around them. This condition was termed a *neuroleptic state*, and chlorpromazine was, therefore, the first neuroleptic drug. Because of these effects, chlorpromazine was tried in the treatment of patients who were suffering from mental illness, and it was found to be effective in ameliorating schizophrenic episodes as well as in preventing relapse. Thus, for the first time, a drug had been found to specifically alter the clinical manifestations of the psychotic process itself. Although it did not provide a permanent cure, its use in conjunction with supportive therapy allowed thousands of patients, who would otherwise be hospitalized permanently, to return to their communities.

Chlorpromazine was introduced into the United States in 1955. At about the same time, another antipsychotic agent—reserpine (Serpasil)—which is unrelated to chlorpromazine structurally (Figure 10.2), was dis-

---

*Although we have a high discharge rate of schizophrenics from institutions, we must be concerned about the ultimate functioning of these persons in society. Many fail to continue their medication and function poorly as a result. It has been estimated that as many as 50 percent of our adult homeless population may, indeed, suffer from inadequately controlled schizophrenia.

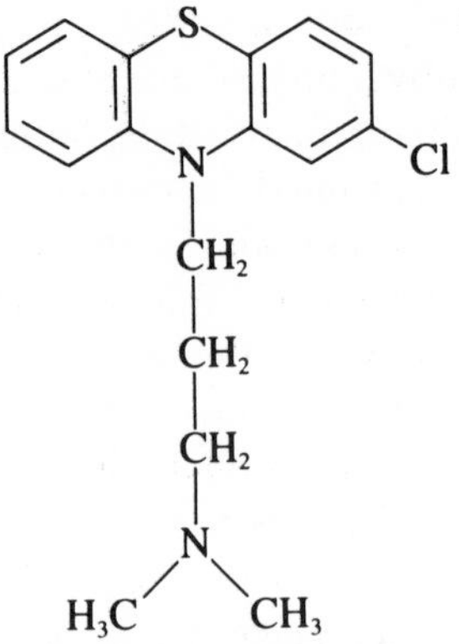

Chlorpromazine (Thorazine)

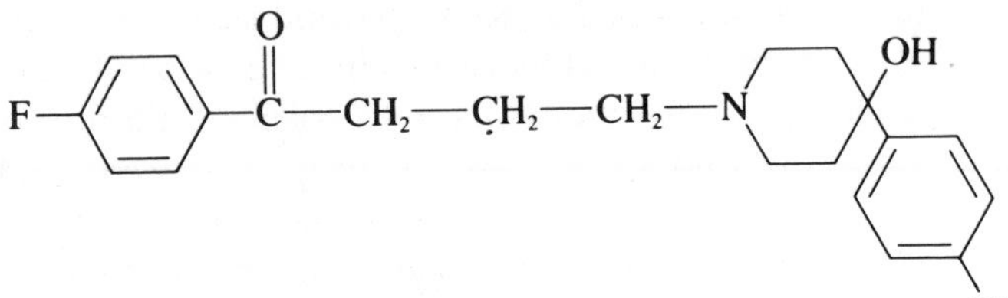

Haloperidol (Haldol)

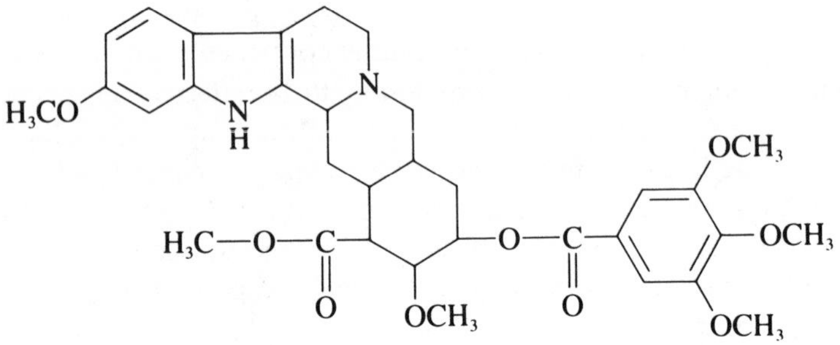

Reserpine (Serpasil)

FIGURE 10.2

Structural formulas of three representative antipsychotic tranquilizers. Chlorpromazine is a representative of the group of phenothiazine tranquilizers; nine other phenothiazine derivatives are available.

covered and introduced into therapy. If chlorpromazine had not been discovered, reserpine would have been the drug of choice for the treatment of psychotic patients, despite the fact that it produces a number of bothersome side effects. Thus, because both drugs were introduced almost simultaneously and both were effective, chlorpromazine—the drug that produced the lower number of side effects—was the one that survived. Reserpine is now rarely used in medicine.

Today, there is renewed interest in developing new neuroleptic drugs that might be superior to chlorpromazine and the other phenothiazines. As a consequence, a class of drugs called *butyrophenones*, which was developed in Belgium during the mid-1960s, is now being used. Two butyrophenones are available in the United States: haloperidol (Haldol) and droperidol (Inapsine). Neither seems to have a significant advantage over the phenothiazines, but haloperidol is used occasionally for patients who cannot tolerate the phenothiazines.

During the 1970s and 1980s, there were continuing efforts to develop neuroleptic drugs that would be effective therapeutically without causing the severe side effects (see the following discussion) that are observed in patients who take phenothiazines and butyrophenones. Early agents included loxapine (Loxitane) and molindone (Moban), neither of which separates the efficacy of these drugs from their principal side effects (parkinsonism-like, involuntary, extrapyramidal motor movements, discussed below). Currently, clozapine (Clozaril) is drawing a great deal of interest because its potential for inducing parkinsonism-like side effects is low, and it seems to be effective in patients who are refractory to other neuroleptics.

Although these drugs are not the curative "wonder drugs" they were thought to be during the 1950s, antipsychotic drugs have had a remarkable impact on psychiatry—an impact that can legitimately be called revolutionary.

Biological Theories of Schizophrenia

The etiology of schizophrenia remains obscure. As noted previously, a strong, but by no means invariable, hereditary factor exists.[2,3]

The Altered Amine Theory

The altered amine theory of schizophrenia (an older theory) is based on evidence that some schizophrenic patients excrete abnormal products of amine metabolism in their urine—products that are not found in the urine of normal patients. These altered substances are thought to be methylated metabolites of dopamine. The relation of these methylated metabolites of dopamine to schizophrenia may be based, in part, on the fact that some methylated products of normally occurring biological amines are hallucinogenic (Chapter 11). For example, mescaline and dimethyltryptamine (DMT) are methylated derivatives of dopamine and serotonin, and they can induce a behavioral state that resembles a psychosis. It is not yet clear, however, whether a drug-induced psychosis is related to schizophrenia or, indeed, if schizophrenics produce a common methylated amine that underlies the disorder. Thus, evidence in support of this theory is very weak.

The Inherited Gene Theory

A second theory of schizophrenia asserts that this disease is a specific *inherited* disease that results from a single mutant, inherited gene. It has been hypothesized that an as yet undiscovered metabolic error leads to schizophrenic illness. Evidence in favor of this theory is based on the fact that the incidence of schizophrenia in the general population is approximately 1 percent but increases to 7 to 16 percent in children who have one schizophrenic parent and to 40 to 68 percent in children who have two schizophrenic parents. In studies of identical twins, the incidence of schizophrenia in both monozygotic persons, when they are reared separately, is about the same as that for twins who are reared together. Although no specific genetic deficit has been identified yet, a predisposition to schizophrenia almost certainly is inherited. Currently investigators are examining the amino acid composition and genetic makeup of dopamine receptors that have been isolated from the brain tissue of schizophrenics.

The Dopamine Theory

The leading hypothesis concerning the biological basis of schizophrenia—the dopamine theory—is based on the fact that all neuroleptic drugs can antagonize the actions of dopamine and that this action is responsible for most of their clinical effects.[4] Thus, a state of functional overactivity of dopamine or, what is more likely, an increased sensitivity of dopamine receptors may occur in selected neuronal pathways of schizophrenic patients. Very likely, postsynaptic receptor sites (on which dopamine neurons synapse) are hypersensitive to ordinary amounts of dopamine.[5] This theory is based on pharmacological evidence; drugs that block a subgroup of dopamine receptors (dopamine-2 receptors) are clinically useful, in a dose-related manner, in the treatment of patients who suffer from schizophrenia (Figure 10.3). What is missing, however, is clear evidence that the neurochemistry of dopamine is altered in the brains of schizophrenic persons. Evidence in favor of this theory includes the fact that schizophrenic persons have more dopamine-binding sites than normal persons.[5] Also, it has been demonstrated that an abnormally high amount of dopamine is found in postmortem tissue that has been taken from the amygdala (left side only!) of schizophrenic persons. As stated:

> This finding accords with other evidence suggesting asymmetry in the neurological abnormality in schizophrenia (e.g., the frequent occurrence of left-sided temporal lobe epilepsy in schizophrenic patients) and is the clearest evidence so far of a primary disturbance of dopamine metabolism in schizophrenia.[2]

Referring to a more complicated mechanism that involves the subdivision of dopamine receptors into two types (dopamine-1 and dopamine-2):

> Other evidence for a change in dopamine function is a small increase in the number of dopamine (D-2) receptors. . . . Most evidence suggests that the abnormality in schizophrenia is related to D-2 rather than D-1 . . . receptors, though the two subtypes have a very similar distribution in the brain. The increase in receptor binding appears to be confined to D-2 receptors, and the antischizophrenic effect of various drugs relates more closely to their activity on D-2 than D-1 receptors.[2]

Indeed, almost all of the currently available neuroleptic drugs have an exceedingly high affinity for dopamine-2 receptors in direct relation to their antischizophrenic effects,[4] and their clinical potency correlates best with their affinity for dopamine-2 receptors. As recently stated:

> It has been suggested that psychoses result from excessive dopamine-2 receptor-mediated activity and that the therapeutic effects of the clinically employed antipsychotic drugs are produced by blockade or chronic adaptive . . . alteration . . . of these receptors.[1,6]

In contrast to the older neuroleptic drugs, the newer drug clozapine differs in that it has an affinity for dopamine-1 receptors, and the blockade of these receptors underlies its effectiveness as an anti-

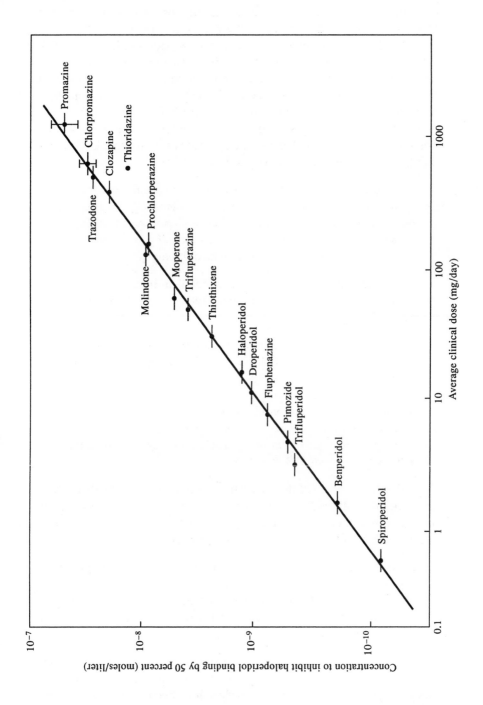

psychotic medication.[7] Further, a blockade of serotonin receptors might also contribute to its effect.[1] Clozapine has a very much lower affinity for dopamine-2 receptors.[8,9,10] Thus, by using clozapine, we can block dopamine-1 receptors to provide relief from symptoms of schizophrenia while minimizing the neuroleptic (parkinsonism-like, extrapyramidal) motor effects (which are presumably caused by the blockade of dopamine-2 receptors). As stated by Cohen:

> It has been shown that Type I schizophrenics, a syndrome associated with hallucinations, delusions, and overactivity, have increased numbers of dopamine-2 receptors. Type II schizophrenics, manifested by flattened affect, regression, withdrawal and, at times, cerebral atrophy, have no dopamine-2 receptor increase. It is likely that Type I schizophrenia is an early phase of the disorder, and that by the time that Type II symptoms appear, the dopamine receptor disturbance has subsided, and chronic residual symptoms remain. The drugs that are used in the treatment of the schizophrenic syndrome are more effective for the Type I disorder.[5]

Here, Dr. Cohen appears to be referring to the traditional neuroleptic drugs. Clozapine, with dopamine-1 blocking activity, is more effective in treating patients who suffer from refractory, type II schizophrenia. It is less useful for patients who suffer from type I schizophrenia and exhibit a low incidence of the motor-movement side effects that are characteristic of neuroleptic drugs that block dopamine-2 receptors.[11,12]

Dopamine receptors are located at several sites within the brain (Appendix III). Neuroleptic drugs block dopamine receptors in the following areas: (1) the limbic and frontal cortical areas of the brain, which correlates with the therapeutic action of neuroleptic drugs; (2) the extrapyramidal system, which correlates with many of the motor dysfunctions that are produced by these drugs; (3) the hypothalamic–pituitary axis, which correlates with the hormonal alterations that are induced by these agents; and (4) certain centers of the brain stem (especially the chemoreceptor trigger zone of the medulla), which correlates with the antivomiting effect.

FIGURE 10.3

Correlation between the clinical potency and receptor-binding activities of neuroleptic drugs. Clinical potency is expressed as the daily dose that is used in treating schizophrenia, and binding activity is expressed as the concentration needed to produce 50 percent inhibition of haloperidol binding. [From H. P. Rang and M. M. Dale,[2] Figure 22.1, p. 501.]

Thus, antagonism of dopamine neurotransmission appears to underlie both the therapeutic effects and most of the side effects of these drugs. The phenothiazines represent the primary class of drugs whose actions cause a blockade of dopamine receptors, and they are the primary class of drugs used to treat schizophrenic patients. Conversely, drugs that have actions that result in *potentiation* of dopamine neurotransmission will produce conditions in patients that closely resemble schizophrenia. Currently, amphetamine-induced psychosis (Chapter 6) provides the best available model for acute paranoid schizophrenia. Thus, schizophrenia is probably associated with excessive, or hyperactive, neurotransmission at dopamine synapses, possibly at a specific subdivision.[13,14] Whether this *association* can be extended to *causation* is still obscure.

Classification of Antipsychotic Drugs

All drugs that are currently used to ameliorate schizophrenic episodes also produce prominent neurological side effects. These side effects result in alterations of motor behavior that closely resemble those observed in patients who have Parkinson's disease. To date, movement disorders cannot reasonably be separated from the therapeutic effects. These disorders consist of rigidity, tremor, slowed movements, and restlessness. Some of these symptoms disappear when the medication is discontinued, but persistent or permanent motor disorders also occur (described later).

It has been a goal of pharmacologists to find antipsychotic drugs that would be effective therapeutically in the treatment of schizophrenia without causing this neuroleptic syndrome. Some progress has been seen in patients who take the drug clozapine, in whom the motor disorders tend to be minimized while therapeutic effectiveness (even in refractory schizophrenia) is maintained (see the following discussion). Thus, eventually, perhaps, the term *neuroleptic* will refer to the older, more traditional antipsychotic drugs (which are dopamine-2 receptor blockers), and newer, clozapine-like antipsychotic drugs will be developed that are devoid of blocking effects on dopamine-2 receptors and of parkinsonism-like actions. Ideally, antipsychotic drugs would then be classified as (1) neuroleptic antipsychotic drugs and (2) nonneuroleptic antipsychotic drugs. For now, however, we will continue to use the more inclusive term *neuroleptic* as a description of most of the drugs that are currently available.

Phenothiazine Derivatives

The phenothiazines are the most widely used neuroleptic antipsychotic drugs. However, they are also used extensively for other purposes, for example, in the treatment of nausea and vomiting, for preanesthetic sedation, to delay ejaculation, for relief of severe itching, in the treatment of alcoholic hallucinosis and hallucinations that are induced by psychedelic agents (see Chapter 11), and in the treatment of intractable hiccups.[1]

Table 10.1 lists ten phenothiazine derivatives that are available for clinical use. However, this discussion focuses on the prototype agent of this class—chlorpromazine (Thorazine)—because it is the most widely known and the best investigated agent in this group. As discussed previously, its mechanism of action involves antagonism of dopamine-2 receptors in various locations within the brain. The locations that are pertinent to this discussion are the reticular formation of the brain stem, the hypothalamus, the limbic system, and the basal ganglia. By examining the consequences of blocking dopamine-2 receptors in each of these structures, we can explain the pharmacological effects of these drugs.

Pharmacokinetics

The phenothiazines are absorbed erratically and unpredictably from the gastrointestinal tract. However, because patients usually take these drugs for long periods of time (even for a lifetime), the oral route of administration is still effective and commonly used. Intramuscular injection of phenothiazines is also quite effective; it increases the effectiveness of the drug by about four to ten times that achieved with oral administration. Once these drugs are in the bloodstream, the phenothiazines are rapidly distributed throughout the body. The levels of phenothiazines that are found in the brain are low compared with those that are found in other body tissues; the highest concentrations are found in the lungs, liver, adrenal glands, and spleen.

The phenothiazines have half-lives of 24 to 48 hours, and they are slowly metabolized in the liver. The clinical effects of a single dose persist for at least 24 hours. Thus, a daily dose that is taken at bedtime will often minimize certain side effects (such as excessive sedation). The phenothiazines become extensively bound to body tissues, which partially accounts for their slow rate of drug elimination. Indeed, metabolites of some of the phenothiazines can be detected for as long as several months after the drug has been discontinued. Such slow elimination

TABLE 10.1

Antipsychotic drugs.

Chemical classification	Drug name Generic (trade)	Dose equivalent (mg)	Sedation	Autonomic side effects*	Involuntary movement
PHENOTHIAZINE	Chlorpromazine (Thorazine)	100	High	High	Moderate
	Prochlorperazine (Compazine)	15	Moderate	Low	High
	Fluphenazine (Prolixin)	2	Low	Low	High
	Trifluoperazine (Stelazine)	5	Moderate	Low	High
	Perphenazine (Trilafon)	8	Low	Low	High
	Acetophenazine (Tindal)	20	Moderate	Low	High
	Carphenazine (Proketazine)	25	Moderate	Low	High
	Triflupromazine (Vesprin)	25	High	Moderate	Moderate
	Mesoridazine (Serentil)	50	High	Moderate	Low
	Thioridazine (Mellaril)	100	High	Moderate	Low
THIOXANTHENE	Thiothixene (Navane)	4	Low	Low	High
	Chlorprothixene (Taractan)	100	High	High	Moderate
BUTYROPHENONE	Haloperidol (Haldol)	2	Low	Low	High
	Droperidol (Inapsine)	NA[†]	Low	Low	High
MISCELLANEOUS	Lozapine (Loxitane)	10	Moderate	Low	Moderate
	Molindone (Moban)	10	Moderate	Moderate	Moderate

*Autonomic side effects include dry mouth, blurred vision, constipation, urinary retention, and reduced blood pressure.   [†]NA, not available.

may also contribute to the slow rate of recurrence of psychotic episodes following the cessation of drug therapy.

Pharmacological Effects

Although it is clear that antipsychotic efficacy and parkinsonism-like side effects result from a blockade of dopamine-2 receptors, the neuroleptics that are currently available also block acetylcholine, serotonin, histamine, and norepinephrine receptors nonspecifically. Indeed, each of the effects of phenothiazines can be explained in terms of the blockade of certain of these various receptors.

Blockade of acetylcholine receptors results in dry mouth, dilated pupils, blurred vision, constipation, urinary retention, and tachycardia (rapid heart rate).

Blockade of norepinephrine receptors results in orthostatic (postural) hypotension and sedation. Haloperidol (a non-phenothiazine neuroleptic) produces a lower incidence of orthostatic hypotension and sedation than do the phenothiazines, because it blocks fewer norepinephrine receptors.

Blockade of histamine receptors results in sedation as well as the production of antivomiting properties.

The consequences of blocking serotonin receptors by neuroleptic drugs are unclear. In a recent review, Meltzer[8] attempted to correlate such blockade with antipsychotic action. Indeed, such an action might account for the efficacy of antipsychotic drugs in partially ameliorating some of the hallucinogenic effects of LSD—a psychedelic drug that acts by stimulating serotonin receptors (Chapter 11). It is thought that the blockade of serotonin receptors is closely linked to the blockade of dopamine receptors, and the interaction between these two mechanisms in schizophrenic patients is unclear.

The remainder of the pharmacological effects of chlorpromazine and other phenothiazines follows from the blockade of dopamine-2 receptors at the various sites where such receptors are located in the CNS. As stated previously, such sites include (1) the limbic and frontal–cortical areas, (2) the extrapyramidal system (basal ganglia), (3) the hypothalamic–pituitary system, and (4) the brain stem.

LIMBIC SYSTEM   Dopamine-secreting neurons that are located in the central midbrain portion of the brain stem send axonal projections to those parts of the limbic system that are involved in the regulation of emotion and emotional expression as well as to the limbic forebrain areas, where thought and emotions are integrated. Indeed, it is thought that an increased sensitivity of dopamine receptors in those areas may underlie schizophrenia and, further, that those receptors are the sites of the antipsychotic action of neuroleptic drugs. In patients who exhibit this mechanism, chlorpromazine and other phenothiazines induce a syndrome that is characterized by psychomotor slowing, indifference to sensory stimuli, emotional quieting, and reduction of initiative. These drugs tend to decrease paranoia, fear, hostility, and agitation; and they reduce the intensity of schizophrenic delusions and hallucinations. The phenothiazines do not produce euphoria, and the psychological syndrome that is induced by these drugs is not usually considered to be particularly pleasant. The agitation, restlessness, and hyperactivity of a person who is experiencing an acute schizophrenic attack are often dramatically relieved by treatment. The delusions and hallucinations that are associated with an acute paranoid attack are particularly sensitive to such treatment. Slightly less susceptible to phenothiazine treatment are the apathy and withdrawal states that are observed in certain psychotic persons.

BRAIN STEM   Through their actions on the brain stem, the phenothiazines suppress the centers that are involved both in behavioral arousal (the ascending reticular activating center) and in vomiting (the chemoreceptor trigger zone). By suppressing activity in the reticular formation, the phenothiazines induce an indifference to external stimuli, reducing the inflow of sensory stimuli that would otherwise reach higher brain centers. Thus, greater levels of sensory input are necessary to alert or arouse a person who is being treated with phenothiazines. In the chemoreceptor trigger zone, the phenothiazines exert a marked protective action against nausea and vomiting, making them some of the best antinauseants available. Again, this reflects a dopamine-2 receptor blocking action.

BASAL GANGLIA   Neuroleptic drugs produce two main kinds of motor disturbances, which comprise perhaps the most bothersome and most serious side effects associated with the use of these agents. The two syndromes are (1) parkinsonism-like symptoms and (2) tardive (late) dyskinesia.

The basal ganglia (caudate nucleus, putamen, and globus pallidus) are rich in dopamine neurons and, when these decrease in number to about 20 percent of normal, parkinsonism-like symptoms become clinically evident. This disorder is usually characteristic of aging. Patients exhibit a rhythmic tremor of the hands, drooling, cogwheel rigidity, loss of spontaneous and associated movements, a blank stare, dulled facial expressions, and a stooped posture. Acute symptoms of this kind occur in a large proportion of patients who are treated with neuroleptic drugs. The symptoms are closely related to the dose that is used; they develop quite rapidly; and they are reversible. As stated previously, clozapine causes less dopamine-2 blocking activity, so it produces fewer movement disorders.

Tardive dyskinesia is a much more puzzling and serious form of movement disorder.[2] Patients who experience this syndrome exhibit involuntary movements, often of the face and tongue, but also of the trunk and limbs, which can be severely disabling. More characteristic are sucking and smacking of the lips, lateral jaw movements, and darting, pushing, or twisting of the tongue. Choreiform movements of the extremities are frequent. The syndrome appears a few months to several years after neuroleptic treatment has been started (hence, the description, *tardive*) and is usually permanent. The incidence has been estimated to include more than 10 percent of patients who are treated with neuroleptic drugs, but this depends greatly on the dosage, the age of the patient (it is most common in patients older than 50) and, partly, the particular drug that is used. Adequate control of these dyskinesias may necessitate restarting the neuroleptic medication or increasing the dosage, which is a problem if parkinsonism-like side effects are troublesome. Baldessarini reviews these effects at length.[15]

HYPOTHALAMUS–PITUITARY   There are known pathways of dopamine-secreting neurons that extend from the hypothalamus to the pituitary gland. The hypothalamus is intimately involved in the emotions, in eating and drinking, and in sexual behavior as well as in controlling the secretion of some pituitary hormones. By suppressing the function of the hypothalamus, phenothiazines interrupt these functions. By suppressing the appetite, food intake may be reduced. By suppressing the temperature-regulating centers of the hypothalamus, body temperature will fall in a cold room and rise in a hot room (poikilothermy). In addition, several body hormones are affected. Dopamine is likely the prolactin-release–inhibiting hormone of the hypothalamus. Thus, when dopamine receptors are blocked, the hormone prolactin is released, which often causes breast enlargement in males and lactation in females. Phenothiazines also reduce the release of sex hormones from the pituitary gland (Chapter 14). Thus, in men, ejaculation may be blocked, and in women, libido may be decreased, ovulation may be blocked, and normal menstrual cycles may be suppressed, resulting in infertility.

Side Effects and Toxicity

The phenothiazines cause a variety of side effects, which, in general, are direct extensions of their pharmacological actions (listed previously). Some of these effects invariably accompany the therapeutic use of these drugs (Table 10. 1).

Phenothiazines produce a variety of disturbances of movement, including tremors, muscle rigidity, walking disorders, and involuntary movements. Other side effects include increased heart rate, dry mouth, blurred vision, orthostatic (postural) hypotension, and constipation. More serious, but much less common, side effects include altered pigmentation of the skin, pigment deposits in the retina, permanently impaired vision, decreased pituitary function, menstrual disorders, and allergic (or hypersensitivity) reactions, which include liver dysfunction and blood disorders. These side effects can cause significant clinical problems, because nonhospitalized patients tend to stop taking their medicine in order to avoid them and inevitably suffer a return of psychotic symptoms. Thus, patient *compliance* is a significant problem. These drugs are relatively nonlethal, even when a massive overdose is taken.

Tolerance and Dependence

One of the positive attributes of the phenothiazines is that they are not behaviorally reinforcing, so, therefore, they are not prone to abuse. They do not produce tolerance, physical dependence, or psychological dependence. Psychotic patients may take phenothiazines for years without necessarily having to increase their dose because of tolerance; if a dose is increased, it is usually done to accomplish better control of psychotic episodes. Discontinuation of a phenothiazine is not followed by symptoms of withdrawal, possibly because it may take many months for the drug and its metabolites to be excreted completely.

Haloperidol

In 1967, haloperidol (see Figure 10.2) was introduced to the United States as the first of a series of compounds that are referred to as *butyrophenone derivatives*. A second compound, droperidol, has subsequently been introduced, and it is used in anesthesia for its antivomiting properties.

Pharmacologically, haloperidol is remarkably similar to the phenothiazines. Haloperidol produces sedation and an indifference to external stimuli; it reduces initiative, anxiety, and activity. It is well absorbed orally and has a moderately slow rate of metabolism and excretion. Indeed, stable blood levels can be seen for up to 3 days following discontinuation of the drug. It takes approximately 5 days for 40 percent of a single dose to be excreted by the kidneys.[16]

The mechanism of the antipsychotic action of haloperidol is like that of the phenothiazines—blockade of dopamine-2 receptors. Haloperidol does not produce most of the serious toxicities that are occasionally observed in patients who are taking phenothiazines (jaundice, blood abnormalities, and so on), but it causes parkinsonism-like motor movements that are even more pronounced. It does not usually produce sedation. In general, however, haloperidol is an interesting, effective drug for the treatment of psychotic patients; and it offers an alternative for those patients who may not respond to the phenothiazines.

Reserpine

As stated earlier, reserpine (Serpasil) was identified during the early 1950s as an effective drug to treat psychotic patients, but its significant side effects made the phenothiazines preferable. Therefore, it is used rarely today. Its side effects include severe mental depression, significant depression of blood pressure, and severe diarrhea. However, reserpine is of interest both historically and mechanistically, because it depletes dopamine by preventing its entrance into the presynaptic vesicles that protect it from the enzyme monoamine oxidase (MAO) (Appendix III). In other words, it blocks the uptake of dopamine from inside the presynaptic nerve terminal into the storage granules, thus exposing it to the enzyme MAO, which metabolizes it rapidly.

Miscellaneous (Atypical) Antipsychotic Drugs

The phenothiazines, reserpine, and haloperidol are the traditional, historical, or typical drugs for the pharmacological management of schizophrenic patients. A variety of other agents either have been tried

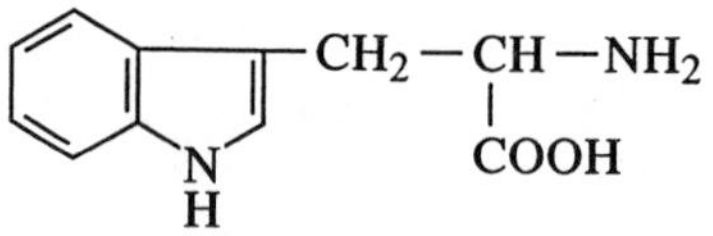

Tryptophan

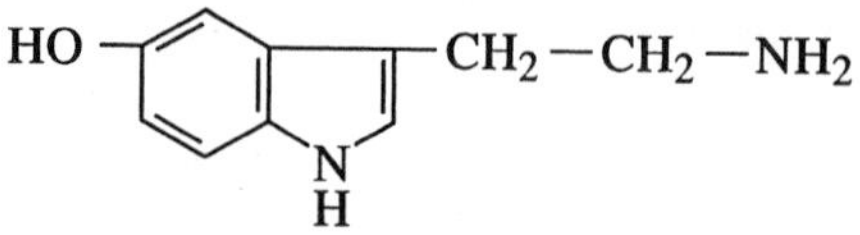

Serotonin

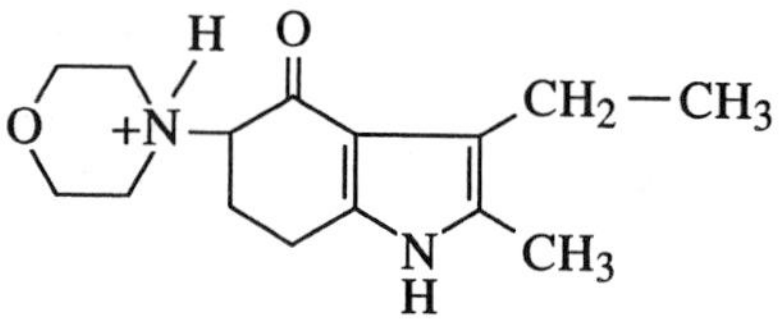

Molindone
(Moban)

FIGURE 10.4

Structures of molindone, serotonin, and tryptophan.

or are currently available. These agents may be classified conveniently as *atypical* antipsychotic drugs.[18] Three of these drugs, which are currently available for clinical use, will be discussed briefly. Many others are available for experimental use, and perhaps in the future some of them will become available clinically.

Molindone (Moban) is structurally unique as an antipsychotic medication. It resembles the neurotransmitter serotonin and its precursor, tryptophan (Figure 10.4). Molindone is effective in the treatment of both schizophrenia and acute, active psychoses. It produces moderate sedation, increased motor activity, and, possibly, euphoria. Abnormal motor movements that occur resemble those that are observed in patients who take phenothiazines. Molindone is rapidly absorbed

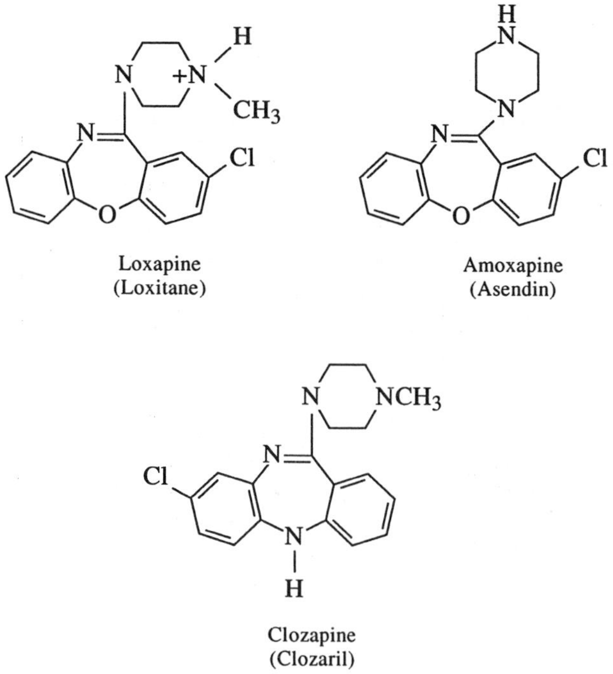

FIGURE 10.5

Structures of loxapine, amoxapine, and clozapine.

when it is taken orally, and it is metabolized before it is excreted. Clinical effects following a single dose of molindone persist for about 24 to 36 hours.

Loxapine (Loxitane) is an antipsychotic drug that has a unique structure (Figure 10.5). It resembles somewhat the tricyclic antidepressants [especially amoxapine (Asendin), Chapter 8]. However, its actions differ little from those of the older antipsychotic drugs. It has antipsychotic, antiemetic, and sedative properties; and it causes abnormal motor movements as side effects. It lowers convulsive thresholds and, therefore, must be used with caution in epileptic patients. Loxapine is well absorbed when it is taken orally, and it is metabolized and excreted within about 24 hours.

Clozapine (Clozaril) is an antipsychotic drug that is closely related structurally to loxapine (Figure 10.5). Reference has already been made to clozapine, emphasizing its unique ability to exert antipsychotic effects without inducing the parkinsonism-like side effects that are associated with the blockade of dopamine-2 receptors. (Clozapine is thus the first specific dopamine-1 blocker.) An extensive review of clozapine may be found in papers from a recent symposium[18] and in recent reviews.[17,19] The primary limitation to its wider use is the appearance of a potentially fatal blood dyscrasia. To receive the drug, one must be entered into a strict monitoring protocol that involves both the manufacturer and an affiliated hospital. The yearly costs of clozapine (including the required weekly blood monitoring) are estimated to be $9000 to $12,000. The receptor specificity of clozapine demonstrates that antipsychotic effects can be separated from motor-movement abnormalities.

Other agents are currently under investigation. Despite some initial reports of modest efficacy, *carbamazepine (Tegretol)* does not appear to be effective in the treatment of schizophrenia.[20] Hollister[21] briefly reviews a variety of experimental drugs that affect a variety of subtypes of dopamine and serotonin receptors.

STUDY QUESTIONS

1. How are the terms *neuroleptic* and *antipsychotic* alike? How do these terms differ?
2. What is a nonneuroleptic antipsychotic drug? How might such an agent be expected to differ from a traditional antipsychotic drug?
3. Describe the overall appearance of a schizophrenic person. Describe the overall appearance of a schizophrenic patient who has been treated with chlorpromazine.
4. Discuss the meaning of the term *tranquilizer*.
5. What is the difference between a major tranquilizer and a sedative-hypnotic antianxiety agent?
6. The major tranquilizers have been called "chemical straightjackets." Do you agree or disagree?
7. Discuss the mechanism of action of neuroleptic antipsychotic drugs.
8. Discuss the major side effects of phenothiazines.

9. Discuss the consequences of reducing the numbers of institutionalized schizophrenic patients.

10. Compare and contrast *clozapine* and *chlorpromazine*.

NOTES

1. American Medical Association, *Drug Evaluations, Annual 1991* (Milwaukee, Wis.: American Medical Association, 1990), pp. 233–255.

2. H. P. Rang and M. M. Dale, "Neuroleptic Drugs," in H. P. Rang and M. M. Dale, eds., *Pharmacology* (Edinburgh: Churchill Livingstone, 1987), pp. 499–512.

3. K. S. Kendler, "The Genetics of Schizophrenia: A Current Perspective," in H. Y. Meltzer, ed., *Psychopharmacology: The Third Generation of Progress* (New York: Raven Press, 1987), pp. 705–713.

4. P. Seeman, "Dopamine Receptors and the Dopamine Hypothesis of Schizophrenia," *Synapse* 1 (1987): 133–152.

5. S. Cohen, *The Chemical Brain: The Neurochemistry of Addictive Disorders* (Irvine, Calif.: Care Institute, 1988), pp. 22–23.

6. E. K. G. Syvalahti, "Dopamine Receptors and Psychiatric Drug Treatment," *Annals of Clinical Research* 20 (1988): 340–347.

7. D. M. Coward, A. Imperato, S. Urwyler, and T. G. White, "Biochemical and Behavioral Properties of Clozapine," *Psychopharmacology* 99, Supplement (1989): s6–s12.

8. H. Y. Meltzer, "Clinical Studies on the Mechanisms of Action of Clozapine: the Dopamine–Serotonin Hypothesis of Schizophrenia," *Psychopharmacology* 99, Supplement (1989): s18–s27.

9. L. Ereshefsky, M. D. Watanabe, and T. K. Tran-Johnson, "Clozapine: An Atypical Antipsychotic Agent," *Clinical Pharmacy* 8 (1989): 691–709.

10. H. Y. Meltzer, B. Bastani, K. Y. Kwon, L. F. Ramirez, S. Burnett, and J. Sharpe, "A Prospective Study of Clozapine in Treatment-Resistant Schizophrenic Patients. I. Preliminary Report," *Psychopharmacology* 99, Supplement (1989): s68–s72.

11. H. Helmchen, "Clinical Experience with Clozapine in Germany, *Psychopharmacology* 99, Supplement (1989): s80–s83.

12. L. Farde, F. A. Wiesel, A.-L. Nordstrom, and G. Sedvall, "D1- and D2-Dopamine Receptor Occupancy During Treatment with Conven-

tional and Atypical Neuroleptics," *Psychopharmacology* 99, Supplement (1989): s28–s31.

13. M. E. Lickey and B. Gordon, *Drugs for Mental Illness* (New York: W. H. Freeman and Co., 1983), p. 119.

14. S. H. Snyder, "Dopamine Receptors, Neuroleptics, and Schizophrenia," *American Journal of Psychiatry* 138 (1981): 460–463.

15. R. J. Baldessarini, "Drugs and the Treatment of Psychiatric Disorders," in A. G. Gilman, T. W. Rall, A. S. Nies, and P. Taylor, eds., *Goodman and Gilman's The Pharmacological Basis of Therapeutics,* 8th ed. (New York: Pergamon, 1990), pp. 395–400.

16. B. K. Colasanti, "Antipsychotic Drugs," in C. R. Craig and R. E. Stitzel, eds., *Modern Pharmacology,* 3d ed. (Boston: Little, Brown, 1990), pp. 461–472.

17. C. A. Tamminga and J. Gerlach, "New Neuroleptics and Experimental Antipsychotics in Schizophrenia," in H. Y. Meltzer, ed., *Psychopharmacology: The Third Generation of Progress* (New York: Raven Press, 1987), pp. 1129–1140.

18. Scientific Update Meeting, "Clozapine (Leponex/Clozaril)," *Psychopharmacology* 99, Supplement (1990).

19. P. Stephens, "A Review of Clozapine: An Antipsychotic for Treatment-Resistant Schizophrenia," *Comprehensive Psychiatry* 31 (1990): 315–326.

20. W. T. Carpenter, R. Kurz, B. Kirkpatrick, T. E. Hanlon, A. T. Summerfelt, R. W. Buchanan, R. W. Waltrip, and A. Breier, "Carbamazepine Maintenance Treatment in Outpatient Schizophrenics," *Archives of General Psychiatry* 48 (1991): 69–72.

21. L. E. Hollister, "On the Horizon: New Psychotherapeutic Drugs," *Pharmacy and Therapeutics* 16(1991): 195–209.

Psychedelic Drugs

Mescaline, LSD, and Other "Mind-Expanding" Agents

Psychedelic drugs comprise a group of heterogeneous compounds that induce visual, auditory, or other hallucinations and cause the persons who use them to separate from reality. These agents may induce disturbances in cognition and perception and, in some instances, may produce behavior that is similar to some aspects of that observed in psychotic patients. Because of this wide range of psychological effects, a single term cannot be used to classify these agents adequately.

The term *hallucinogen* has been widely used for psychedelic drugs, because most of these agents can induce hallucinations if the dose that is taken is high enough. However, that term appears to be somewhat inappropriate, because it does not adequately describe the range of pharmacological actions that are caused by this diverse group of substances. The term *psychotomimetic* has been assigned to these compounds because of their alleged ability to mimic psychoses or induce psychotic states. However, careful analysis of the action of these drugs indicates that their effects do not produce the same behavioral patterns that are observed in persons who experience psychotic episodes.

Because neither of those terms comprehensively, yet briefly, characterizes the pharmacology of these drugs, we must rely on a descriptive term, such as *phantasticum* (proposed by Lewin in 1924) or *psychedelic* (proposed by Osmond in 1957), to imply that these agents all have the ability to alter sensory perception and, therefore, may be considered to be "mind expanding."

The psychedelic agents have a long and colorful history. Indeed, many are derived from plants, so they are natural in origin. Today, however, many psychedelic agents are synthetically produced in laboratories, many of which are clandestine and, therefore, unregulated.

Psychedelic drugs have been used for thousands of years. Because of the effects of these naturally occurring drugs on sensory perception, they have frequently been ascribed magical, religious, or mystical properties, and they have been used as sacraments in religious rites. For many years, the compounds were primarily restricted to local religious rituals, and most persons were barely aware of their existence. During the late 1960s and 1970s, however, the psychedelic agents were "discovered," and strongly advocated by certain members of modern society. These agents were used to enhance perception, expand reality, promote personal awareness, and stimulate or induce comprehension of the spiritual or supernatural. As stated by Jaffe:

> There is heightened awareness of sensory input, often accompanied by an enhanced sense of clarity, but a diminished control over what is experienced. Frequently there is a feeling that one part of the self seems to be a passive observer (a "spectator ego") rather than an active organizing and directing force, while another part of the self participates and receives the vivid and unusual sensory experiences. The attention of the user is turned inward, preempted by the seeming clarity and portentous quality of his own thinking processes. In this state the slightest sensation may take on profound meaning. Commonly, there is a diminished capacity to differentiate the boundaries of one object from another and of the self from the environment. Associated with the loss of boundaries there may be a sense of union with "mankind" or the "cosmos."[1]

Classification

Because the psychedelic drugs differ widely in chemical structure, it would be difficult to classify them on that basis. However, their structures do resemble those of certain neurotransmitters. Thus, it is possible

TABLE 11.1

Classification of psychedelic drugs.

Anticholinergic psychedelic drugs
  Atropine
  Scopolamine

Catecholamine-like psychedelic drugs
  Mescaline
  DOM (STP), MDA, MMDA, TMA, DMA, MDMA
  Myristin, elemicin

Serotonin-like psychedelic drugs
  Lysergic acid diethylamide (LSD)
  Dimethyltryptamine (DMT)
  Psilocybin, psilocin, bufotenin
  Ololiuqui (morning glory seeds)
  Harmine

Psychedelic anesthetic drugs
  Phencyclidine (Sernyl)
  Ketamine (Ketalar)

to classify them according to the transmitters that they most closely resemble or according to the transmitter receptors that are thought to be their sites of action (Table 11.1). As discussed in previous chapters, several synaptic transmitters are prominently involved in the actions of psychoactive drugs. These transmitters include acetylcholine, two catecholamines (norepinephrine and dopamine), and serotonin. Interestingly, each of the psychedelic drugs is structurally related to one of these four transmitters.

Anticholinergic psychedelic drugs comprise a small group of compounds that produce intoxication, delirium, and amnesia by blocking postsynaptic acetylcholine receptors (Figure 11.1).

As discussed in Chapter 6, the behavioral stimulation that is induced by amphetamines and cocaine results from increased dopamine and norepinephrine neurotransmission. In high doses, these drugs can induce a paranoid psychosis, which may be accompanied by delusions, hallucinations, and disturbances in sensory perception. Thus, amphetamines and cocaine might well have been classified as psychedelic agents in addition to being classified as behavioral stimulants. Amphetamines and cocaine might be classified (with similar compounds) as *catecholamine-like psychedelic drugs* (Figure 11.2). Similar compounds include mescaline, DOM (also called STP), TMA, MDA, MMDA, DMA, and certain drugs that are obtained from nutmeg (myristin and

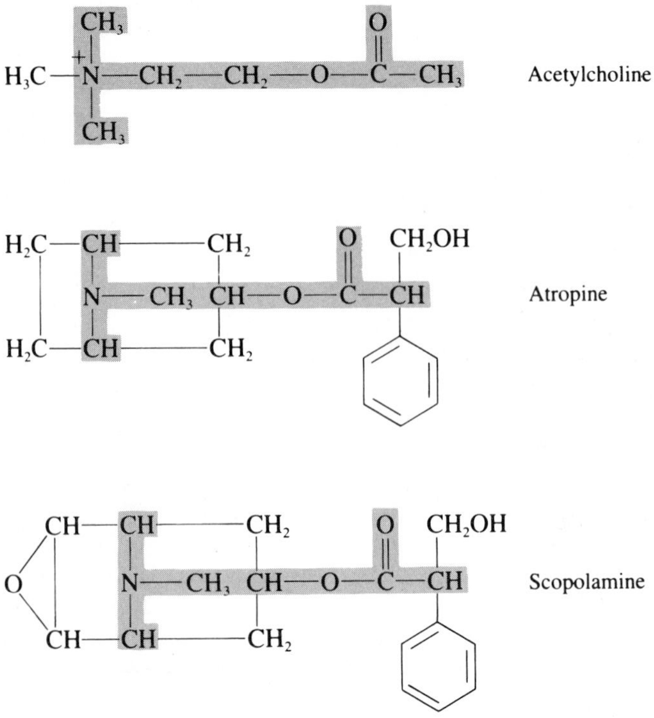

FIGURE 11.1

Structural formulas of acetylcholine (a chemical transmitter) and the anticholinergic psychedelic drugs atropine and scopolamine. Atropine and scopolamine act by blocking acetylcholine receptors. The shaded portion of each molecule illustrates structural similarities, which presumably contribute to receptor "fit."

elemicin). However, all these compounds differ from one another as well as from amphetamines and cocaine in terms of their greater intensity of psychedelic action and their lesser intensity of behavioral stimulation. Because amphetamines and cocaine produce more behavioral stimulation than psychedelic action, they are classified as stimulant drugs rather than as psychedelic drugs.

Serotonin inhibits activity and behavior; it increases sleep time; and it reduces feeding, aggression, play, and sexual activity.[2] The synthesis of lysergic acid diethylamide (LSD) and the discovery of its hallucinogenic properties, as well as its structural resemblance to

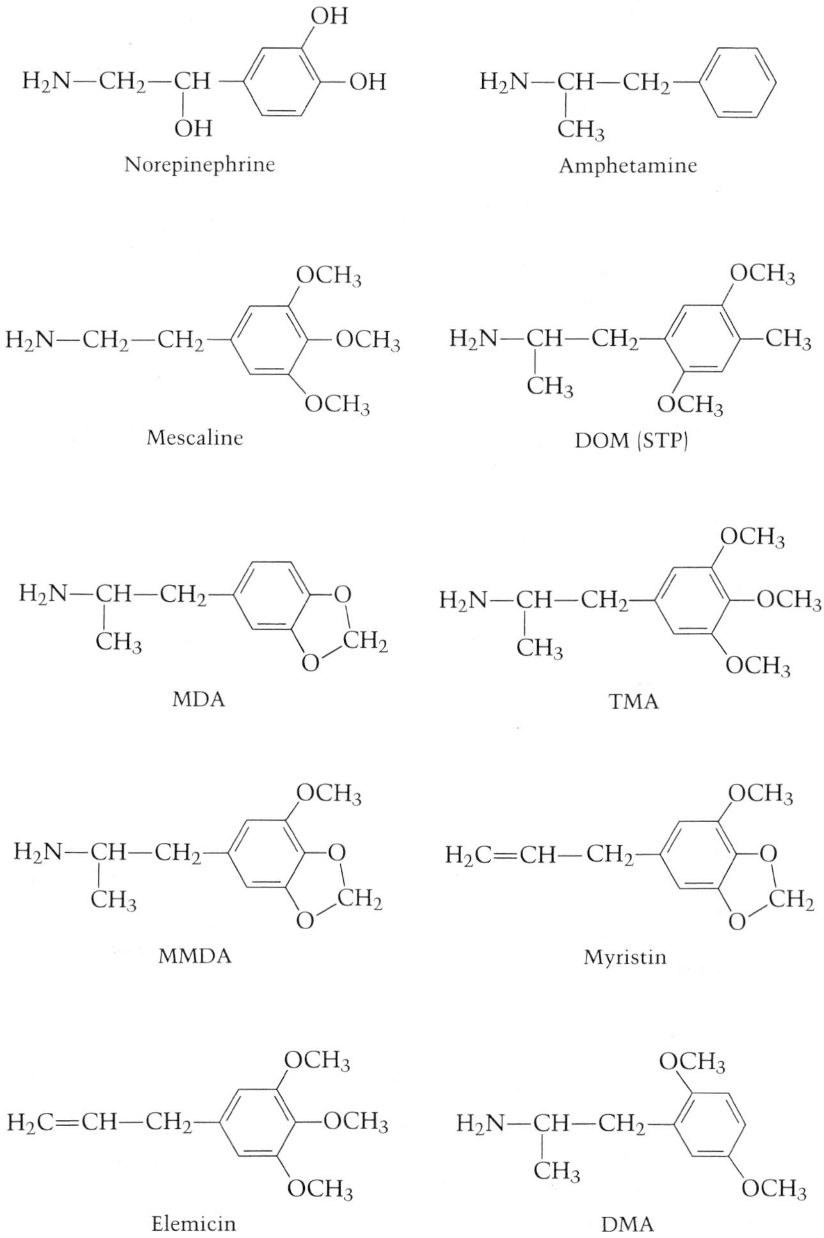

FIGURE 11.2

Structural formulas of norepinephrine (a chemical transmitter), amphetamine, and eight catecholamine-like psychedelic drugs. These eight drugs are structurally related to norepinephrine and are thought to exert their psychedelic actions through alterations of transmission at norepinephrine synapses in the brain.

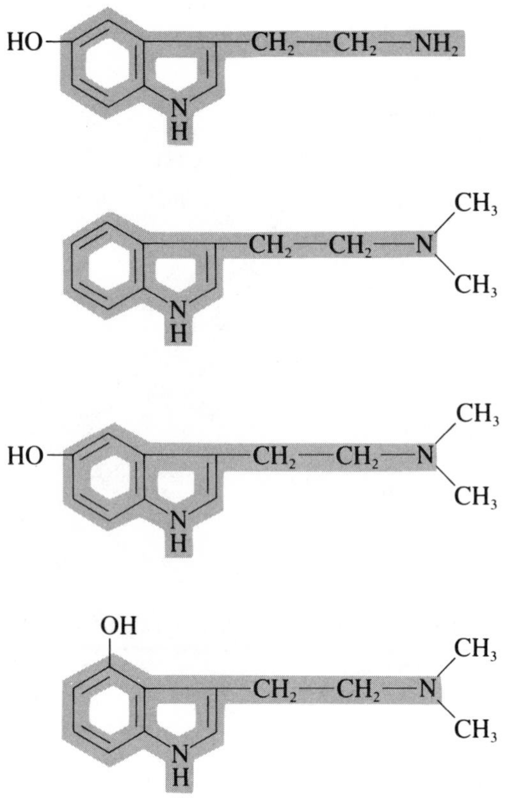

Serotonin
(5-hydroxytryptamine)

DMT
(dimethyltryptamine)

Bufotenin
(5-hydroxy-DMT)

Psilocin
4-hydroxy-DMT)

FIGURE 11.3

Structural formulas of serotonin (a chemical transmitter) and six serotonin-like psychedelic drugs. These six drugs are structurally related to serotonin (as indicated by the shading) and are thought to exert their psychedelic actions through alterations of serotonin synapses in the brain. Although LSD is structurally much more complex than serotonin, the basic similarity of the two molecules is apparent.

serotonin, brought recognition of a class of psychedelic drugs—the *serotonin-like psychedelic drugs* (Figure 11.3). This group of drugs includes psilocybin and psilocin (both from the magic mushroom, *Psilocybe mexicana*), dimethyltryptamine (DMT), and bufotenin.

Finally, phencyclidine and ketamine are referred to as *psychedelic anesthetic drugs* (Figure 11.4). These agents are unrelated structurally to the other psychedelic compounds. To date, the receptors on which these drugs exert their activity have not been identified. Both the

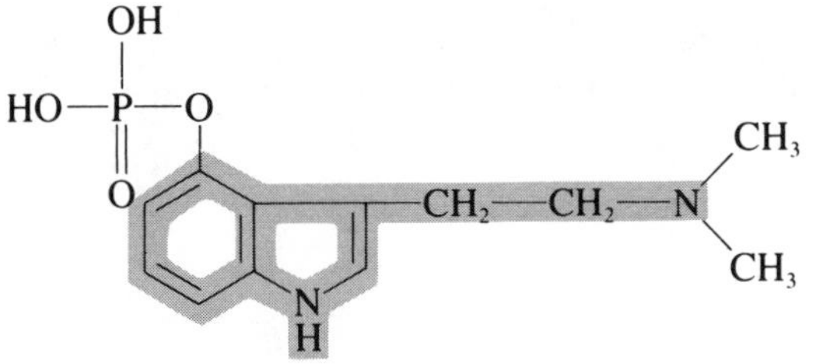

Psilocybin
(4–phosphoryl-DMT)

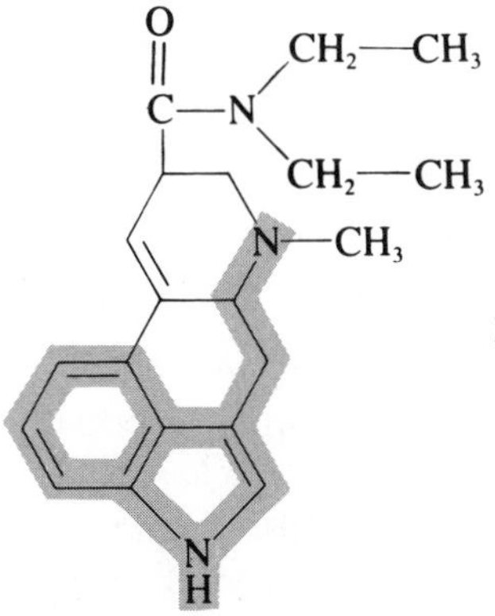

LSD

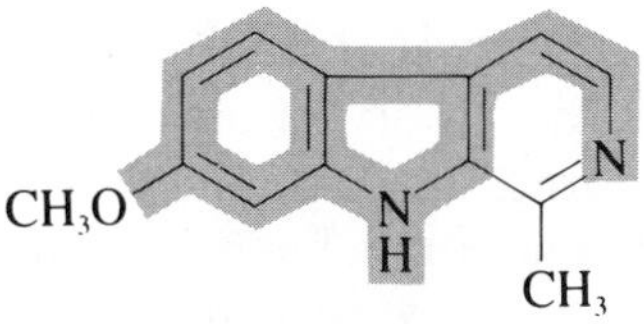

Harmine

FIGURE 11.3 (continued)

opioid sigma receptor (Chapter 9) and a specific amino acid receptor have been postulated as the sites of action of these drugs (discussed in the following text).

Anticholinergic Psychedelic Drugs

Intoxicating drugs classified as anticholinergic psychedelic drugs all appear to exert their effects secondary to blocking postsynaptic acetylcholine receptors. Atropine and scopolamine are examples of such drugs. They attach to and occupy acetylcholine receptor sites, but they do not activate them. Thus, they block the access of the

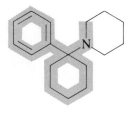
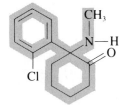

Phencyclidine (Sernyl)   Ketamine (Ketalar)

FIGURE 11.4

Structural formulas of the psychedelic anesthetic drugs phencyclidine and ketamine.

neurotransmitter acetylcholine to its receptors, and thereby prevent synaptic transmission.

Historical Background

The history of atropine and scopolamine is long and colorful. Both drugs are distributed widely in nature; they are found in especially high concentrations in the plant that is known as *belladonna,* or *deadly nightshade (Atropa belladonna).* These drugs are also found in *Datura stramonium* (Jamestown weed, jimsonweed, stinkweed, thorn apple, or devil's apple) and in *Mandragora officinarum* (mandrake). Both professional and amateur poisoners of the Middle Ages frequently used deadly nightshade as a prime source of poison. In fact, the plant's name, *Atropa belladonna,* is derived from *Atropos* (the Greek goddess who supposedly cuts the thread of life). *Belladonna* means "beautiful woman," which refers to its pupil-dilating properties when it is applied topically to the eyes (eyes with widely dilated pupils were presumably a mark of beauty).

Plants that contain atropine and scopolamine have been used and misused for centuries. For example, the delirium that is caused by these substances may have persuaded certain persons that they had the ability to fly—that they were witches. More recently, cigarettes that are made from the leaves of *Datura stramonium* and *Atropa belladonna* are smoked occasionally to induce intoxication. Such cigarettes were sold in pharmacies until recently as a form of treatment for asthma. Throughout the world, leaves of plants that contain atropine or scopolamine are still used to prepare intoxicating beverages; and marijuana and opium preparations from the Far East have, in the past, been fortified with plant material from *Datura stramonium.*

Pharmacological Effects

Atropine and scopolamine act on the peripheral nervous system to depress salivation (causing dry mouth), reduce sweating, increase body temperature, dilate the pupils, blur vision, and markedly increase heart rate. Because these drugs inhibit the secretion of acid into the stomach, they have been used in the medical treatment of ulcers. However, their effectiveness is limited, and better drugs have been developed for this purpose.

In the CNS, low doses of scopolamine produce drowsiness, mild euphoria, profound amnesia, fatigue, delirium, mental confusion, dreamless sleep, and loss of attention. Atropine, however, must be given in much larger doses to produce these effects, because it does not cross the blood-brain barrier easily. Rather than expanding consciousness, awareness, and insight, these drugs cloud consciousness and produce amnesia; they do not expand sensory perception.

When large doses of atropine are taken, a behavioral state that resembles a toxic psychosis occurs. Delirium, mental confusion, sedation, and amnesia dominate CNS effects; and superimposed on these effects are peripheral actions—tachycardia, blurred vision, and dry mouth. All these effects can convey a sense of excitement and loss of control to the user. However, the clouding of consciousness and the absence of any memory of the episode render these compounds unattractive as psychedelic drugs. Indeed, it would be more appropriate to refer to them as somewhat dangerous intoxicant drugs rather than as psychedelic drugs.

Catecholamine-like Psychedelic Drugs

In earlier chapters, norepinephrine and dopamine synapses were identified as the sites action for cocaine, amphetamines, the antidepressants, and lithium. These synapses are also important sites of action for a large group of psychedelic drugs that are structurally similar to both catecholamine neurotransmitters and amphetamines (Figure 11.2). Such psychedelic agents include mescaline, DOM (also called STP), TMA, MDA, MMDA, DMA, myristin, and elemicin. All of these agents exhibit actions that differentiate them from amphetamines (classified in Chapter 6 as behavioral stimulants, despite the fact that they can cause hallucinations and a state that resembles a major psychosis).

If we examine the structures of these psychedelic drugs in relation to amphetamines and catecholamine neurotransmitters,[3] we might presume that their pharmacological effects would occur as a result of actions at catecholamine synapses. Although this presumption is probably correct,[4] the end result behaviorally and pharmacologically is an alteration of serotonin neurotransmission, which results in LSD-like effects.[5] Further, we now understand that the mechanisms by which serotonin· and catecholamine neurons function are tightly intertwined and that an alteration of the activity of one system affects the other as well (Appendix III). The mechanisms producing the psychedelic syndrome and the contribution of altered neuronal functioning to this effect have not yet been explained. Possible mechanisms of psychedelic drug action will be further discussed when we examine the mechanism of action of LSD.

Mescaline (Peyote)

Peyote *(Lophophora williamsii)* is a plant that is common to the southwestern United States and Mexico. It is a spineless cactus that has a small crown, or "button," and a long root. When it is used for psychedelic purposes, the crown is cut from the cactus and dried, which causes a hard brown disc to form. This disc, which is frequently referred to as a *mescal button,* may later be softened in the a person's mouth and swallowed.

HISTORICAL BACKGROUND   The use of peyote extends back to pre-Columbian times, when it was used in the religious rites of the Aztecs and other Mexican Indians. Currently, peyote is available legally for use as a sacrament. Peyote is an important part of the religious practice of the Native American Church of North America—an organization that claims some 250,000 members from Indian tribes throughout North America. Members of the Native American Church regard peyote as a sacrament, in the same way that members of Christian churches regard bread and wine as sacraments. The use of peyote for religious purposes is not considered to be "abuse." Indeed, peyote is seldom abused by members of the Native American Church. Today, the federal government and 23 states permit sacramental use of peyote. Recently, however, the U.S. Supreme Court, which had earlier ruled that no federal control will interfere with freedom of religion, ruled that states may ban even religious uses of peyote without violating the constitutional right of free religious exercise. Thus, the controversy continues!

PHARMACOLOGICAL EFFECTS   The initial research on the active ingredients of the peyote cactus was carried out near the end of the nineteenth century by German pharmacologists. In 1896, mescaline (Figure

11.2) was identified as the active ingredient in peyote. The chemical structure of mescaline was elucidated in 1918, and the compound was then produced synthetically. More recently, because of its structural resemblance to norepinephrine, a wide variety of synthetic mescaline derivatives has been synthesized, and all have methoxy (—OCH₃) groups or similar additions on their benzene rings (Figure 11.2). Why methoxylation of the benzene ring adds psychedelic properties to the drug is not clear, but it is thought that at higher doses (for example, at doses higher than those that exert amphetamine-like behavioral stimulation), these molecules "fit" the presynaptic serotonin receptors better and, thus, exert LSD-like psychedelic effects.

When it is taken orally, mescaline is rapidly and completely absorbed, and significant concentrations are usually achieved in the brain within 30 to 90 minutes. The effects of a single dose of mescaline persist for approximately 10 hours. The drug does not appear to be metabolized before it is excreted.

Presumably because of its resemblance to norepinephrine, low doses of mescaline (2 to 3 mg/kg) produce effects that are similar to those observed in patients during the fight/flight/fright syndrome. These effects include dilation of the pupils, increased blood pressure and heart rate, an increase in body temperature, EEG and behavioral stimulation, and other excitatory symptoms. These symptoms are all similar to the effects that are produced by amphetamines. However, such actions are not the primary effects that are sought by persons who use mescaline. As one writer stated:

> Interest in mescaline centers on the fact that it causes unusual psychic effects and visual hallucinations. The usual oral dose (5 mg/kg) in the average normal subject causes anxiety, sympathomimetic effects, hyperreflexia of the limbs, static tremors, and vivid hallucinations that are usually visual and consist of brightly colored lights, geometric designs, animals and occasionally people; color and space perception is often concomitantly impaired, but otherwise the sensorium is normal and insight is retained.[6]

Synthetic Amphetamine Derivatives

DOM, MDA, TMA, MMDA, and DMA are structurally related to mescaline and, as might be expected, they produce effects that are similar to those produced by mescaline. They have moderate amphetamine-like effects at low doses, but LSD-like effects tend to dominate. They are considerably more potent and more toxic than mescaline.

DOM (STP, Serenity-Tranquility-Peace) has effects that are similar to those of mescaline; doses of 1 to 6 mg produce euphoria, which is followed by a 6- to 8-hour period of hallucinations. DOM is 100 times more potent than mescaline, but it is much less potent than LSD. The use of DOM is associated with a high incidence of overdose (because it is potent and street doses are poorly controlled). Acute toxic reactions are common; they consist of tremors that may eventually lead to convulsive movements and prostration, which may be followed by death. Because of the frequency of these effects, the use of DOM is not widespread.

MDA, MMDA, and *TMA* are encountered occasionally as "designer drugs." Producers of these drugs attempt to circumvent legal regulations by producing compounds that have modest structural differences from the FDA-regulated compounds. In general, the effects of these drugs resemble those of mescaline and LSD; they reflect the mix of catecholamine and serotonin interactions.

MDMA ("Ecstasy") resembles MDA in structure, but MDMA may be less hallucinogenic. Psychiatrists proposed clinical use of MDMA as a possible drug to promote empathy and compassion in patients. However, MDMA has been shown to produce irreversible destruction of serotonin neurons in both monkeys and rats. Thus, the compound is potentially too dangerous for human use.

Compounds that are sold on the street as mescaline are often not mescaline at all but, rather, LSD, one of the synthetic mescaline derivatives, or phencyclidine. Users must be careful *(caveat emptor)*, because higher doses of any of these substitute drugs can be dangerous and some may even be neurotoxic.

Myristin and Elemicin

Myristin and *elemicin* are active ingredients in nutmeg and mace, and they are responsible for the psychedelic action of these spices. Nutmeg and mace are obtained, respectively, from the dried seed and the seed coat of the nutmeg tree (*Myristica fragans*). Nutmeg and mace are occasionally used as drugs, and abuse of these substances occurs when no other compounds are available. Ingestion of large amounts (between 1 and 2 teaspoons, usually brewed in tea) may, after a delay of 2 to 5 hours, induce euphoria and changes in sensory perception, including visual hallucinations, euphoria, acute psychotic reactions, and feelings of depersonalization and unreality.

Considering the close structural resemblance of myristin and elemicin to mescaline (Figure 11.2), these psychedelic actions are not unexpected. However, both drugs produce many unpleasant side effects, including vomiting, nausea, and tremors. After nutmeg or mace has been taken to produce its psychedelic action, the side effects usually dissuade users from trying these agents a second time.

Serotonin-like Psychedelic Drugs

As discussed previously, serotonin is a neurotransmitter that is actively involved in the regulation of body temperature, sleep, and sensory perception. Numerous serotonin-secreting neurons originate in the brain stem and project to all major areas of the brain (Appendix III). Some theories arose during the late 1950s asserting that some types of mental illness could be caused by abnormalities of the transmission between serotonin neurons. Those theories were supported by the observation that several hallucinogenic compounds resemble serotonin structurally. Figure 11.3 shows that dimethyltryptamine (DMT), bufotenin, psilocin, psilocybin, and LSD resemble the structure of serotonin in much the same way that amphetamine, mescaline, myristin, and the synthetic mescaline derivatives resemble the structures of catecholamine neurotransmitters.

Because the structure of LSD is similar to that of serotonin, and LSD is a potent *antagonist* of the peripheral actions of serotonin, an *early* hypothesis asserted that the psychedelic effects of LSD might be related to the antagonism of serotonin in the CNS. Support for this postulate increased when it was found that LSD decreases the discharge rate of serotonin neurons.[7] However, psychedelic effects persist after these serotonin neurons are destroyed, which suggests that the effect must be exerted directly on the postsynaptic receptors for serotonin. Recently, it has been shown that LSD binds to a specific subtype of serotonin receptor (the serotonin-2 receptor), where LSD acts as an agonist (stimulant).[3] Indeed, a correlation exists between the binding of LSD to this receptor and its potency as a psychedelic agent. In turn, this agonist action at serotonin-2 receptors triggers a series of responses that involve other neurotransmitter systems (especially catecholamine neurons; hence, the overlap between the two classes of psychedelic drugs), which eventually results in a *psychedelic syndrome* that is characteristic of all these drugs.[3] As stated by Cohen, when we attempt to correlate neurophysiological data with behavioral actions:

One speculation about the manner by which hallucinogens manifest their impressive alterations of mood, perception, and thought is that the pontine raphe, a major center of 5-HT [serotonin] activity, serves as a filtering station for incoming sensory stimuli. It screens the flood of sensations and perceptions, eliminating those that are unimportant, irrelevant, or commonplace. A drug like LSD may disrupt the sorting process, allowing a surge of sensory data and an overload of brain circuits. Dehabituation, in which the familiar becomes novel, is noted under LSD. It may also be caused by lowering the sensory gates by inhibition of the raphe activity.[5]

Such brain-stem filtering of sensory input was first postulated in the mid-1950s,[8] which is certainly a reflection on the intuitive and deductive abilities of neuropharmacologists of that time.

Because LSD-like psychedelics appear to act by stimulating serotonin-2 receptors, drugs that block serotonin receptors might be useful in ameliorating or antagonizing the effects of psychedelic drugs. Indeed, the neuroleptic drugs (Chapter 10) exert their antipsychotic action by blocking receptors for dopamine and serotonin, and these drugs have been used successfully to treat patients who are experiencing an LSD-induced psychosis. However, the neuroleptics may cause additional problems, so they are not clinically useful in this regard. However, they are still used in the treatment of otherwise uncontrollable persons who are suffering from psychedelic drug intoxication. In milder cases of intoxication, patient reassurance and protection are used until the effects of the drug subside.

Lysergic Acid Diethylamide (LSD)
During the 1960s and early 1970s, lysergic acid diethylamide (LSD) became one of the most remarkable and controversial drugs known. LSD, in doses that are so small that they might even be considered infinitesimal, is capable of inducing remarkable psychological changes in a person, while causing relatively few alterations in the general physiology of the body.

HISTORICAL BACKGROUND   LSD was first synthesized in 1938 by Albert Hoffman, a Swiss chemist, as part of an organized research program that was established to investigate possible therapeutic uses of compounds that are obtained from ergot. Ergot is a natural product that is derived from a fungus *(Claviceps purpurea)*, which grows as a parasite on rye in grainfields of Europe and North America. The active products that are extracted from ergot are derivatives of lysergic acid. The pharmacological actions of these lysergic acid derivatives do not usually include hallucinations, but they do include constriction of blood vessels and increased contractions of the uterus. Therapeutically, ergot alkaloids are used in the treatment of migraine headaches and to control postpartum hemorrhages. Further discussion of ergot derivatives, which are used as stimulants for dopamine receptors to manage patients who have symptoms of Parkinson's disease, is presented in Chapter 13.

Early pharmacological studies of LSD in animals failed to reveal anything unusual, and the compound was almost forgotten. The psychedelic action was neither sought nor expected, because most derivatives of ergot are not psychoactive. Thus, LSD remained on the laboratory shelf unnoticed from 1938 until 1943, when Dr. Hoffmann had an unusual experience. He later described that experience:

> In the afternoon of 16 April, 1943, . . . I was seized by a peculiar sensation of vertigo and restlessness. Objects, as well as the shape of my associates in the laboratory, appeared to undergo optical changes. I was unable to concentrate on my work. In a dreamlike state I left for home, where an irresistible urge to lie down overcame me. I drew the curtains and immediately fell into a peculiar state similar to drunkenness, characterized by an exaggerated imagination. With my eyes closed, fantastic pictures of extraordinary plasticity and intensive color seemed to surge toward me. After two hours this state gradually wore off.[9]

Hoffmann correctly suspected that his experience must have resulted from an accidental ingestion of LSD. He decided to ingest some of the compound under controlled conditions and to describe the experience more completely. Using the dose of other drugs as a guide, he administered what seemed to be a minuscule dose (only 0.25 milligram, orally). However, we now know that this dose is many times that required to induce psychedelic effects in most persons. As a result of this miscalculation, his response was quite spectacular:

> After 40 minutes, I noted the following symptoms in my laboratory journal: slight giddiness, restlessness, difficulty in concentration, visual disturbances, laughing. . . . Later, I lost all count of time. I noticed with dismay that my environment was undergoing progressive changes. My visual field wavered and everything appeared deformed as in a faulty mirror. Space and

time became more and more disorganized and I was overcome by a fear that I was going out of my mind. The worst part of it being that I was clearly aware of my condition. My power of observation was unimpaired. . . . Occasionally, I felt as if I were out of my body. I thought I had died. My ego seemed suspended somewhere in space, from where I saw my dead body lying on the sofa. . . . it was particularly striking how acoustic perceptions, such as the noise of water gushing from a tap or the spoken word, were transformed into optical illusions. I then fell asleep and awakened the next morning somewhat tired but otherwise feeling perfectly well.[10]

These descriptions of the original LSD trip that Hoffman experienced are probably the most lucid and exciting observations that have ever been presented, possibly because the chemist had no preconceived notions about what to expect.

For several years, LSD remained something of a laboratory and clinical curiosity. In 1949, the first North American study of LSD in humans was conducted, and, during the 1950s, large quantities of LSD were distributed to pharmacologists and physicians throughout the world for research purposes. A significant impetus to that research was the notion that the effects of LSD might constitute a model for psychosis, which would provide some insight into the biochemical or physiological processes of mental illness and its treatment.

Subsequently, it was demonstrated that LSD mimicked the transmitter action of serotonin—an observation that led to the hypothesis that serotonin might somehow be involved in mental illness. Thus, throughout the 1950s, LSD was regarded as a tool that might be useful in acquiring an understanding of psychoses. LSD has been used as an adjunct to psychotherapy by some therapists to help patients verbalize their problems and gain some insight into the underlying causes of their problems. However, the effectiveness of that approach to treatment is still much debated.

This early work with LSD on human volunteers was conducted at large medical centers, so the experiments introduced the LSD experience to college campuses and, from there, to a wider audience.

The drug reached its peak in popularity during the late 1960s, after which its use decreased markedly. It is not used much today. Considering the long history of other psychedelic drugs, it is unlikely that the recreational use of LSD will ever disappear completely. It is quite clear, however, that the use of LSD in medicine and in psychotherapy is limited. In the laboratory, these agents will continue to be used to help neuroscientists unravel some of the mysteries of the brain, especially those that are associated with the role of serotonin in synaptic transmission.

PHARMACOKINETICS   LSD is usually taken orally, and it is rapidly absorbed. Because the doses of LSD are so small that several doses could be placed on the head of a pin, the drug is often added to other substances, such as pieces of paper or sugar cubes, which can be handled more easily. LSD is distributed rapidly and efficiently throughout the body; it diffuses easily into the brain; and it readily crosses the placenta. It appears that the largest amounts of LSD in the body may be found in the liver, where the compound is metabolized before it is excreted. Relatively small amounts of the drug are found in the brain, although the compound is so potent that only a few micrograms (for example, 25 micrograms, or one-millionth of an ounce) are needed to induce psychedelic effects.

When it is taken orally, LSD has a rapid onset of action (between 30 and 60 minutes), and its effects persist for approximately 10 or 12 hours. The half-life of LSD is about 3 hours.

Because of its extreme potency, the small number of available metabolites, and the fact that most LSD is excreted in bile into the intestinal tract, only minuscule amounts can be detected in urine. Thus, conventional urine screening tests are inadequate to detect LSD. When the use of LSD is suspected, urine is collected (up to 30 hours after ingestion), and an ultrasensitive radioimmunoassay is performed to verify its presence.

PHYSIOLOGICAL EFFECTS   Although the LSD experience is characterized primarily by psychological alterations (see the following discussion), subtle physiological changes also occur. Persons who take LSD may experience a slight increase in body temperature, dilation of the pupils, a slightly increased heart rate and blood pressure, increased levels of glucose (sugar) in the blood, and dizziness, drowsiness, nausea, and other effects that, although noticeable, seldom interfere with the psychedelic experience. LSD is known to possess a low level of toxicity. Deaths that occur as a direct result of an LSD overdose have not been reported, although fatal accidents and suicides are known to occur when persons are intoxicated by LSD. The use of LSD during pregnancy is certainly unwise, because of possible adverse effects on the fetus.[11]

PSYCHOLOGICAL EFFECTS   Although the physiological alterations that are produced by LSD are usually quite mild, the psychological effects are intense. The exact response that a person may have to using LSD is unpredictable. It is influenced by a variety of factors, including the personality of the user, his or her expectation of the effects that the drug will produce, previous experience with LSD and other psychoactive drugs, attitudes toward the use of LSD or any other illicit drug, motivations for using the drug, the setting in which the drug is administered, and the persons with whom the user interacts during the LSD experience.

Because of these variables, it is difficult to predict the exact psychological experience that a person might have on any given occasion. Thus, it is quite difficult to describe the experience that occurs as a result of using LSD by listing the variety of responses. Nevertheless, these responses include alterations in mood and emotion, in which laughter or sorrow may be evoked easily and even simultaneously. Both euphoria and dysphoria can be experienced, even by the same person during the same "trip." The principal psychological effects involve perceptual changes, especially visual hallucinations and distortions.

Hitner describes the LSD-induced psychedelic state by dividing it into three phases:

(1) The *somatic phase* occurs initially after absorption and consists of CNS stimulation and autonomic changes which are predominantly sympathomimetic in nature; (2) the *sensory phase* is characterized by sensory distortions and pseudohallucinations, which are the effects desired by the drug user; and (3) the *psychic phase* signals a maximum drug effect where disruption of thought processes, depersonalization, true hallucinations, and psychotic episodes may occur. Experiencing the latter phase would be considered a "bad trip."[3]

Similarly, Jaffe describes the second and third phases as follows:

In the second or third hour, visual illusions, wavelike recurrences of perceptual changes (e.g., micropsia, macropsia), and affective symptoms may occur. Afterimages are prolonged, and the overlapping of present and preceding perceptions occurs. Some subjects recognize these confluences, whereas others elaborate them into hallucinations. In contrast to naturally occurring psychoses, auditory hallucinations are rare. Synesthesias, the overflow from one sensory modality to another, may occur. Colors are heard and sounds may be seen. Subjective time is also seriously altered, so that clock time seems to pass extremely slowly. The loss of boundaries and the fear of fragmentation create a need for a structuring or supporting environment and experienced companions. During the "trip," thoughts and memories can vividly emerge under self-guidance or unexpectedly, to the user's distress. Mood may be labile, shifting from depression to gaiety, from elation to fear. Tension and anxiety may mount and reach panic proportions. After about 4 to 5 hours, if a major panic episode does not occur, there may be a sense of detachment and the conviction that one is magically in control.[12]

TOLERANCE AND DEPENDENCE   *Tolerance* (a need to increase the dose to obtain the same effect) of both the psychological and physiological alterations that are induced by LSD readily develops, and *cross-tolerance* occurs between LSD and most other psychedelic agents. Cross-tolerance between LSD and marijuana has not been demonstrated.

Physical dependence on LSD does not develop, even when the drug is used repeatedly for a prolonged period of time. In fact, most heavy users of the drug say that they ceased using LSD because they tired of it, had no further need for it, or have had enough. Even when the drug is discontinued because of concern about bad trips or about physical or mental harm, withdrawal signs are not exhibited.

ADVERSE REACTIONS AND TOXICITY   The adverse reactions and toxicities that are attributed to LSD generally fall into four categories: (1) the effects on the psychological state of the user; (2) the possibility of permanent damage to the brain; (3) the possible effects on the fetus when the drug is taken by a pregnant woman; and (4) the deleterious effects upon society in general as a result of widespread use.

Concerning effects on the psychological state of the user:

> Unpleasant experiences with LSD are relatively frequent and may involve an uncontrollable drift into confusion, dissociative reactions, acute panic reactions, a reliving of earlier traumatic experiences, or an acute psychotic hospitalization. Prolonged non-psychotic reactions have included dissociative reactions, time and space distortion, body image changes, and a residue of fear or depression stemming from morbid or terrifying experiences under the drug. . . . With the failure of usual defense mechanisms, the onslaught of repressed material overwhelms the integrative capacity of the ego, and a psychotic reaction results. It appears that this [LSD-induced] disruption of long-established patterns of adapting may be a lasting or semipermanent effect of the drug.[13]

LSD reduces a person's normal ability to control emotional reactions, and drug-induced alterations in perception can become so intense that they overwhelm his or her ability to cope.

Whether long-term, frequent, high-dose use of LSD results in discernible damage to the brain has not been determined, but it is generally agreed that occasional use of LSD for experimental purposes does not induce physical damage. Because LSD can eliminate normal defense (or coping) mechanisms, it may precipitate psychotic episodes that normally would have been suppressed.

There is also the possible problem of persistent flashbacks, which may recur weeks or even months later. The mechanism that underlies flashbacks is unknown, but it may involve a long-lasting impairment of psychological defense mechanisms, which causes a periodic emergence of repressed feelings.[14] As stated:

> Recurrences of drug effects without the drug—"flashbacks"—are a puzzling phenomenon; they occur in more than 15 percent of users. Commonly precipitated by use of marihuana, anxiety, fatigue, or movement into a dark environment, "flashbacks" may persist intermittently for several years after the last exposure to LSD. They are exacerbated by the use of phenothiazines. In some individuals the use of psychedelics can precipitate serious depressions, paranoid behavior, or prolonged psychotic episodes. Whether such episodes would have occurred without the drug is not clear. Prolonged psychotic episodes following repeated use of LSD tend to resemble naturally occurring schizophreniform psychotic states, and the prognosis appears to be similar. . . . It is possible that repeated use of LSD can induce subtle deficits in the capacity for abstract thinking.[12]

As summarized by Rang and Dale:

> There has been much concern over reports that LSD and other psychotomimetic drugs, as well as causing potentially dangerous "bad trips," can lead to more persistent mental disorders. There are recorded instances in which altered perception and hallucinations have lasted for up to 3 weeks following a single dose of LSD, and also reports of a persistent state resembling paranoid schizophrenia, which responds to antipsychotic drugs but may recur later. It is not at all clear whether this is due to a long-term effect of LSD, or whether LSD-taking is more likely in subjects destined to develop schizophrenia. The cautious view must be that LSD is causative. This, coupled with the fact that the occasional

"bad trip" can result in severe injury through violent behavior, means that LSD and other psychotomimetics must be regarded as highly dangerous drugs.[4]

Possible hazards to the fetus when a pregnant woman takes LSD are also unknown. Laboratory evidence indicates that *extremely high* doses of LSD may cause chromosome breakage. However, doses of LSD that are usually encountered do not appear to increase the rate of chromosome breakage. In fact, clinical data indicate that the incidence of fetal abnormalities in offspring of LSD users is the same as that in the normal population. Although there is *some* evidence of an increased incidence of structural abnormalities in infants born of parents who use LSD, those same parents tend to take a variety of other drugs as well, which makes it impossible to blame one specific compound.

Fears of long-term damage to *society* as a result of widespread use of LSD appear to be unsubstantiated. Use of LSD has decreased markedly. Further, even though some users experience psychological dependence, most persons eventually cease taking LSD and return to less potent drugs. Thus, despite the extreme potency and unusual psychedelic effects of LSD, the social use of other psychoactive drugs that have potent behavioral reinforcing properties (such as alcohol, nicotine, cocaine, amphetamine, and the opiates) should cause more concern.[15]

LSD-like Tryptamine Derivatives

Dimethyltryptamine (DMT) is a naturally occurring psychedelic compound that is structurally related to serotonin. It is capable of producing LSD-like effects in the user, and like LSD, DMT has been shown to bind to serotonin-2 receptors.[3]

DMT is used widely throughout much of the world. It is an active ingredient of various types of South American snuff, such as cohoba (prepared from the beans of the *Piptadenia peregrina*) and yopo (a similar product from the West Indies). DMT is partly responsible for the hallucinations and confusional syndrome that follow inhalation of these powders, but the presence of the drug bufotenin (5-hydroxy-DMT) also contributes to the effect. Unlike LSD, DMT is not absorbed when it is taken orally. Therefore, it must be smoked or sniffed to be effective.

The psychedelic properties of DMT appear to result predominantly from alterations in visual perception or the occurrence of true hallucinations. Euphoria and behavioral excitability often accompany the sensory alterations. The duration of action of DMT is extremely short—usually only about 1 hour (hence its slang name, "businessmen's LSD").

Psilocybin (4-phosphoryl-DMT) and *psilocin (4-hydroxy-DMT)* are two psychedelic agents that are found in at least 15 species of mushrooms that belong to the genera *Psilocybe, Panaeolus,* and *Conocybe.* These mushrooms grow throughout much of the world, including Central America and the northwestern portion of the United States.[16] *Psilocybe mexicana* (also referred to as *Teonanacatl,* or "God's Flesh") has a long and colorful history of use as a religious sacrament throughout Central America.

Psilocin and psilocybin are approximately 200 times less potent than LSD. Unlike DMT, psilocin and psilocybin are absorbed effectively when they are taken orally; the mushrooms are eaten raw to induce psychedelic effects. There is great variation in the concentration of psylocybin and psilocin among the different species of mushrooms as well as significant differences between mushrooms of the same species. For example, the usual oral dose of *Psilocybe semilanceata* ("Liberty Caps") may occur in a range of 10 to 40 mushrooms, while the dose for *Psilocybe cyanescens* may be found in only 2 to 5 mushrooms. Thus, the species must be properly identified to determine the proper dose. In addition, some extremely toxic species of mushrooms are not psychoactive, but they bear a superficial resemblance to the mushrooms that contain psilocybin and psilocin. Thus, to avoid unpleasant experiences, one must be familiar with all hallucinogenic and poisonous species of mushrooms.

For a long time, psilocin and psilocybin were both thought to be pharmacologically active. However, as Figure 11.3 shows, the only difference between the two compounds is that psilocybin contains a molecule of phosphoric acid. After the mushroom has been ingested, phosphoric acid is apparently removed from psilocybin, which produces psilocin, the active psychedelic agent.

Although the psychedelic effects of *Psilocybe mexicana* have long been part of Indian folklore, *Psilocybe* intoxication was not described until 1955, when Gordon Wasson, a New York banker, traveled through Mexico. He mingled with native tribes and was allowed to participate in a *Psilocybe* ceremony, in which he consumed the "magic" mushroom. Wasson said:

> It permits you to travel backwards and forward in time, to enter other planes of existence, even to know God. . . . Your body lies in the darkness, heavy as lead, but your spirit seems to soar and leave the hut, and with the speed of thought to travel where it listeth, in

time and space, accompanied by the shaman's singing . . . at least you know what the ineffable is, and what ecstasy means. Ecstasy! The mind harks back to the origin of that word. For the Greeks, *ekstasis* meant the flight of the soul from the body. Can you find a better word to describe this state?[17]

The hallucinations and distortions of time and space that are caused by psilocybin are similar to those produced by LSD. However, the duration of action is only between 2 and 4 hours. Cross-tolerance occurs between psilocybin, LSD, and mescaline.

Psilocybin binds to serotonin-2 receptors, but it is not as potent as LSD, and it is somewhat easier to adjust the dose to reach a desired effect. Low doses of psilocybin (up to 4 or 5 milligrams) induce a pleasant experience that causes mental relaxation. Higher doses (up to 15 milligrams) induce perceptual alterations with occasional hallucinations. Another description of the experience that follows ingestion of the psilocybin mushroom is offered by Weil.[18]

Ololiuqui (morning glory seeds) is yet another naturally occurring agent that is used by Central and South American Indians both as an intoxicant and as a hallucinogen. The drug is used ritually as a means of communicating with the supernatural, as are extracts of most plants that contain psychedelic drugs. The use of ololiuqui seeds in Central and South America was first described by the Spaniard Hernandez, who stated that:

> When the priests wanted to commune with their Gods . . . [they ate ololiuqui seeds and] a thousand visions and satanic hallucinations appeared to them.[19]

The seeds were analyzed in Europe by Albert Hoffmann, who identified several ingredients. One ingredient was lysergic acid amide (not lysergic acid diethylamide, LSD). The lysergic acid amide that Hoffmann identified is approximately one-tenth as active as LSD as a psychoactive agent. However, considering the extreme potency of LSD, lysergic acid amide is still quite potent.

Accompanying the psychedelic action of ololiuqui are the usual side effects of serotonin psychedelic drugs: nausea, vomiting, headache, increased blood pressure, dilated pupils, sleepiness, and so on. These side effects are usually quite intense and serve to limit the recreational use of ololiuqui. Ingestion of 100 or more seeds produces sleepiness, distortion of perception, hallucinations, and confusion. Flashbacks have been reported, but they are infrequent.

Harmine is a psychedelic agent that is obtained from the seeds of *Peganum harmala*, which is a native plant in the Middle East. These seeds have been used for centuries. Intoxication by harmine is usually accompanied by nausea and vomiting, sedation, and, finally, sleep. The psychic excitement that users experience consists of visual distortions that are similar to those induced by LSD.

Psychedelic Anesthetics

Phencyclidine, which was developed in 1956, is a potent analgesic and amnestic agent. It was used briefly as an anesthetic in humans during the late 1950s. However, despite its potential use as an analgesic–amnestic agent, patients who were given this drug reported quite bizarre reactions, including agitation, excitement, disorientation, delirium, and "hallucinatory" phenomena. The perception of body changes, disorganized thought, suspiciousness, confusion, and lack of cooperation that were exhibited resemble a schizophrenic state that consisted of both production (positive) and deficit (negative) symptoms.

Phencyclidine is no longer used in humans. It is now being marketed as a veterinary anesthetic, primarily for use in primates as an immobilizing agent. Another compound, ketamine, which is related structurally to phencyclidine (see Figure 11.4), has subsequently been found to induce a similar state of anesthesia. However, the psychedelic effects of ketamine are much less severe. Ketamine is still available for use in humans as a specialized anesthetic agent.

In 1967, small amounts of phencyclidine became available in the "drug culture," and, during that year, it was referred to as the "PeaCe Pill" (PCP). Between the years 1971 and 1975, most PCP was available as a component of various illicit drug mixtures. In 1975, however, a resurgence in the use of illicit phencyclidine occurred, and it became one of the most abused drugs in the United States. By the 1980s, the use of PCP had peaked, and it has now decreased markedly.

Phencyclidine has appeared on the illicit market in the form of powder, tablets, leaf mixtures, and 1-gram "rock" crystals. When the powder or a leaf mixture of phencyclidine is found on parsley, mint, or other leaves, it is usually prepared in the form of a cigarette, a "joint." Phencyclidine is commonly sold as "crystal," "angel dust," "hog," "PCP," "THC," "cannabinol," or "horse tranquilizer." The most persistent misrepresentation is "THC." When it is sold as "crystal" or "angel dust" (terms also used for methamphetamine), the drug is usually available in concentrations that vary between 50 and 100 percent. When it is purchased under other names or in concoctions, the amount of phencyclidine falls to a range of 10 to 30 percent. Phencyclidine can be taken orally; it can be smoked or snorted; or it can be injected intravenously. Powdered forms are usually sprinkled on "joints" or, sometimes, snorted.

PCP is well absorbed, whether it is taken orally or smoked. When it is smoked, peak effects occur in about 15 minutes, when about 40 percent of the dose appears in the user's bloodstream. Oral absorption is slower; maximum blood levels are not reached until about 2 hours after the drug has been taken. The elimination half-life of PCP averages about 18 hours, but it varies widely.

About 90 percent of PCP is metabolized, and its metabolites are excreted in the urine. A positive urine assay for PCP is assumed to indicate that PCP was used within the previous week. Blood and saliva tests for PCP can also be done. False-positive test results for PCP are common and, therefore, a positive assay requires secondary confirmation.

The pharmacology of phencyclidine is complicated. This compound and its close relative, ketamine, are frequently referred to as *dissociative anesthetics*, because patients may feel dissociated from themselves and from their environment. In humans, phencyclidine appears to be unique among all the anesthetic drugs that have been studied. This drug induces an unresponsive state with intense analgesia and amnesia, although the patient's eyes remain open (blank stare), and he or she may even appear to be awake. Significant depression of either respiration or blood pressure is rarely observed. When it is used illicitly, low doses of phencyclidine produce mild agitation, euphoria, disinhibition, or excitement in a person who appears to be grossly "drunk" and exhibits a blank stare. The subject may be rigid and unable to speak. In many cases, however, the patient may be communicative, although he or she does not respond to pain. When patients are given high doses, a state of coma or stupor is induced. Blood pressure usually becomes elevated, but respiration does not become depressed. The patient may recover from this state within 1 to 4 hours, although a state of confusion may last for 8 to 72 hours.

Massive oral "overdoses," involving up to 1 gram of street-purchased material, have been reported to result in prolonged periods of stupor or coma. This state may last for several days and may be marked by a depression of respiration that is potentially lethal, intense seizure activity, and increased blood pressure. Following this period of stupor, a prolonged recovery phase, which is marked by confusion and delusions, may last as long as 2 weeks. In some persons, this state of confusion may be followed by a psychosis that lasts several weeks to a few months.

Chronic users of phencyclidine frequently present themselves in hospital emergency rooms with psychiatric problems such as paranoid psychosis, severe depression, anxiety, or concern about brain damage. Regarding treatment of overdosage:

> *Treatment* of overdosage is symptomatic and is directed at protecting the patient and others from the effects of impaired behavior and judgment and at supporting vital functions. Hastening excretion by continuous gastric suction and acidification of the urine can substantially shorten the half-life of the drug but can also increase the risk of renal failure. . . . Hypersalivation may require suction, respiratory depression may require artificial ventilation, and fever may require external cooling. Convulsions have been treated with diazepam and hypertension with hydralazine. Clinicians advise isolation of patients from external stimuli to the degree compatible with support of vital functions and control of violent or self-destructive behavior. . . . Coma may be preceded or followed by delirium, paranoia, and assaultive behavior, and clinical arrangements must take this into consideration. . . . A psychotic phase may last for several weeks after a single dose of phencyclidine.[20]

The major risks that are associated with the use of PCP result from behavioral problems or toxic reactions. Behavioral problems include falling, drowning, burns, driving accidents, aggressive or violent behavior, and so on. These problems seem to occur as a result of impaired perception, delusional beliefs, or acute schizophrenic-like behavior. A tendency toward violence may occur. The toxic reactions to PCP are manifested as acute intoxication, acute psychosis, or coma that occurs when an overdose is taken. The intoxicated state is manifested by agitation, confusion, excitement, a "blank stare," violent behavior, analgesia, and amnesia.

Self-inflicted injuries and injuries that are sustained during the application of physical restraints are frequent, because intoxicated persons are not aware of their surroundings and sometimes are not aware of, or unresponsive to, pain. Such injuries account for many of the injuries and deaths that are associated with PCP intoxication. Respiratory depression, generalized seizure activity, and pulmonary edema have all been implicated. PCP has been implicated in a number of deaths by drowning, sometimes in very shallow water. Other reported causes of death include violent behavior, automobile accidents, and suicide. For additional readings on phencyclidine, recent volumes are recommended.[21-23]

The mechanisms that cause the psychedelic, analgesic, and amnestic effects of phencyclidine and ketamine are not clear. Phencyclidine interacts with several transmitter systems, including those of acetylcholine, dopamine, serotonin, and norepinephrine neurons. More uniquely, phencyclidine binds to certain neuronal receptors in the limbic system (particularly in the frontal cortex and the hippocampus). These receptors seem to be of two types. The first type of receptor may be the sigma opioid receptor[24] (which is also thought to mediate the dysphoric effects of mixed agonist–antagonist opioids as well as the analgesic and psychotomimetic actions of phencyclidine). The second type of receptor may be an excitatory amino acid (N-methyl-D-aspartate) receptor that has been shown to be inhibited by phencyclidine.[25-28] It is not known why such a receptor might exist. One might speculate that the presence of a "PCP receptor" would necessitate the existence of an endogenous chemical (perhaps an "endopsychosin") which, when present in excess, might produce schizophrenic behavior.[29]

This multiplicity of actions provides researchers with a most interesting tool for studying the mechanisms of mental illness. Although the personality changes that are associated with the use of LSD are somewhat similar to those induced by phencyclidine, many of the other features of phencyclidine-induced psychosis are not common in persons who take other psychedelic drugs. In addition, phencyclidine (more than any other drug) produces psychic disturbances that resemble those observed in schizophrenic patients. This pattern suggests that a possible relation might exist between the cellular effects of phencyclidine and the biochemistry of schizophrenia.

STUDY QUESTIONS

1. What is a psychedelic drug?
2. What differentiates a psychedelic drug from a behavioral stimulant, such as amphetamine or cocaine?
3. List four different types (classes) of psychedelic drugs.

4. Differentiate between mescaline and LSD.
5. What is a "designer drug"?
6. How does LSD exert psychedelic actions?
7. What is the psychedelic syndrome?
8. What are some of the problems that are associated with the use of LSD?
9. How does phencyclidine differ from a nonselective CNS depressant? How does phencyclidine differ from LSD?
10. Phencyclidine is used as an animal tranquilizer or immobilizer. What properties of phencyclidine contribute to this use?

NOTES

1. J. H. Jaffe, "Drug Addiction and Drug Abuse," in A. G. Gilman, T. W. Rall, A. S. Nies, and P. Taylor, eds., *Goodman and Gilman's The Pharmacological Basis of Therapeutics*, 8th ed. (New York: Pergamon, 1990), p. 553.

2. S. Cohen, *The Chemical Brain: The Neurochemistry of Addictive Disorders* (Irvine, Calif.: Care Institute, 1988), p. 29.

3. H. W. Hitner, "Psychotomimetic Drugs," in J. R. DiPalma and G. J. DiGregorio, eds., *Basic Pharmacology in Medicine*, 3d ed. (New York: McGraw-Hill, 1990), pp. 242–244.

4. H. P. Rang and M. M. Dale, *Pharmacology* (Edinburgh: Churchill Livingstone, 1987), pp. 575–577.

5. S. Cohen, *The Chemical Brain: The Neurochemistry of Addictive Disorders* (Irvine, Calif.: Care Institute, 1988), pp. 66–67.

6. S. G. Potkin, F. Karoum, L. W. Chuang, et al., "Phenethylamine in Paranoid Chronic Schizophrenia," *Science* 206 (1979): 470.

7. R. B. McCall, "Neurophysiological Effects of Hallucinogens on Serotonergic Neuronal Systems," *Neuroscience and Biobehavioral Reviews* 6 (1982): 509–514.

8. E. K. Killam, "Pharmacology of the Reticular Formation," in D. H. Efrom, ed., *Psychopharmacology: A Review of Progress 1957–1967*, U.S. Public Health Service Publication No. 1836 (Washington D.C.: U.S. Government Printing Office, 1968), pp. 411–445.

9. *Interim Drug Report of the Commission of Inquiry into the Nonmedical Use of Drugs*, Gerald LeDain, chairman (Ottawa: Information Canada, 1970), p. 58.

10. *Interim Drug Report of the Commission of Inquiry into the Nonmedical Use of Drugs*, Gerald LeDain, chairman (Ottawa: Information Canada, 1970), pp. 58–59.

11. L. P. Finnegan and K. O'B. Fehr, "The Effects of Opiates, Sedative-Hypnotics, Amphetamines, Cannabis, and Other Psychoactive Drugs on the Fetus and Newborn," in O. J. Kalant, ed., *Research Advances in Alcohol and Drug Problems*, vol. 5 (New York: Plenum Press, 1980), pp. 653–723.

12. J. H. Jaffe, "Drug Addiction and Drug Abuse," in A. G. Gilman, T. W. Rall, A. S. Nies, and P. Taylor, eds., *Goodman and Gilman's The Pharmacological Basis of Therapeutics*, 8th ed. (New York: Pergamon, 1990), p. 556.

13. G. G. Dimijian, "Contemporary Drug Abuse," in A. Goth, ed., *Medical Pharmacology*, 11th ed. (St. Louis: Mosby, 1984), p. 356.

14. G. G. Dimijian, "Contemporary Drug Abuse," in A. Goth, ed., *Medical Pharmacology*, 11th ed. (St. Louis: Mosby, 1984), p. 357.

15. R. A. Wise, "The Role of Reward Pathways in the Development of Drug Dependence," *Pharmacology and Therapeutics* 35 (1987): 227–263.

16. J. Ott, *Hallucinogenic Plants of North America* (Berkeley: Wingbow Press, 1979).

17. M. E. Crahan, "God's Flesh and Other Pre-Columbian Phantastica," *Bulletin of the Los Angeles County Medical Association* 99 (1969): 17.

18. A. Weil, *The Marriage of the Sun and the Moon* (Boston: Houghton Mifflin, 1980).

19. Quoted in E. M. Brecher and Consumer Reports editors, *Licit and Illicit Drugs* (Mt. Vernon, N.Y.: Consumers Union, 1972), p. 345.

20. J. H. Jaffe, "Drug Addiction and Drug Abuse," in A. G. Gilman, T. W. Rall, A. S. Nies, and P. Taylor, eds., *Goodman and Gilman's The Pharmacological Basis of Therapeutics*, 8th ed. (New York: Pergamon, 1990), p. 558.

21. D. H. Clouct, ed., *Phencyclidine: An Update*, National Institute of Drug Abuse, Research Monograph No. 64, Department of Health and Human Services, Publication No. (ADM) 86-1443 (Washington, D.C.: U.S. Government Printing Office, 1986).

22. D. O. Clardy, R. H. Cravey, B. J. MacDonald, S. J. Wiersema, D. S. Pearce, and J. L. Ragle, "The Phencyclidine-Intoxicated Driver," *Journal of Analytical Toxicology* 3 (November–December 1979): 238–241.

23. E. F. Domino, "Neurobiology of Phencyclidine—An Update," in R. C. Peterson and R. C. Stillman, eds., *PCP Phencyclidine Abuse: An Appraisal*, National Institute on Drug Abuse (Washington, D.C.: U.S. Government Printing Office, 1978), pp. 18–43.

24. R. S. Zukin and S. R. Zukin, "A Common Receptor for Phencyclidine and the *Sigma* Opiates," in J. M. Kamenka, E. F. Domino, and P. Geneste, eds., *Phencyclidine and Related Arylcyclohexylamines: Present and Future Applications* (Ann Arbor: NPP Books, 1983), pp. 107–124.

25. S. R. Lukin and D. C. Javitt, "Mechanisms of Phencyclidine (PCP)-N-methyl-D-aspartate (NMDA) Receptor Interaction: Implications for Drug Abuse Research," in L. S. Harris, ed., *Problems of Drug Dependence 1989*, NIDA Research Monograph No. 95 (Washington D.C.: U.S. Government Printing Office, 1989), pp. 247–254.

26. J. L. Junien and B. E. Leonard, "Drugs Acting on Sigma and Phencyclidine Receptors: A Review of Their Nature, Function, and Possible Therapeutic Importance," *Clinical Neuropharmacology* 12 (1989): 353–374.

27. K. M. Johnson and S. M. Jones, "Neuropharmacology of Phencyclidine: Basic Mechanisms and Therapeutic Potential," *Annual Review of Pharmacology and Toxicology* 30 (1990): 707–750.

28. J. Church and D. Lodge, "Anticonvulsant Actions of Phencyclidine Receptor Ligands: Correlation with N-methylaspartate Antagonism in Vivo," *General Pharmacology* 21 (1990): 165–170.

29. P. C. Contreras, J. B. Monahan, T. H. Lanthorn, L. M. Pullan, D. A. DiMaggio, G. E. Handelmann, N. M. Gray, and T. L. O'Donohue, "Phencyclidine. Physiological Actions, Interactions with Excitatory Amino Acids and Endogenous Ligands," *Molecular Neurobiology* 1 (1987): 191–211.

Marijuana

The Ancient Drug of Cannabis

This ancient drug has sedative, euphoriant, and (in large doses) hallucinogenic properties. The hemp plant *Cannabis sativa* grows throughout the world and flourishes in most temperate and tropical regions. It is one of humanity's oldest cultivated nonfood plants. The earliest written reference to *Cannabis sativa* dates from approximately 2700 B.C. The active compound, delta-9-tetrahydrocannabinol (hereafter referred to as *THC*), is most concentrated in the resin that is obtained from the flowers of the female plant.

Names for *Cannabis* products include *marijuana, hashish, charas, bhang, ganja,* and *sinsemilla.* Hashish and charas, which consist of the dried resinous exudate of the female flowers, are the most potent preparations. The THC content in charas and hashish averages about 7 to 8 percent in a range tht extends up to about 14 percent.[1] Ganja and sinsemilla refer to the dried material that is found in the tops of the female plants, where the THC content averages about 4 to 5 percent, (rarely over 7 percent). Bhang and marijuana are low-grade preparations that are taken from the dried remainder of the plant. The THC content of bhang and marijuana is about 1 percent. Thus, marijuana products that are commercially available vary in THC concentration from about 1 percent to about 4 to 7 percent and only rarely to higher concentrations. The usual range of potency for marijuana seems to be 2 to 5 percent. This concentration has not changed remarkably during the past decade or so. (Note that THC is the active ingredient in each product; only the concentration and purity of THC vary.)

Classification

Tetrahydrocannabinol (THC) is a difficult compound to classify. At low-to-moderate doses, THC is a mild sedative-hypnotic agent. Its pharmacological effects resemble those of alcohol and the antianxiety agents. Unlike the sedative-hypnotic compounds, however, higher doses of THC may (in addition to sedation) produce euphoria, hallucinations, and heightened sensations—effects that are similar to a mild LSD experience. Further, high doses of THC do not produce anesthesia, coma, or death (also unlike the sedatives). Little cross-tolerance occurs between THC and LSD or between THC and the sedative-hypnotic compounds.

THC exerts multiple actions on several neurotransmitter receptors, but no effect has yet been shown to dominate. Like the general anesthetics, it may interact with neuronal membranes to increase membrane fluidity (an action that has not been correlated with psychedelic action). It blocks acetylcholine receptors, which probably contributes to its mild amnestic property, and it is mildly analgesic. The analgesic action of THC is possibly exerted through specific brain receptors and may involve the inhibition of a specific enzyme, adenyl cyclase.[2] Its euphoriant action may follow an involvement with dopamine or serotonin receptors.

The courts often classify the products of *Cannabis sativa* with the opioids as narcotics. However, THC is not a narcotic; it is quite distinct from opioids pharmacologically. Further, only high doses of THC (greater than 10 to 20 percent THC) will cause pharmacological effects that resemble those of the psychedelic drugs. Thus, at least for this discussion, THC will be classified as a unique psychoactive drug. The structure of THC does not resemble that of any known or suspected chemical transmitter.

History

The history of *Cannabis sativa* from about 2700 B.C. until the nineteenth century still remains obscure. Marijuana is used primarily as a mild intoxicant. It is somewhat milder than alcohol and much less useful for religious and psychedelic experiences than the naturally occurring psychedelic drugs. Although products from *Cannabis sativa* have been claimed to have a wide variety of medical uses, none of those uses seemed to persist for very long, and, even today, few are documented.

Cannabis sativa is rather new to Western culture. During the American colonial period, in the 1700s, the plant was grown widely in Virginia, presumably for its fiber, which was used for rope. Even George Washington grew hemp for fiber and, possibly, for its medicinal and other properties.

Hemp cultivation flourished in the United States for many years, but then it declined when more profitable crops, such as cotton, were introduced and the importation of cheap hemp from the Far East began. Periodically, however, hemp is still grown commercially in this country. During World War II, for example, cultivation of hemp was expanded when imports became severely limited. However, hemp need not be cultivated, because *Cannabis sativa* grows wild and does not need to be tended.

Marijuana—at least until the beginning of the twentieth century—was not used widely either for medical or recreational purposes. Its psychoactive properties had been discovered, but they had not attracted the attention of most persons. The use of marijuana was restricted primarily to the "less desirable" element in society. During the early 1920s, the news media portrayed marijuana as being evil and as being a part of "underground" activities. In 1926, a New Orleans newspaper exposed the "menace of marijuana," claiming that an association existed between marijuana and crime; and laws were subsequently passed in Louisiana to outlaw its use. Slowly, during the next 5 years, others took up the call; and more states began to pass laws against the use of marijuana.

Probably the greatest impetus to the outlawing of marijuana was provided during the early 1930s. The Commissioner of Narcotics, Harry Anslinger, had an intense interest in encouraging the states and the Bureau of Narcotics to enforce vigorously the laws against using marijuana. During the next few years, marijuana began to be looked on as a narcotic—an agent that was responsible for crimes of violence and a great danger to public safety. These attitudes were popularized

TABLE 12.1

Percentage of high-school seniors nationwide responding to a confidential question-naire who said they had used drugs within the past 30 days.

	'75	'76	'77	'78	'79	'80	'81	'82	'83	'84	'85	'86
Marijuana, hashish	27.1	32.2	35.4	37.1	36.5	33.7	31.6	28.5	27.0	25.2	25.7	23.4
Cocaine	1.9	2.0	2.9	3.9	5.7	5.2	5.8	5.0	4.9	5.8	6.7	6.2
Alcohol	68.2	68.3	71.2	72.1	71.8	72.0	70.7	69.7	69.4	67.2	65.9	65.3

Source: University of Michigan Institute for Social Research. Conducted for the National Institute on Drug Abuse, 1987.

throughout the 1930s by numerous news articles, which convinced the public that marijuana was, indeed, evil. By approximately 1940, the country was convinced that marijuana was a "killer drug" and a potent narcotic that (1) induced people to commit crimes of violence, (2) led to heroin addiction, and (3) was a great social menace.

The campaign against marijuana and the emotion that it generated continued throughout the 1950s. At that time, the use of marijuana was still primarily restricted to persons who were in the lower classes of society. Then, during the late 1950s and early 1960s, marijuana and other psychoactive drugs became extremely popular among middle- and upper-class youths. Throughout the 1960s, the use of marijuana by American youths increased steadily. However, the rate of experimenta-tion with marijuana did not explode with the same rapidity as that of LSD, and its widespread use did not really develop until the late 1960s and early 1970s, when the use of LSD and other potent psychedelic drugs had begun to decline.

It has been estimated that by 1972, at least 2 million Americans used marijuana daily. The use of marijuana often exceeded the use of alcohol by young adults. Then the number of persons who used marijuana increased steadily throughout the 1970s. In 1977, a national survey on drug use showed that young adults (persons between 18 and 25 years old) used marijuana the most and that the extent of use declined precipitously among persons who were older than 35 years of age. If we take these percentages of *Cannabis* users and extrapolate them to the general population, we find that 43 million Americans had tried marijuana by the spring of 1977.

A 1986 survey (Table 12.1) noted that the percentage of high-school seniors who smoke marijuana has been declining steadily since the peak period of use—from 1977 to 1979. Disquieting, however, was the confirmation that the number of students who smoke cigarettes has not declined; use of alcohol has only slightly declined; and use of cocaine has increased dramatically. Marijuana is still used rarely by persons who are over the age of 50. Also, daily use of marijuana by high-school seniors has declined from a peak of 11 percent in 1978 to less than 4 percent currently.[3] About 6 to 10 million Americans currently smoke marijuana at least once every week.

Thus, the escalation in the use of marijuana that was noted during the 1970s has decreased, but it has probably reached a plateau. Those persons who exhibit chronic use of marijuana may not change their habits markedly in the near future. Further, the combined effects of alcohol and marijuana have caused a major problem in terms of traumatic incidents (vehicular or otherwise) that involve young adults.[4]

Pharmacokinetics

As stated previously, most marijuana that is available in the United States has a THC content that rarely exceeds 7 percent and usually averages about 2 to 4 percent. These percentages are important in terms of the pharmacological effects of *Cannabis* (see the next section).

In the United States, THC is usually administered in the form of a hand-rolled marijuana cigarette (the average marijuana cigarette contains between 1 and 2 grams of plant material). Thus, if a marijuana cigarette contains 1.5 grams of plant material with a THC content of 3 percent, the cigarette contains approximately 0.045 gram (45 milligrams) of THC. Because THC is usually administered by smoking marijuana, the quantity of drug that is actually absorbed into the bloodstream varies considerably with the previous smoking experience of the user, the amount of time that the smoke is held in the lungs, and the number of other persons who are smoking the same cigarette.

Usually, persons who have previously smoked marijuana several times can hold the smoke in their lungs longer than can novices, which allows a longer period of time for the THC to be absorbed into the bloodstream before the smoke is exhaled. Similarly, persons who have a habit of inhaling the smoke of tobacco cigarettes usually can hold marijuana smoke in their lungs longer than can nonsmokers. Further, the fewer persons who share a marijuana cigarette, the more THC is available to each smoker. In general, approximately one-fourth to one-half of the THC that is present in a marijuana cigarette is actually available in the smoke. Thus, if a cigarette contains 45 milligrams of THC, about 11 to 22 milligrams are available in the smoke. It is extremely unlikely, however, that even a single person smoking one cigarette would be able to absorb 100 percent of the THC that is available in that cigarette. In practice, the amount of THC that is absorbed into the bloodstream as a result of the social smoking of one marijuana cigarette is probably much lower—in a range of 2 to 20 percent (0.4 mg to 10 mg).[5]

As discussed in Chapter 1, the absorption of inhaled drugs is rapid and complete. The onset of action of THC usually occurs within minutes after smoking begins, and peak concentrations in plasma are reached within 10 to 30 minutes. Unless more is smoked, the effects seldom last longer than 2 or 3 hours. THC is also absorbed when it is administered orally, but the absorption is slow and incomplete. When THC is administered orally, the onset of action usually takes 3 to 60 minutes, with peak effects occurring 2 to 3 hours after ingestion. Its effects persist for 3 to 5 hours or even longer. THC is approximately three times more effective when it is smoked than when it is taken orally. Because marijuana products are crude preparations and are not soluble in water, they should not be administered by injection. Indeed, injection of any product of *Cannabis sativa* or any other plant is extremely dangerous. It should be noted that when a product is sold illicitly as "THC," it virtually never contains THC but, rather, it may contain any of a number of other psychedelic agents.

Once THC is absorbed, it is distributed to the various organs of the body—especially those that have significant concentrations of fatty material. Thus, THC readily penetrates the brain; the blood-brain barrier does not appear to hinder its passage. Similarly, THC readily crosses the placental barrier and reaches the fetus. It is almost completely metabolized to an active product (11-hydroxy-delta-9-THC) that is converted to an inactive metabolite and then excreted.[5]

After the initial period of intoxication, THC levels fall rapidly for about 1 hour to a low level (due to a high solubility of THC in body fat) that persists for days. The metabolism of THC is quite slow; an elimination half-life of about 30 hours is generally accepted, although some report half-lives of about 4 days.[6] Thus, THC persists in the body for several days or even weeks. Such a delay tends to prolong and intensify the activity of subsequently smoked marijuana, which may at least partially explain why regular users achieve a "high" more quickly, more easily, and with a smaller amount of the drug than do intermittent users (a phenomenon that was formerly, and probably mistakenly, called "reverse tolerance").

Because only minute quantities of THC are found in the urine of persons who use the drug, detection tests for THC focus primarily on isolating its metabolites. Such detection tests are complex and involve specialized chemical techniques, such as immunoassay, chromatography, or spectrometry. Although acute or occasional use is detected for about 1 to 3 days, chronic smokers (even if they only smoke two to three times weekly) will have persistently positive urine tests for THC metabolites. A heavy smoker who stops smoking may show positive urine tests for about 1 month after cessation. Thus, a positive urinalysis can indicate recent use as well as that which might have occurred several weeks earlier. Multiple sampling may be necessary to differentiate the results. As stated by Hawks and Chiang:

> A single positive urine test does not mean that the person was under the influence of marijuana at the time the urine specimen was collected. A true-positive urine test means only that the person providing the specimen used marijuana in the recent past, which could be hours, days, or weeks depending on the specific use pattern.[7]

Pharmacological Effects

In animals, THC induces sedation, and it decreases spontaneous motor activity as well as behavioral responses to painful stimuli. THC decreases body temperature, calms aggressive behavior, potentiates the effects of barbiturates and other sedatives, blocks convulsions, and depresses reflexes. In primates, specifically, THC produces sedation, decreases aggression, decreases the ability to perform complex behavioral tasks, seems to induce hallucinations, and appears to cause temporal distortions. THC causes the animal to increase the frequency of its social interactions. High doses can depress ovarian function, lower the concentration of female sex hormones, decrease ovulation, and, perhaps, decrease sperm production.[5]

In humans, THC affects the functioning of both the cardiovascular system and the CNS. Increases in pulse rate and slight increases in blood pressure are commonly encountered. Blood vessels of the cornea become dilated, which results in the bloodshot eyes that are usually observed in persons who indulge in alcohol. THC users frequently report increased appetite, dry mouth, occasional dizziness, increased visual and auditory perception, and nausea. Taste, touch, and smell may be enhanced; time perception may be altered; and an increased sense of well-being, mild euphoria, relaxation, and relief from anxiety occur.

The usual subjective effects of normal, social doses of marijuana consist of subtle mood alterations that resemble daydreaming or mild sedative-hypnotic drug intoxication—alterations that are frequently imperceptible to the novice or the nonsmoking observer. At higher doses of THC (several cigarettes or moderate doses of hashish taken orally), the user will experience an intensification of emotional responses and alterations in sensation, which resemble mild sensory distortions or even mild hallucinations. Few persons who currently smoke marijuana socially are seeking these effects. Only a small percentage of persons who smoke marijuana use it to induce a pronounced state of sensory distortion. As described by Jaffe, for usual doses of marijuana:

> Most commonly there is an increased sense of well-being or euphoria, accompanied by feelings of relaxation and sleepiness when subjects are alone; where users can interact, sleepiness is less pronounced and there is often spontaneous laughter. . . . Short-term memory is impaired, and the capacity to carry out tasks requiring multiple mental steps deteriorates. This effect on memory-dependent, goal-directed behavior has been called "temporal disintegration," and is correlated with a tendency to confuse past, present, and future, and with depersonalization—a sense of strangeness and unreality about the self.
>
> Balance and stability of stance are affected even at low doses, effects that are more apparent when the eyes are closed. Decreases in muscle strength and hand steadiness can be demonstrated. Performance of relatively simple motor tasks and simple reaction times are relatively unimpaired until higher doses are reached. More complex processes, including perception, attention, and information processing, which are involved in driving and flying, are impaired by doses equivalent to one or two cigarettes; the impairment persists for 4 to 8 hours, well beyond the time that the user perceives the subjective effects of the drug. . . . The impairment produced by alcohol is additive to that induced by marihuana.
>
> Marihuana smokers frequently report increased hunger, dry mouth and throat, more vivid visual imagery, and a keener sense of hearing. Subtle visual and auditory stimuli previously ignored may take on a novel quality, and the nondominant senses of touch, taste, and smell seem to be enhanced. Yet, in usual social doses, marihuana decreases empathy and the perception of emotions in others. . . . Altered perception of time is a consistent effect of cannabinoids. Time seems to pass more slowly—minutes may seem like hours.[5]

Psychotoxic doses of THC induce delusions, paranoia, hallucinations, confusion and disorientation, depersonalization, altered sensory perception, and increasing anxiety. As doses are increased further, these drug effects intensify, causing more vivid hallucinations, delusions, and increasing disorientation. Jaffe discusses the effects of such doses:

> Higher doses of THC can induce frank hallucinations, delusions, and paranoid feelings. Thinking becomes confused and disorganized; depersonalization and altered time sense are accentuated. Anxiety reaching panic proportions may replace euphoria, often as a result of the feeling that the drug-induced state will never end. With high enough doses, the clinical picture is that of a toxic psychosis with hallucinations, depersonalization, and loss of insight. . . . Most users are able to regulate their intake in order to avoid the excessive dosage that produces these unpleasant effects. . . . Use of marihuana may also cause an acute exacerbation of symptomatology in stabilized schizophrenics, and it is an independent risk factor for the development of schizophrenia.[5]

Although chronic smoking of marijuana is now quite common, the chronic use of tobacco is much more prevalent. Because inhalation is by far the most common route of administration, knowledge about the gaseous and particulate components of both marijuana and tobacco smoke (Table 12.2)[7] is particularly relevant. Note that with the exception of the presence of THC in marijuana and nicotine in tobacco, both inhalants are remarkably similar. However, marijuana smoke contains about 50 percent more carcinogens. In determining the significance of the higher content of carcinogens in marijuana smoke, we must remember that the amount of tobacco used by the average cigarette smoker is 10 to 20 times the amount of marijuana used by the average marijuana smoker. On the other hand, when a person smokes marijuana, he or she inhales more deeply and holds the smoke in the lungs longer. Thus, chronic use of marijuana should be expected to cause a profound affect on the lungs.

A chronic smoker of marijuana maintains a constant state of intoxication. Such behavior, by itself, causes particular risks. As Cohen states:

> Being stoned during much of one's waking hours is particularly undesirable during the formative years when critical coping techniques should be mastered. When preadolescents and adolescents use marijuana, and not just marijuana, to distance themselves from

TABLE 12.2

Comparison of gaseous and particulate components of marijuana and tobacco smoke.

	Marijuana cigarette	Tobacco cigarette
Gas phase analysis		
Carbon monoxide (vol %)	3.99	4.58
(mg)	17.6	20.2
Carbon dioxide (vol %)	8.27	9.38
(mg)	57.3	65.0
Ammonia (μg)	228	178
HCN (μg)	532	498
Isoprene (μg)	83	310
Acetaldehyde (μg)	1200	980
Acetone (μg)	443	578
Acrolein (μg)	92	85
Acetonitrile (μg)	132	123
Benzene (μg)	76	67
Toluene (μg)	112	108
Dimethylnitrosamine (ng)	75	84
Methylethylnitrosamine (ng)	27	30
Particulate matter analysis		
Phenol (μg)	76.8	138.5
o-Cresol (μg)	76.8	24
	17.9	24
m-,p-cresol (μg)	54.4	65
2,4- and 2,5-dimethylphenol (μg)	6.8	14.4
Cannabidiol (μg)	190	—
Δ^9THC (μg)	820	—
Nicotine	—	2850
Naphthalene (ng)	3000	1200
1-methylnaphthalene (ng)	6100	3650
2-methylnaphthalene (ng)	3600	1400
Benzo(a)anthracene (ng)	75	43
Benzo(a)pyrene (ng)	31	22.1

Source: D. Hoffman, K. D. Brunemann, G. B. Gori, and E. L. Wynder.[7]

the problems and frustrations of their existence, they do themselves a substantial disservice. They deprive themselves of learning time and may, as a result, never learn the strategies for living this admittedly difficult life.[8]

Therapeutic Uses

Currently, there is one approved and several possible therapeutic uses for THC and its various derivatives. *Dronabinol* (Marinol) and *nabilone*

(Cesamet) are THC derivatives. These drugs are available for use in the treatment of nausea and vomiting that are associated with chemotherapy in cancer patients.[9,10] THC also exhibits mild analgesic properties, decreases epileptic seizures, decreases the pressure of fluid within the eyes, and decreases the resistance of airways in the lungs. Thus, marijuana is potentially useful in treating pain, epilepsy, glaucoma, and asthma, although other drugs exist that are more effective. It is unlikely that marijuana or THC will be approved by the FDA for these purposes.

At present, marijuana must still be considered a remarkably nonlethal compound. No deaths have been reported that can be attributed directly to its use, although deaths can certainly follow the intravenous injection of nonsterile preparations of marijuana or hashish (which may be unrelated to the THC content). Such use of marijuana products is certainly to be condemned.

Side Effects and Toxicity

Behavioral alterations that occur as a result of intoxication are a major side effect. Marijuana alters a person's ability to drive an automobile safely,[4,11-13] and the impairment of driving ability that occurs resembles that observed in persons who abuse alcohol. As summarized:

> The impairment persists for 4–8 hours, well beyond the time that the user perceives the subjective effects of the drug. The impairment is apparent to trained observers: 94% of subjects failed a roadside sobriety test 90 minutes after smoking marijuana; 60% still failed after 150 minutes.[5]

Similarly, Soderstrom et al.[4] studied patients who were injured in motor vehicle accidents (67 percent) or from nonvehicular trauma (33 percent). Marijuana was detected in 35 percent of subjects, and alcohol was present in 33 percent. The person's sex (male) and age (younger than 30 years) correlated with an increased incidence of marijuana use. A combination of both marijuana and alcohol were present in 16.5 percent of subjects: marijuana alone was present in 18.3 percent, alcohol alone was present in 16.1 percent, and neither drug was present in 49.1 percent.

The effects of marijuana and alcohol on a person's driving ability are additive. Thus, persons who drive should be concerned about the deterioration in driving ability that occurs when marijuana is used along with other drugs. Nearly 50 percent of regular marijuana users drink alcoholic beverages when using marijuana.[14] The combined use of these two drugs produces a greater impairment in the performance of complex tasks than does the use of either drug by itself.

Although few adverse health consequences are associated with the *acute* use of marijuana, it now appears that *chronic* use is associated with significant toxicity. The impact of these toxicities (and potential toxicities) has been examined (so far) on the lungs, the heart, the brain, and the endocrine and reproductive systems.[12]

Reports of altered *lung function* show evidence of bronchial irritation and inflammation, airway narrowing with increased reactivity to irritants (as in asthma), reduced macrophage and ciliary activity (leading to a reduced ability to clear the lungs of inhaled particulate matter), and signs of early stages of emphysema.[15] These pulmonary changes should not be surprising, because they result from the persistent and repetitive inhalation of the gases and particulate products that comprise marijuana smoke (Table 12.2). When marijuana is taken orally, the pulmonary effects are absent and the THC even seems to act beneficially by relaxing the smooth muscles of the lungs.

Aside from its irritant effects, the obvious question is whether marijuana smoke causes lung cancer. Currently, no direct evidence shows that chronic marijuana smoking causes lung cancer. However, cancers of the upper respiratory tract and tongue have been noted in persons who smoke marijuana.[16] Also, it is possible that marijuana smokers are in a prodromal phase of *Cannabis*-induced lung cancer. Cellular changes that are consistent with early cancerous stages are found in biopsies of the bronchial tubes in heavy marijuana smokers and in a variety of animal models.[17]

Of some concern is the possibility that marijuana adversely affects the *heart*. A significant increase in heart rate occurs after smoking, which has been well documented, but this increase appears to be free of adverse consequences. Patients who exhibit an existing impairment of heart function may find that the use of marijuana will precipitate chest pain (angina pectoris). Because most persons who use marijuana are younger than 35 years of age (Figure 12.1), those who suffer from impaired heart function are rare. In the future, this finding may prove to be very significant if the use of marijuana increases to include older persons or if today's younger users continue to use this drug as they progress into middle age. For now, however, it seems prudent to warn patients who may have impaired heart function not to use marijuana.

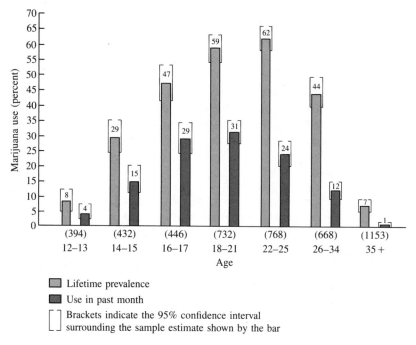

FIGURE 12.1

Marijuana (or hashish) experience by age: lifetime prevalence and use in past month, 1977. [From Secretary of Health, Education, and Welfare,[21] p. 6.]

Neither physiological nor anatomical abnormalities of the *brain* have been demonstrated convincingly in chronic users of marijuana. One persistent concern is that it leads to a gradually developing state of apathy, underachievement, loss of the work ethos, and a possible loss of goal direction. Such concerns arose during the early 1970s, when it was observed that some American armed-forces enlisted men, who used high doses of hashish on a chronic basis, exhibited apathy, dullness, impaired judgment, loss of interest in personal appearance, poor hygiene, and some loss of memory. Such effects were reversed when use of the drug was discontinued. Today, this situation, which arises from long-term, high-dose use of *Cannabis,* is called *amotivational syndrome,* or *burnout,* and is characterized by mental dulling, emotional blunting, and loss of drive and goal directedness. Although marijuana is not the only factor involved, it most likely contributes.

As stated by Cohen:

That some people become ambitionless and sluggish under the influence of a considerable amount of *Cannabis* should not be surprising. THC is a CNS depressant and chronic daytime intoxication with any sedative will demotivate people. The fact that it takes weeks to years for the process to reverse itself is more difficult to explain, and the long retention time of THC in lipids like brain tissue does not directly resolve the issue.[18]

As stated by Jaffe:

Chronic marihuana users may exhibit apathy; dullness; impairment of judgment, concentration, and memory; and loss of interest in personal appearance and pursuit of conventional goals. This has been called the "amotivational syndrome." It is clear that this may be due in part to factors other than the use of cannabis, and it is difficult to know the contribution of drug use in any given case. Cessation may lead to gradual improvement over a period of several weeks. At present there is no evidence to suggest that any personality changes are due to irreversible organic brain damage. However, the possibility of an adverse effect of frequent or chronic low levels of intoxication on developing personality cannot be dismissed.[5]

The fact that some juveniles are often heavy users of marijuana causes increased concern. Certainly, if heavy, long-term marijuana use is linked to the formation of complex social, psychological, and behavioral changes in young persons, then it is only one of many contributing factors.

Evidence has implicated long-term marijuana use with a degree of *immunosuppression*, which may render the smoker susceptible to infections, diseases, or cancer.[19,20] Although data in this area are controversial and implications have not been proved, marijuana smoking, in some circumstances, can partially suppress immunity. The clinical significance of this occurrence is not known, but it should be noted also that other depressant drugs, such as alcohol, barbiturates, benzodiazepines, and anticonvulsants, share this immunosuppressive action.

Evidence of *Cannabis*-induced suppression of *sexual function* and *reproduction* is being gathered. The chronic use of marijuana by males can reduce levels of the hormone testosterone and inhibit sperm formation.[5] Reductions in male fertility and sexual potency, however, have not been reported. Alcohol also reduces testosterone levels. In females, the hormones FSH (follicle stimulating hormone) and LH (luteinizing hormone) are reduced by marijuana. Menstrual cycles can be affected and anovulatory cycles have been reported. Because marijuana freely crosses the placenta, it probably should not be used during pregnancy.

Tolerance and Dependence

It was previously thought that physical dependence on THC did not develop, and, indeed, this appears to be true for recreational users of the drug.[21] However, drug withdrawal symptoms are observed in persons who use high doses repeatedly. Abrupt discontinuation of cannabinoids after chronic use of high doses is followed by

> irritability, restlessness, nervousness, decreased appetite, weight loss, insomnia, rebound increase in REM sleep, tremor, chills, and increased body temperature. Overall the syndrome is relatively mild, begins within a few hours after cessation of drug administration, and lasts about 4 to 5 days.[5]

Tolerance to *Cannabis* is well substantiated and is thought to result from an adaptation of the brain to the continuous presence of the drug rather than from an increased rate of elimination. Soldiers who returned from the Far East demonstrated that experienced marijuana users could tolerate quantities of the drug that were toxic to persons who were accustomed to using less. Thus, experienced, frequent users of marijuana experience less pronounced physiological and psychological changes at a constant level of use than would less-experienced users. This finding leaves little doubt that under conditions of heavier, more regular use, tolerance to THC does develop. Such heavy, long-term use is, however, still only infrequently encountered in this country. Thus, as Szara states:

> I think it is justified to conclude at this point that the development of *Cannabis*-type tolerance and physical dependence—as different from the opiate type—is a theoretical possibility, but its practical significance in a naturalistic setting (if any) is probably slight. . . . In conclusion, the results of studies presented in this volume [*The Pharmacology of Marijuana*] appear to justify the position taken by the *Fourth Marijuana and Health Report*:

"Occasional use may impair perception, cognition, and driving ability but does not lead to detectable physical or mental health consequences. Everyday light use is already suspected of producing some deleterious effects and heavy daily use undoubtedly has some consequences in the function of pulmonary, hormonal, and central nervous systems. Exactly what these consequences are and how significant remain the subject of further extensive investigations."[22]

The daily use of low doses of marijuana does not produce a clinically significant degree of tolerance, even though tolerance has been observed in persons who use high doses regularly. Some degree of cross-tolerance between alcohol and THC has been observed in rats, but no cross-tolerance occurs between THC and the psychedelic drugs.

As with other psychoactive drugs, the definition of marijuana dependence contains three critical elements:[23] (1) preoccupation with the acquisition of marijuana, (2) compulsive use of marijuana, and (3) relapse to, or recurrent use of, the drug. To date, marijuana dependence is usually observed in persons who exhibit poly-drug abuse, so few treatment programs are oriented solely toward marijuana abuse.[24-26] A twelve-step program that might be a useful approach for treating persons who exhibit marijuana dependence has been discussed.[27]

Marijuana and Public Safety

The first reports that causally linked the use of marijuana to aggression, violence, and crime appeared during the 1930s. It was felt (with little factual basis) that marijuana led to antisocial acts, to crimes of violence and aggression, and even to the use of opiates. As the Commission on Marijuana and Drug Abuse stated in 1972:

In the absence of adequate understanding of the effects of the drug . . . largely unsubstantiated stories profoundly influenced public opinion and gave birth to the stereotype of the marijuana user as physically aggressive, lacking in self-control, irresponsible, mentally ill and, perhaps most alarming, criminally inclined and dangerous. . . . Now, more than 30 years later many observers are skeptical about the existence of a cause–effect relationship between marijuana use and antisocial conduct.[21]

Major government reports conclude that there is no scientific proof that the use of marijuana, by itself, is responsible for criminal behavior. There appears to be little or no relation between marijuana and violent crime. Marijuana is much less likely than alcohol to precipitate aggressive behavior. If there is any relation between drug use and crime, other psychoactive drugs that produce aggressive behavior (such as alcohol or the amphetamines) are more likely responsible. As the National Commission on Marijuana and Drug Abuse pointed out:

> In essence, neither informed current professional opinion nor empirical research, ranging from the 1930s to the present, has produced systematic evidence to support the thesis that marijuana use, by itself, either invariably or generally leads to or causes crime, including acts of violence, juvenile delinquency, or aggressive behavior. Instead the evidence suggests that sociolegal and cultural variables account for the apparent statistical correlation between marijuana use and crime or delinquency.[28]

Conclusions

Based on the previous discussion, how should society respond to the known pharmacology of marijuana? There is now enough information on the pharmacological and toxicological effects of marijuana to begin formulating a new legal policy. Many states, in fact, have already done this by removing felony penalties for simple possession of small amounts. As the National Commission on Marijuana and Drug Abuse reported in 1972, "The State is obliged to justify restraints on individual behavior."[29] Therefore, if the state is to maintain harsh marijuana laws, it should justify their severity.

Perhaps the most conservative course of action might be for society to oppose the widespread use of marijuana as part of an attempt to discourage the use of all psychoactive drugs (at least insofar as they might endanger others), and refrain from punishing those who use marijuana (or at least mete out less severe punishment). Such a course of action was proposed by the National Commission on Marijuana and Drug Abuse, which recommended only the following changes in federal law:

> Possession of marijuana for personal use would no longer be an offense, but marijuana possessed in public would remain contraband subject to summary seizure and forfeiture.

Casual distribution of small amounts of marijuana for no remuneration, or insignificant remuneration not involving profit, would no longer be an offense.[30]

The Commission further recommended that a plea of marijuana intoxication shall not be a defense to any criminal act that was committed when a person was under its influence, nor shall proof of such intoxication constitute a negation of specific intent.[31]

These changes would essentially "decriminalize" the possession of small amounts of marijuana in all states, and persons who are apprehended with small quantities would no longer be subject to a punishment that many regard as more severe than the offense. The product would not be legalized, and the state would continue to discourage its use; but those in possession of small amounts would not be subject to punishment. The call for the legalization of marijuana was recently restated in a popular business magazine in an article that discusses the Dutch experience with controlled legalization of marijuana. It argues that

the importance of a legal market for marijuana is that it could help steer young people away from hard drugs by breaking the connection between marijuana smokers and drug pushers.[32]

Although marijuana is not a "killer weed," it is *not* an innocuous substance that is devoid of toxicity. The legal statutes should protect users, nonusers who might be affected by intoxicated users, and juveniles who might not be able to make rational decisions concerning the risks and benefits of the drug. It is up to society to determine the extent and mechanism through which protection is offered.

The explosive increase in marijuana use that occurred during the 1970s now appears to have leveled off, and it may be reaching a point of social acceptance or tolerance. States that have not yet decriminalized the possession of marijuana are recognizing the reality of its widespread use and are considering decriminalization. It is also becoming clear that little evidence supports the contention that the use of marijuana will displace the use of alcohol and other psychoactive drugs. Persons who use marijuana are also likely to use alcohol, often simultaneously.[14] The more heavily the user smokes marijuana, the greater the likelihood that he or she has used or will use other drugs. Such drug use may be related to a "drug-use proneness" and an involvement with other drug users rather than to the characteristics of marijuana per se.

It appears, then, that society is accepting and tolerating (although not yet approving) the social use of marijuana as a recreational drug. Legal guidelines for recreational use and limitations, however, are still far from decided.

STUDY QUESTIONS

1. Describe the range of potencies (concentrations) of THC in various preparations of marijuana.

2. How are the effects of THC similar to those of the nonselective depressants? How are the effects of THC dissimilar to those of the nonselective depressants?

3. How are the effects of THC similar to those of the psychedelic drugs? How are the effects of THC dissimilar to those of the psychedelic drugs?

4. How does the half-life of THC in the body reflect a person's ability to become intoxicated more easily and with a smaller amount of the drug after repeated use of marijuana?

5. Organize and discuss some of the concerns and toxicities that are associated with varying degrees of marijuana use by young adults.

6. Discuss the involvement of marijuana use in traumatic incidents and crimes of violence.

7. Organize and discuss the concerns about long-term toxicities that may possibly be associated with chronic use of marijuana.

8. Discuss the development of tolerance to and dependence on the use of marijuana?

9. How might a treatment program be organized for persons who are dependent on marijuana?

10. What do you think society's response would be to the continued illicit use of marijuana?

NOTES

1. O. Ray and C. Ksir, *Drugs, Society, and Human Behavior*, 5th ed. (St. Louis: Times Mirror/Mosby, 1990), pp. 324–325.

2. A. C. Howlett, M. R. Johnson, and L. S. Melvin, "Classical and Nonclassical Cannabinoids: Mechanism of Action—Brain Binding," in P. T. K. Pham and K. Rice, eds., *Drugs of Abuse: Chemistry, Pharmacology, Immunology, and AIDS*, NIDA Research Monograph 96 (Washington, D.C.: U.S. Government Printing Office, 1990), pp. 100–111.

3. T. R. Okrie, "Three Positive Shifts Away from Marijuana Use, 1979–1988," *Journal of School Health* 59 (1989): 34–36.

4. C. A. Soderstrom, A. L. Trifillis, B. S. Shankar, and W. E. Clark, "Marijuana and Alcohol Use Among 1023 Trauma Patients, A Prospective Study," *Archives of Surgery* 123 (1988): 733–737.

5. J. W. Jaffe, "Drug Addiction and Drug Abuse," in A. G. Gilman, T. W. Rall, A. S. Nies, and P. Taylor, eds., *Goodman and Gilman's The Pharmacological Basis of Therapeutics*, 8th ed. (New York: Pergamon, 1990), pp. 549–553.

6. E. Johansson, M. M. Halldin, S. Agurell, and L. E. Hollister, "Terminal Elimination Plasma Half-Life of Delta-1-tetrahydrocannabinol in Heavy Users of Marijuana," *European Journal of Clinical Pharmacology* 37 (1989): 273–277.

7. D. I. Hoffman, K. D. Brunemann, G. B. Gori, and E. L. Wynder, "On the Carcinogenicity of Marijuana Smoke," *Recent Advances in Phytochemistry* 9 (1975): 63–81.

8. S. Cohen, "Adverse Effects of Marijuana: Selected Issues," in R. B. Millman, P. Cushman, Jr., and J. H. Lowinson, eds., *Research Developments in Drug and Alcohol Use, Annals of the New York Academy of Sciences* 362 (1981): 120.

9. M. Pomeroy, J. J. Fennelly, and M. Towers, "Prospective Randomized Double-Blind Trial of Nabilone versus Dronabinol in the Treatment of Cytotoxic-Induced Emesis," *Cancer Chemotherapy and Pharmacology* 17 (1986): 285–288.

10. M. Manzo, "Dronabinol and Nabilone Ease Cancer Chemotherapy," *Nursing* 18 (1988): 81.

11. D. H. Gieringer, "Marijuana, Driving, and Accident Safety," *Journal of Psychoactive Drugs* 20 (1988): 93–101.

12. L. E. Hollister, "Health Aspects of *Cannabis*," *Pharmacological Reviews* 38 (1986): 1–20.

13. L. E. Hollister, "*Cannabis*—1988," *Acta Psychiatry Scandinavia* 78, Supplement 345(1988): 108–118.

14. U.S. Department of Health and Human Services, *National Survey on Drug Abuse: Main Findings, 1982* (Washington, D. C.: U. S. Government Printing Office, 1983), pp. 27–42.

15. H. Gong, Jr., S. Fligiel, D. P. Tashkin, and R. G. Barbers, "Tracheobronchial Changes in Habitual, Heavy Smokers of Marijuana with and without Tobacco," *American Review of Respiratory Disease* 136 (1987): 142–149.

16. G. A. Caplan and B. A. Brigham, "Marijuana Smoking and Carcinoma of the Tongue: Is There an Association?" *Cancer* 66 (1990): 1005–1006.

17. U.S. Department of Health and Human Services, *The Health Consequences of Smoking: The Changing Cigarette. A Report of the Surgeon General* (Washington, D.C.: U.S. Government Printing Office, 1981), pp. 81–85.

18. S. Cohen, "Adverse Effects of Marijuana: Selected Issues," in R. B. Millman, P. Cushman, Jr., and J. H. Lowinson, eds., *Research Developments in Drug and Alcohol Use, Annals of the New York Academy of Sciences* 362 (1981): 123.

19. M. D. Yahya and R. R. Watson, "Immunomodulation by Morphine and Marijuana," *Life Sciences* 41 (1987): 2503–2510.

20. L. E. Hollister, "Marijuana and Immunity," *Journal of Psychoactive Drugs* 20 (1988): 3–8.

21. Secretary of Health, Education, and Welfare, *Marihuana and Health, 7th Report to the U.S. Congress* (Washington, D.C.: U.S. Government Printing Office, 1977).

22. S. Szara, in M. C. Braude and S. Szara, eds., *The Pharmacology of Marihuana*, vol. 2 (New York: Raven Press, 1976), p. 690.

23. N. S. Miller and M. S. Gold, "The Diagnosis of Marijuana (*Cannabis*) Dependence," *Journal of Substance Abuse Treatment* 6 (1989): 183–192.

24. N. S. Miller, M. S. Gold, and B. M. Belkin, "The Diagnosis of Alcohol and *Cannabis* Dependence in Cocaine Dependence," *Advances in Alcohol and Substance Abuse* 8 (1990): 33–42.

25. A. M. Washton, "Structured Outpatient Treatment of Alcohol vs. Drug Dependencies," *Recent Developments in Alcoholism* 8 (1990): 284–304.

26. R. L. Hubbard, "Treating Combined Alcohol and Drug Abuse in Community-Based Programs," *Recent Developments in Alcoholism* 8 (1990): 273–283.

27. N. S. Miller, M. S. Gold, and A. C. Pottash, "A 12-Step Treatment Approach for Marijuana (*Cannabis*) Dependence," *Journal of Substance Abuse Treatment* 6 (1989): 241–250.

28. National Commission on Marihuana and Drug Abuse, *Marihuana: A Signal of Misunderstanding*, R. P. Shafer, chairman (New York: Signet, 1972), p. 94.

29. National Commission on Marihuana and Drug Abuse, *Marihuana: A Signal of Misunderstanding*, R. P. Shafer, chairman (New York: Signet, 1972), p. 159.

30. National Commission on Marihuana and Drug Abuse, *Marihuana: A Signal of Misunderstanding*, R. P. Shafer, chairman (New York: Signet, 1972), p. 85.

31. National Commission on Marihuana and Drug Abuse, *Marihuana: A Signal of Misunderstanding*, R. P. Shafer, chairman (New York: Signet, 1972), p. 191.

32. A. Kupfer, "What to Do About Drugs," *Fortune*, June 20, 1988, pp. 39–41.

Drugs for Neurological Disorders

Earlier chapters focused on drugs that are classified as psychoactive, and, therefore, are either subject to abuse or used therapeutically for the treatment of psychiatric diseases. However, because there is an increasing interest in the broader scope of drugs that act on the CNS, this chapter extends our discussion of neuropsychopharmacology to cover five additional classes of drugs that affect the nervous system. These agents include antiepileptic drugs, antiparkinsonian drugs, drugs that are used to treat spasticity and muscle spasms, nonnarcotic analgesic–anti-inflammatory drugs, and local anesthetics.

Antiepileptic Drugs

Seizures are manifestations of electrical disturbances that occur in the brain. The term *epilepsy* refers to CNS disorders that are characterized by seizures that have a rapid onset, a relatively brief duration of action, and a tendency toward chronic recurrences. Most seizure disorders do

TABLE 13.1

Classification of epileptic seizures.

Seizure type	Characteristics
Partial seizures (focal, local seizures)	
Simple partial seizures	Various manifestations, without impairment of consciousness, including convulsions confined to a single limb or muscle group (*Jacksonian motor epilepsy*), specific and localized sensory disturbances (*Jacksonian sensory epilepsy*), and other limited signs and symptoms depending on the particular cortical area producing the abnormal discharge
Complex partial seizures	Attacks of confused behavior, with impairment of consciousness, with a wide variety of clinical manifestations, associated with bizarre generalized EEG activity during the seizure but with evidence of anterior temporal lobe focal abnormalities even in the interseizure period in many cases
Partial seizures secondarily generalized	
Generalized seizures (convulsive or nonconvulsive)	
Absence seizures	Brief and abrupt loss of consciousness associated with high-voltage, bilaterally synchronous, 3-per-second spike-and-wave pattern in the EEG, usually with some symmetrical clonic motor activity varying from eyelid blinking to jerking of the entire body, sometimes with no motor activity
Atypical absence seizures	Attacks with slower onset and cessation than is usual for absence seizures, associated with a more heterogeneous EEG
Myoclonic seizures	Isolated clonic jerks associated with brief bursts of multiple spikes in the EEG
Clonic seizures	Rhythmic clonic contractions of all muscles, loss of consciousness, and marked autonomic manifestations
Tonic seizures	Opisthotonus, loss of consciousness, and marked autonomic manifestations
Tonic-clonic seizures (grand mal)	Major convulsions, usually a sequence of maximal tonic spasm of all body musculature followed by synchronous clonic jerking and a prolonged depression of all central functions
Atonic seizures	Loss of postural tone, with sagging of the head or falling

Source: T. W. Rall and L. S. Schleifer,[4] p. 437.

TABLE 13.2

Antiepileptic drugs that are available in the United States.

Year introduced	Generic name	Trade name
1912	Phenobarbital	Luminal
1935	Mephobarbital	Mebaral
1938	Phenytoin	Dilantin
1946	Trimethadione	Tridione
1947	Mephenytoin	Mesantoin
1949	Paramethadione	Paradione
1951	Phenacemide	Phenurone
1952	Metharbital	Gemonil
1953	Phensuximide	Milontin
1954	Primidone	Mysoline
1957	Methsuximide	Celontin
1957	Ethotoin	Peganone
1960	Ethosuximide	Zarontin
1968	Diazepam	Valium
1974	Carbamazepine	Tegretol
1975	Clonazepam	Klonopin
1978	Valproic acid	Depakene
1981	Clorazepate	Tranxene
	Lorazepam	Ativan

Source: Modified from R. M. Julien, "Antiepileptic Drugs," in N. T. Smith and A. N. Corbascio, eds., *Drug Interactions in Anesthesia*, 2d ed. (Philadelphia: Lea & Febiger, 1986), p. 246.

not disappear spontaneously, and they are rarely amenable to surgical therapy. Thus, drug therapy is the only widely applicable mode of treatment. To aid in determining the most effective drug treatment, the various types of seizure disorders are broadly classified into two groups: generalized seizures and partial seizures, with multiple subdivisions of each group (Table 13.1). Indeed, it is imperative that the type of seizure be characterized accurately, because drug therapy for epilepsy is quite selective.

Table 13.2 lists the antiepileptic drugs that are available and the year in which each one was introduced. Although the exact mechanisms of action of antiepileptic drugs remain obscure, these drugs might exert their antiepileptic actions in two general ways. First, the drug might act directly at a site of abnormal electrical activity within a person's brain to decrease its excitability. Second, the drug might act on adjacent non-epileptic neurons to limit their involvement in a spread of seizure activity that might occur at a distant site. Most antiepileptic drugs that are currently available appear to act primarily (or at least in part) by the second mechanism; that is, they limit the spread of epileptic activity in the brain. Postulated mechanisms of action include stabilizing the membranes of normal neurons and reinforcing the activity of inhibitory neurons, which serve to increase the inhibitory functions of the brain. Indeed, a dysfunction of inhibitory functions exacerbates the development and spread of seizure activity.[1,2] Current research that is aimed at developing new antiepileptic drugs is focused on agents that may selectively reinforce or potentiate the functional activity of GABA neurons by a mechanism that is similar to that of the benzodiazepines (Chapter 5). Indeed, certain benzodiazepines are among the more effective antiepileptic drugs that are available.[3]

Structure–Activity Relationships

Most antiepileptic drugs belong to one of a relatively small number of chemical classes, many of which have been discussed in earlier chapters. The *barbiturates* are the oldest of these drugs and, until recent years, these and the *hydantoins* were the most widely used antiepileptic compounds. More recently, several *benzodiazepines* have been found to be exceedingly useful. Older drugs that are structurally similar to either the barbiturates or the hydantoins (but are slightly altered to make them chemically unique) and that are used to treat epilepsy include the *succinimides*, the *oxazoladines*, and *primidone* (Mysoline). Finally, two newer agents, which are structurally dissimilar, are effective in treating seizures: *carbamazepine* (Tegretol) and *valproic acid* (Depakene). Carbamazepine structurally resembles both phenytoin and imipramine. Valproic acid exerts specific actions at GABA synapses. Structures of representative drugs are shown in Figure 13.1.

Plasma levels of antiepileptic drugs are determined by chemical assay, and those levels are correlated with the level of drug at which the seizures are brought under control. Indeed, by measuring drug concentrations in a patient's plasma, a physician may be assisted in finding the optimal pharmacological treatment for controlling that patient's seizures. Continuing progress in this area has enabled physicians to control seizures in approximately 50 percent of epileptic patients, and significant improvement has been attained for at least half of those

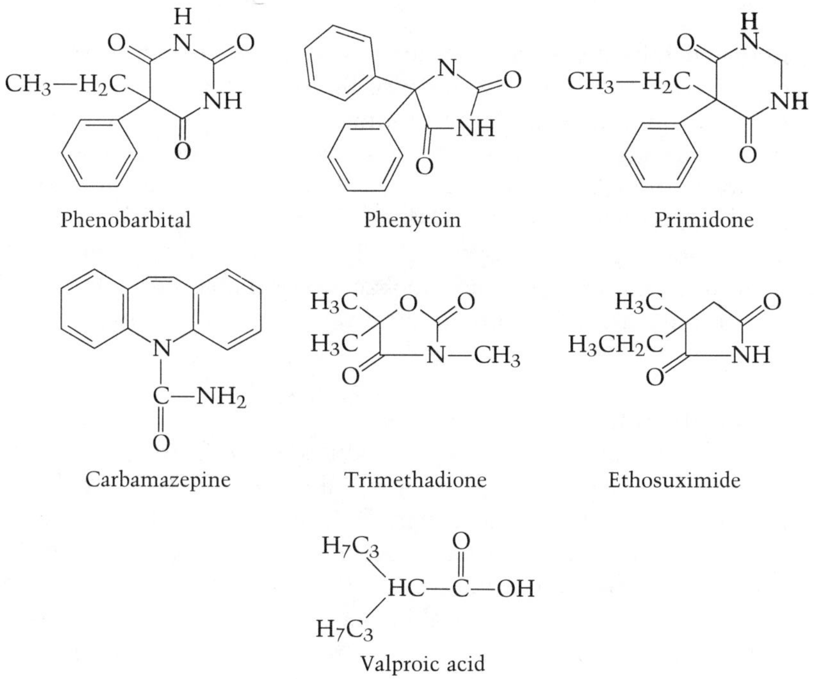

Phenobarbital

Phenytoin

Primidone

Carbamazepine

Trimethadione

Ethosuximide

Valproic acid

FIGURE 13.1

Representative drugs used in the treatment of epilepsy.

remaining. An ongoing search for new drugs and improved techniques for monitoring drug therapy is promising for the treatment of those patients who do not respond to therapies that are currently available.

Barbiturates

The pharmacology of the barbiturates was presented in Chapter 3. The barbiturates presumably exert antiepileptic effects by producing a general non-selective depression of the CNS. Phenobarbital, which was introduced in 1912, was the first widely effective antiepileptic drug. It replaced the more toxic agent, bromide, that had been used for many years. Two other barbiturates are also used occasionally for treating epilepsy: mephobarbital (Mebaral) and metharbital (Gemonil).

Because of their relative lack of toxicity, these drugs are still being used despite the fact that more effective, more specific, and less sedating antiepileptic agents are now prescribed as the drugs of first choice.[1] The barbiturates are primarily useful for treating patients who suffer from generalized seizures; they are much less effective in persons who experience partial seizures. Because the durations of action of these drugs are quite long, doses can be administered only once each day. The primary disadvantages of giving these drugs to children are the adverse neuropsychological reactions (behavioral hyperactivity and interference with learning ability) that follow. Primidone (Mysoline) is an antiepileptic agent that is structurally very similar to phenobarbital (Figure 13.1). Primidone is metabolized to phenobarbital, which might well be the major active form of the drug.

Hydantoins

Phenytoin (Dilantin), which was introduced in 1938, is the prototype for hydantoin anticonvulsants; and it is still one of the most widely used and effective antiepileptic drugs. It is used primarily for treating generalized major motor seizures. At an effective dose level, phenytoin produces less sedation than occurs with use of barbiturates. Phenytoin appears to act by exerting a stabilizing effect on neuronal membranes, limiting the involvement of those neurons in the spread of seizure activity. The drug is slowly, but completely, absorbed when it is taken orally and has a half-life of about 24 hours. Thus, it can be administered once a day. Daytime sedation can be minimized if the patient takes the full daily dose at bedtime.

Although the decreased sedative effects of phenytoin are preferable to the sedative effects of the barbiturates, other toxicities are significant. Patients who take phenytoin commonly experience ataxia (postural instability with staggering) and nystagmus. The drug can interfere with vitamin-D metabolism, and alterations of calcium metabolism and bone formation may occur. Hypertrophy of the gums occurs and commonly results in gingival and dental problems. Hirsutism (abnormal growth of hair) is also common and can be quite annoying to female patients. If phenytoin is administered to pregnant patients, fetal abnormalities frequently occur. Despite these toxicities, however, phenytoin is widely used and reasonably well tolerated for the long-term control of seizures. When a patient fails to respond to phenytoin at therapeutic blood levels, additional drugs may need to be added to the prescribed regimen.

Benzodiazepines

The pharmacology of the benzodiazepines was presented in Chapter 5. Some of these agents, for example, clonazepam (Klonopin) and clorazepate (Tranxene), are frequently used for the treatment of seizures, especially for patients whose conditions are resistant to drug therapy or for those who suffer from certain types of seizures that are difficult to treat. Diazepam (Valium) and midazolam (Versed) are administered intravenously to rapidly control episodes of status epilepticus (an emergency situation that is characterized by rapidly recurring, intense seizures).

Benzodiazepines inhibit the spread of seizures by facilitating GABA neurotransmission (Chapter 5). Also, the toxicity of benzodiazepines is relatively low. Because these drugs are used frequently for treatment of chronic seizures in children, drug-induced personality changes and learning disabilities must be carefully evaluated.

Miscellaneous Antiepileptic Drugs

Carbamazepine (Tegretol) and *valproic acid* (Depakene) are two of the newest and most useful antiepileptic drugs. Carbamazepine is structurally related to the tricyclic antidepressant imipramine (Chapter 8). It has potent antiepileptic properties and is administered either alone or with other antiepileptic drugs to treat generalized major motor seizures and complex partial seizures. For children, it is often preferred to phenobarbital. Carbamazepine is also quite effective in the treatment of psychomotor types of epilepsy (a type of seizure that does not respond to phenytoin). Possibly because of its structural resemblance to imipramine, its sedative effect is much less intense than that of the other antiepileptic agents. The primary limitations of carbamazepine include rare, but potentially serious, alterations in the cellular composition of blood (reduced numbers of white blood cells), presumably secondary to its effects on bone marrow.

Valproic acid (Depakene, Depakote) is a simple organic compound (Figure 13.1) that suppresses a wide variety of seizures. It is quite effective in the treatment of both petit mal and generalized major motor seizures in children. The drug augments the postsynaptic action of GABA on its receptors in the CNS. Valproic acid is rapidly absorbed, but its short half-life necessitates administration of multiple daily doses. The drug is particularly effective for patients in whom other types of drug therapy have failed; and reductions in the number of seizures have been observed in the majority of such patients. About 75 percent of epileptic patients respond favorably to valproic acid. Serious toxicities that are associated with the use of valproic acid are rare.

Older, seldom used antiepileptic agents include such compounds as acetazolamide (Diamox); the oxazolidinediones, trimethadione (Tridione) and paramethadione (Paradione); and the succinimides, ethosuximide (Zarontin), methsuximide (Celontin), and phensuximide (Milontin).

For the interested reader, general principles regarding the choice of drugs for the treatment of epileptic seizures are listed in the readings that are located at the end of this chapter.[1,4,5]

Antiparkinsonian Drugs

Parkinson's disease is a common neurodegenerative disease that affects approximately 500,000 persons in the United States alone. Most cases occur in persons who are over the age of 55 years. Worldwide, it affects about 1 percent of all adults over the age of 65 years. Although the cause of parkinsonism remains unknown, it is clear that it results from a deficiency in the numbers and function of dopamine-secreting neurons that are located in the basal ganglia of the brain. At the simplest level of analysis, functional activity of the basal ganglia is determined by a balance of dopamine-secreting (inhibitory) neurons and acetylcholine-secreting (excitatory) neurons. In 1960, it was reported that patients who suffered from parkinsonism demonstrated a marked deficiency of dopamine in their basal ganglia. Subsequent work has led to the hypothesis that parkinsonism may be caused by an irreversible degenerative loss of dopamine neurons in the basal ganglia and that symptoms emerge when such depletion has expanded to include more than 80 to 90 percent of the normal level of dopamine neurons. Thus, therapy is aimed at restoration from exogenous sources of the dopamine that is absent. As a result, the excitatory effects of the acetylcholine neurons that remain (with their function unopposed by dopaminergic inhibitory neurons) are antagonized.[6,7]

Pharmacological Treatment of Parkinsonism

LEVODOPA   Because a loss of dopamine is the primary problem in patients who have Parkinson's disease, replacement of the dopamine will ameliorate the symptoms of the disease. However, when dopamine is present in plasma, it does not cross the blood-brain barrier into the brain (Chapter 1). Therefore, dopamine cannot be used therapeutically. However, levodopa (DihydrOxyPhenylAlanine) (Figure 13.2), which is the immediate metabolic precursor of dopamine, *does* cross the blood-

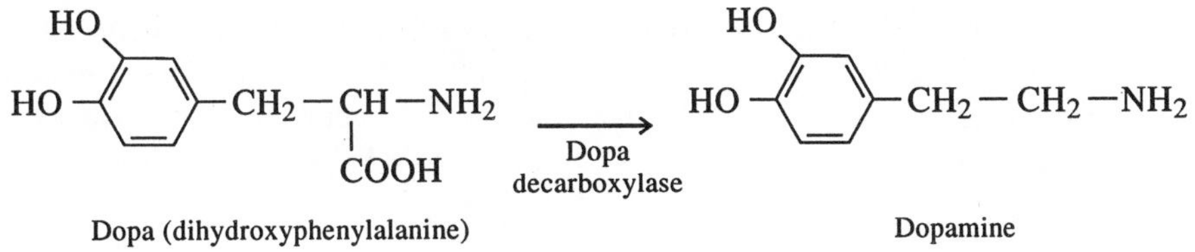

FIGURE 13.2

Decarboxylation of dopa by the enzyme dopa decarboxylase to form dopamine. Levodopa is an isomer of the naturally occurring dopa.

brain barrier and penetrates into the basal ganglia, where it is metabolized into dopamine by the enzyme dopa decarboxylase (discussed in the following text). Administered orally, levodopa is rapidly absorbed into the bloodstream, where most of it (about 95 percent) is converted to dopamine in the plasma. Although only small amounts (about 5 percent) of levodopa cross the blood-brain barrier and are converted to dopamine in the brain, even those small amounts are effective in alleviating the symptoms of parkinsonism. However, the remaining high levels of dopamine in the systemic circulation produce the side effects of nausea, vomiting, cardiac arrhythmias, and alterations in blood pressure. Thus, such therapy, though effective, is obviously not optimal. Some method is needed to reduce the high levels of dopamine in the systemic circulation while maintaining sufficient quantities in the brain.

The biosynthetic pathway of dopamine, which is illustrated in Figure 13.2, shows that the enzyme *dopa decarboxylase* is necessary for the conversion of dopa to dopamine. Thus, by inhibiting this enzyme in the systemic circulation (but not in the brain), systemic biotransformation of the drug should be reduced, with a concomitant reduction in blood levels of dopamine and, therefore, in side effects. In other words, if this dopa-decarboxylase inhibitor did not cross the blood-brain barrier, then the dopa that crossed the blood-brain barrier into the brain could still be converted to dopamine and the symptoms of parkinsonism would still be relieved; but there would be a reduction in the degree of systemic side effects. An example of such a peripherally restricted dopa-decarboxylase inhibitor is the drug *carbidopa*, which is available in combination with levodopa (Sinemet). By combining carbidopa with levodopa, a 75 percent reduction in the effective dose of levodopa can be realized, with a concomitant reduction in side effects and no loss of CNS therapeutic effect. Thus, the current treatment of parkinsonism relies heavily on this combination of levodopa and carbidopa.

Even when administered with carbidopa, levodopa still has adverse side effects. Nausea, vomiting, abnormal involuntary muscle movements, and psychiatric disturbances can occur. The drug must be used with caution in patients who suffer from hypertension or cardiac disease.

Other Drugs for Parkinsonism

AMANTADINE (SYMMETREL)   Amantadine is an antiviral agent that is used primarily to prevent certain types of influenza (flu). Several years ago, it was reported that amantadine would relieve the symptoms of parkinsonism. The mechanism that is responsible for such action is unclear, but the drug probably releases dopamine from whatever dopamine neurons remain in the patient's basal ganglia. Amantadine also appears to potentiate the therapeutic effects of levodopa, although such potentiation is not consistent. Thus, amantadine is much less effective than levodopa for long-term relief of the symptoms of parkinsonism. Adverse effects include slurred speech, ataxia, gastric distress, hallucinations, confusion, and nightmares.

ANTICHOLINERGIC DRUGS   Prior to the introduction of levodopa, use of the anticholinergic drugs was the most effective treatment for the symptoms of parkinsonism. These drugs exert their effect by blocking the excitatory cholinergic (acetylcholine) neurons that persist in the basal ganglia after the inhibitory dopamine neurons have degenerated. Representative agents include trihexyphenidyl (Artane), procyclidine (Kemadrin), and biperiden (Akineton). Significant side effects include blurred vision, constipation, urinary retention, mental confusion, and delirium. Today, these agents are used primarily during the early stages of the disease and for those patients in whom levodopa therapy has failed or has been suboptimal.

DOPAMINE RECEPTOR STIMULANTS (AGONISTS)   Over a period of 1 to 5 years after initiation of levodopa therapy, a gradual loss of responsiveness usually develops. The reason for this loss of effectiveness is unknown, but it may be related to a progressive inability of dopamine neurons to synthesize and store dopamine.[6] To alleviate this problem, attempts have been made to identify specific drugs that will directly stimulate postsynaptic dopamine receptors in the basal ganglia. To date, two such agents are available: bromocriptine (Parlodel) and per-

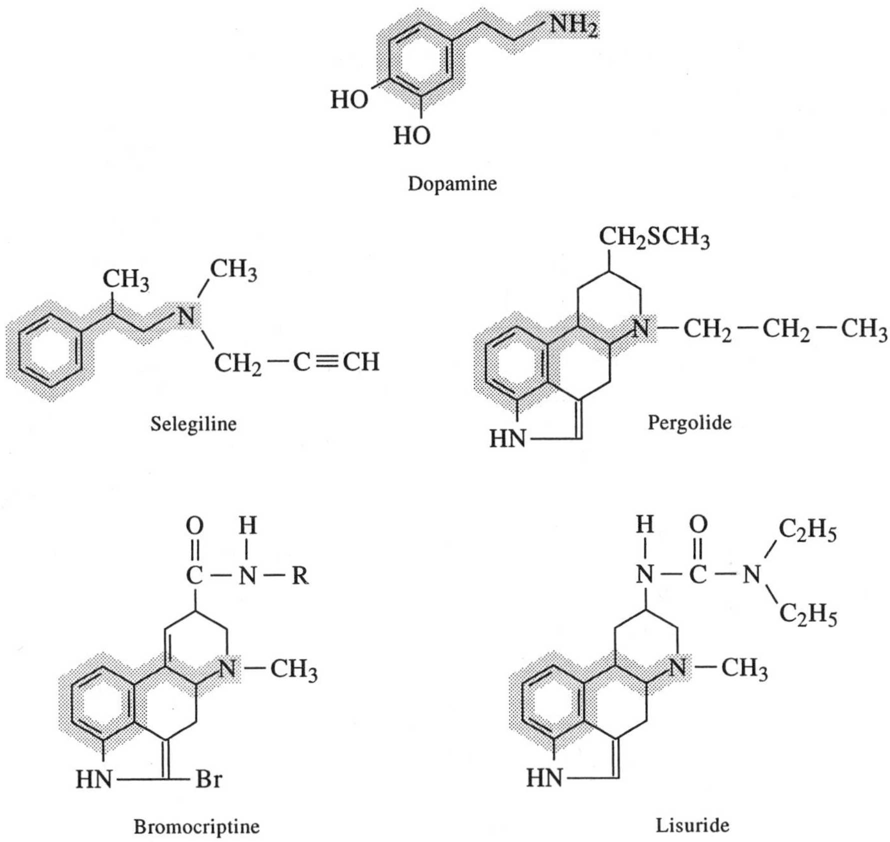

FIGURE 13.3

Structures of dopamine and dopaminergic agonists that are used in the treatment of parkinsonism. The shaded portions, which are shared in common by all these structures, resemble dopamine.

golide (Permax). Both of these drugs are derived from the ergot alkaloid lysergic acid (Chapter 11), and both contain structures that closely resemble that of dopamine (Figure 13.3). A third lysergic acid derivative (lisuride) and several nonergot agonists of dopamine receptors are being studied.[7]

Bromocriptine is a potent agonist of dopamine-2 receptors. It is used as an adjunct to levodopa in patients whose disease is not adequately controlled with levodopa. This combination improves the patient's therapeutic response to a reduced dose of levodopa and thus reduces the side effects of therapy. The efficacy of bromocriptine is often not sustained, however, and this limits its therapeutic usefulness. Wide individual variation occurs in patient responsiveness. Bromocriptine is incompletely absorbed when it is taken orally and has a plasma half-life of about 3 hours. Side effects include nausea, vomiting, hypotension, and mental disturbances, including dreams, delusions, and hallucinations.

Pergolide closely resembles bromocriptine, but it is inherently more potent and has a longer half-life. There are indications that pergolide may be effective following a loss of responsiveness to bromocriptine. Thus, a patient's failure to respond to one dopaminergic agonist may not necessarily rule out a response to another.[6]

Selegiline (Eldepryl) is also used in the treatment of parkinsonism. In Chapter 8, we discussed two subtypes of the enzyme monoamine oxidase (MAO) and the emerging use of selective MAO-A inhibitors as clinical antidepressants. In contrast to MAO-A (which is more closely involved with norepinephrine and serotonin nerve terminals), MAO-B has preferential affinity for dopamine neurons. MAO-B is inhibited by selegiline in a highly selective fashion. Selegiline also appears to inhibit the local breakdown of dopamine, thus preserving the small amounts of dopamine that are present. Both actions enhance the therapeutic effect of levodopa.[7] Selegiline is currently being used increasingly in the treatment of newly diagnosed, younger patients who have Parkinson's disease, because it appears to slow down the early progression of the disease and delays the need for initiating levodopa therapy.[8] Interestingly, selegiline is metabolized to several by-products, including amphetamine and methamphetamine, both of which potentiate dopamine neurotransmission (Chapter 6). Thus, metabolism of this drug provides a third mechanism that helps to alleviate the dopamine deficiency. In summary, selegiline may contribute to therapy for parkinsonism through any of three mechanisms: (1) inhibition of MAO-B, (2) inhibition of the breakdown of dopamine, and (3) metabolism into the active intermediates amphetamine and methamphetamine.

Drugs Used to Treat Spasticity and Muscle Spasms

Spasticity is a term that refers rather broadly to abnormal increases in skeletal muscle tone—increases that result from a dysfunction of motor pathways in the CNS.[9,10] Patients who experience spasticity have hyper-

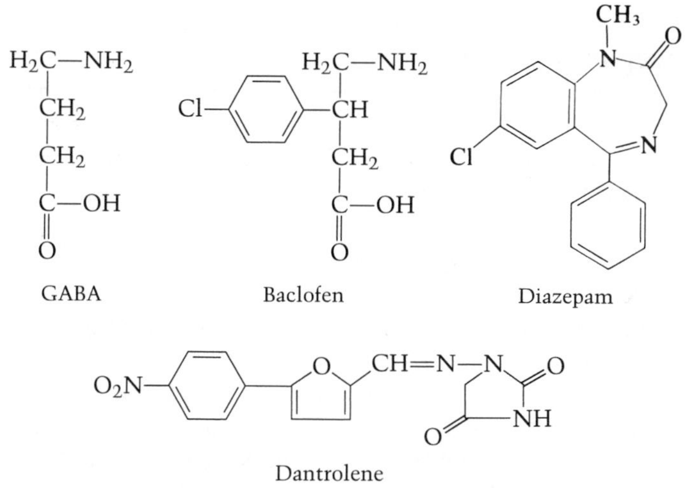

H_2C-NH_2

CH_2

CH_2

$C-OH$

O

GABA

H_2C-NH_2

$Cl-\bigcirc-CH$

CH_2

$C-OH$

O

Baclofen

CH_3

Diazepam

$O_2N-\bigcirc-O-CH=N-N-O$

$-NH$

Dantrolene

FIGURE 13.4

Structure of GABA and three drugs that are used in the treatment of spasticity. Note the resemblance of baclofen to GABA.

active reflexes because their regulation of motor control is lost. There are multiple causes of spasticity, some of which include head injury, stroke, multiple sclerosis, spinal cord trauma, and cerebral palsy. The most effective agents for controlling spasticity include two drugs that act predominantly in the CNS—baclofen (Lioresal) and diazepam (Valium)—and one, dantrolene (Dantrium), which acts directly on skeletal muscles.[10,11]

Baclofen

Baclofen (Lioresal) is a structural derivative of GABA (Figure 13.4). It reduces muscle tone and muscle spasm by altering the transmission of reflexes that travel through the polysynaptic reflex loops that are located in the spinal cord. This action may occur as a result of stimulation of GABA receptors, which inhibits the release of glutamic acid and aspartic acid (two excitatory amino acid transmitters).[12]

Baclofen appears to be more effective than either diazepam or dantrolene in relieving spasms. It is well absorbed when it is taken orally and has a relatively short half-life in plasma, which necessitates multiple daily doses. Side effects include drowsiness, lassitude, dizziness, ataxia, and muscle weakness.

Diazepam (Valium)

As discussed in Chapter 5, diazepam is a benzodiazepine that exerts its effects by facilitating GABA neurotransmission. It is somewhat less effective than baclofen in relieving spasticity. Sedation and ataxia are the primary limiting side effects of diazepam.

Dantrolene (Dantrium)

Dantrolene is unique among the antispastic agents because it acts directly on skeletal muscle.[13] Its site of action is unlike that of the neuromuscular blocking agents, which produce complete muscle paralysis by blocking postsynaptic receptors at the neuromuscular junction. Dantrolene acts at a site that is within the muscle fiber itself. It interferes with the release of calcium ions from the sarcoplasmic reticulum, thus interfering with the primary process of muscle contraction. Unfortunately, this process is not specific for hypertonic (spastic) muscles, and a generalized muscle weakness is produced. Such weakness tends to limit patient compliance in taking the drug, which negates the improvements that the drug can produce (that is, patients who take dantrolene for spasticity generally feel weak, and so they choose to limit the amount of drug that they take). Side effects of dantrolene include muscle weakness, drowsiness, and diarrhea. In rare instances, an allergic-type destruction of the liver can occur, which has been fatal in some cases.

Dantrolene has a life-saving use in general anesthesia, where it alleviates a rare, but previously fatal, syndrome termed *malignant hyperthermia*, which occurs in certain genetically predisposed patients.[14] This syndrome only occurs about once every 10,000 times that an anesthetic is given, and it is triggered by certain anesthetic agents. It involves the drug-induced, massive release of calcium from the sarcoplasmic reticulum—an action that is effectively blocked by an intravenous infusion of dantrolene.

Therapeutic Status

As stated by Cedarbaum and Schleifer:

> No completely satisfactory form of therapy is available for alleviation of skeletal muscle spasticity. While drugs such as baclofen, diazepam and dantrolene are capable of providing variable relief of spasticity in given circumstances, troublesome muscle weakness, adverse effects on gait, and a variety of other side effects minimize their overall usefulness.[11]

Muscle Spasms

In everyday life, a variety of situations can produce acute muscle spasm and pain. Numerous drugs have been employed to provide temporary, symptomatic relief of such discomfort. These drugs include anti-inflammatory analgesics (such as aspirin or ibuprofen), sedative "muscle relaxants" [such as diazepam (Valium), carisoprodol (Soma, Rela), chlorphenesin (Maolate), chlorzaxone (Paraflex), cyclobenzaprine (Flexeril), methocarbamol (Robaxin), orphenadrine (Norflex), and metaxalone (Skelaxin)]. In general, drugs have limited usefulness, but they do provide some relief until the natural healing process occurs. The combination of time, rest, and physical therapy, combined with the pharmacological provision of analgesia and sedation, are all beneficial.

Nonnarcotic Analgesic–Anti-inflammatory Drugs

The nonnarcotic analgesics are a group of chemically unrelated drugs (Figure 13.5) that produce both analgesic and anti-inflammatory effects. They block the generation of peripheral pain impulses by inhibiting the synthesis and release of prostaglandins.[*15,16] These drugs do not bind to opioid receptors. Their effects include (1) reduction of inflammation (anti-inflammatory effect), (2) reduction in body temperature when the patient has a fever (antipyretic effect), (3) reduction in pain without sedation (analgesic effect), and (4) inhibition of platelet aggregation (anticoagulant effect).

Drugs that are classified as nonnarcotic analgesics are numerous and include aspirin and other salicylates, ibuprofen, acetaminophen, indomethacin, phenylbutazone, ketorolac, and several others. Many of these drugs are used to reduce both the inflammation and the pain that are associated with arthritic disease. Gastric irritation serves to limit the long-term usefulness of these compounds.

---

[*]Prostaglandins are autacoids (Chapter 7) that induce local inflammatory responses, which include pain, fever, edema, and erythema (redness). Aspirin-like drugs inhibit the enzyme cyclooxygenase (prostaglandin synthetase), which is responsible for the biosynthesis of certain prostaglandins. In addition, recent studies[17] suggest that prostaglandin synthesis inhibition is only part of aspirin's action; the local anti-inflammatory action also results from aspirin's ability to disrupt white blood cell responsiveness to tissue injury, thus preventing the cellular release of tissue-disruptive enzymes.

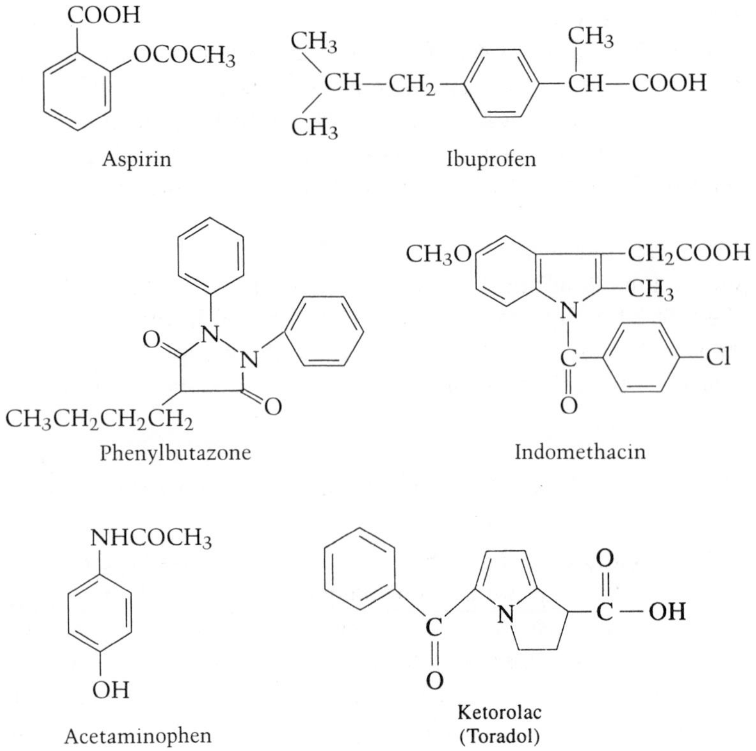

FIGURE 13.5

Chemical structures of anti-inflammatory analgesics.

Aspirin

In the United States, about 10 to 20 thousand tons of aspirin are consumed each year; it is our most popular and most effective analgesic, antipyretic (fever reducing), and anti-inflammatory drug. It is most effective for low-intensity pain (and one should note again that it does not act on opioid receptors within the CNS). The analgesic and anti-inflammatory effects follow peripheral inhibition of both prostaglandin synthesis and white blood cell responsiveness to injury. Its antipyretic effect follows the inhibition of prostaglandin synthesis in the hypothalamus—a structure in the brain that modulates body temperature. However, one caution is necessary regarding the use of aspirin to reduce fever. An association exists between the use of aspirin for the fever that accompanies varicella (chickenpox) or influenza and the subsequent development of Reye's syndrome, including severe liver and brain damage or even death.[18]

Aspirin increases oxygen consumption by the body, which increases carbon-dioxide production—an effect that stimulates respiration. Therefore, an overdose with aspirin is often characterized by a marked increase in respiratory rate, which causes the overdosed person to appear to pant. This occurrence results in other, severe metabolic consequences that are beyond this discussion.

Aspirin exerts important effects on blood coagulation.[17] For blood to coagulate, platelets must first be able to aggregate, which requires the presence of prostaglandins. (Platelets are small components of the blood that adhere to vascular membranes after a vessel injury. They form an initial plug, over which a blood clot eventually forms to limit bleeding from a lacerated blood vessel.) Aspirin can inhibit platelet aggregation and, therefore, reduce the formation of intravascular clots. Low doses of aspirin (for example, one tablet daily) are now widely used for preventing strokes and heart attacks, which can be caused by atherosclerosis, intravascular clotting, or the formation of emboli on either artificial or damaged heart valves.

Side effects of aspirin are common. Gastric upset occurs most frequently. In addition, poisoning by aspirin occurs thousands of times each year and such poisoning can be fatal. Mild intoxication can produce ringing in the ears, auditory and visual difficulties, mental confusion, thirst, and hyperventilation. The serious toxicity that is associated with Reye's syndrome has been discussed already.

Acetaminophen

Acetaminophen (Tylenol) is an effective alternative to aspirin as an analgesic and antipyretic agent. However, its anti-inflammatory effect is minor. It is not clinically useful in the treatment of acute inflammation or in the treatment of arthritis. It is commonly felt that acetaminophen may have fewer side effects than aspirin, and no reports have associated acetaminophen with Reye's syndrome. It should be noted that an acute overdose (either accidental or intentional) may produce severe or even fatal liver damage. Acetaminophen does not inhibit platelet aggregation. Therefore, it is not useful either for preventing vascular clotting or for prophylaxis against heart attacks or stroke.

Side effects of acetaminophen are generally less common than those of aspirin; the drug produces less gastric distress and less ringing in the ears. However, as stated previously, overdose can lead to severe damage to the liver. Alcoholics appear to be especially susceptible to the hepatotoxic effects of even moderate doses of acetaminophen.[19] Indeed, alcoholics should avoid the use of acetaminophen while they persist in heavy consumption of alcohol.

Acetaminophen has been proved to be a reasonable substitute for aspirin when analgesic or antipyretic effectiveness is desired, especially in children and in patients who cannot tolerate aspirin. Candidates for acetaminophen might include patients with peptic ulcer disease or gastric distress or those in whom aspirin is poorly tolerated.

Ibuprofen

Ibuprofen (Advil, Motrin, Nuprin, and Medipren) is an aspirin-like analgesic, antipyretic, and anti-inflammatory agent. Compounds that are similar to ibuprofen include *naproxen* (Naprosyn, Anaprox) and *fenoprofen* (Nalfon). Of these three drugs, only ibuprofen is available without a prescription.

All three of these compounds are effective analgesic, anti-inflammatory, and antipyretic agents. Their effectiveness is comparable to, or greater than, that of acetaminophen, aspirin, codeine, aspirin with codeine, or propoxyphene (Darvon).[16] Their actions presumably occur secondary to drug-induced inhibition of prostaglandin synthesis. The incidence and severity of side effects that are produced by these agents are somewhat lower than those of aspirin, but gastric distress and the formation of peptic ulcers have been reported. Like aspirin and unlike acetaminophen, these compounds inhibit platelet aggregation and, therefore, they interfere with the clotting process. These drugs should be used with caution in patients who suffer from peptic ulcer disease or bleeding abnormalities. At the present time, ibuprofen is not recommended for use by pregnant women. It is not secreted in breast milk.

Phenylbutazone

Phenylbutazone (Butazolidin) is an older, effective anti-inflammatory agent that was used widely at one time to relieve the inflammation that is associated with rheumatoid arthritis. However, significant toxicities have limited its long-term usefulness. Unlike most of the other anti-inflammatory drugs, its half-life is quite long (about 2 days).

Most patients who take phenylbutazone experience some degree of toxicity, usually in the form of gastric distress and skin rashes. More severe toxicities include ulcer formation, allergies, liver and renal dysfunction, and a variety of quite severe abnormalities in various types of blood cells. At the present time, phenylbutazone is considered to be a secondary choice of treatment for the symptoms of rheumatoid arthritis and other similar disorders.

Indomethacin

Indomethacin (Indocin) is an effective anti-inflammatory drug that is used primarily for the treatment of rheumatoid arthritis and similar disorders. Like phenylbutazone, its use is limited because of its toxicities. Indomethacin is an analgesic, antipyretic, and anti-inflammatory agent. Indeed, its clinical effects closely resemble those of aspirin. Side effects occur in about 50 percent of the patients who take indomethacin, with gastric dysfunction being most prominent. Paradoxically, drug-induced headache limits its use in many patients. Other toxicities are rare but potentially serious.

Ketorolac

Ketorolac (Toradol) is a newly introduced analgesic–anti-inflammatory agent. It is the first (and only) of these agents to be available in injectable form for use in the management of pain. Administered intramuscularly, it is quite effective in the short-term postoperative treatment of moderate to severe pain.[20,21] Like the analgesics already discussed, it indirectly inhibits prostaglandin synthesis. Its analgesic potency is comparable to that of low doses of morphine that are administered intramuscularly, and it appears to offer greater anti-inflammatory action. Its half-life is about 4 to 6 hours in most persons, but it is longer in the elderly. Ketorolac is not recommended for use in obstetrics (because it and all other prostaglandin-synthesis inhibitors can adversely affect uterine contraction and fetal circulation).[20]

Local Anesthetics

Local anesthetics are drugs that temporarily interrupt the conduction of electrical impulses in nerve tissue.[22–24] An *ideal* local anesthetic should not irritate the tissues to which it is applied; it should not cause any damage to nerve structures; it should not be toxic after it is absorbed from the site of injection into the bloodstream; and it should have a predictable duration of action. It should be noted that none of the local anesthetics that are available quite meet all these requirements. Also, reversibility of action is mandatory, because normal nerve conduction must be regained after the drug has been removed from the nerve tissue. This latter requirement is met by all local anesthetics that are available.

Mechanism of Action

Local anesthetics block the conduction of nerve impulses by acting directly on nerve-cell membranes. At appropriate concentrations, sensory, autonomic, and motor nerve fibers can all be completely, yet reversibly, blocked. As discussed in Appendix I, the neuronal membrane is a semipermeable, lipid–protein structure that maintains a large difference in the concentration of sodium and potassium ions across the membrane. This separation of ions maintains a resting electrical potential of minus 75 to 90 mV, with the interior side of the membrane negatively charged relative to its exterior side. Transient fluctuations occur in the sodium-ion permeability as electrical impulses are conducted along the axons of the neuron. However, when the axons are at rest, the channels through which the sodium ions travel are blocked by calcium ions. Thus, the prevailing theory holds that local anesthetics act by displacing calcium ions from the inner surface of the neuronal membrane, blocking the sodium channels and preventing the depolarization-induced movement of sodium ions across the membranes. This action blocks the process of depolarization and the propagation of nerve impulses.

Classification

The chemical structure of local anesthetics comprises three parts. Each molecule includes an aromatic ring, an intermediate chain, and a nitrogen-containing (amine) portion (Figure 13.6). The aromatic ring accounts for the fat solubility of the anesthetic, and the amine portion accounts for its water solubility. Changes in either portion alter the fat–water distribution of the drug and thus affect its duration of action. The intermediate chain can be either an ester or an amide. Anesthetics that contain ester intermediate chains are metabolized in the plasma by an enzyme called *plasma cholinesterase,* whereas anesthetics that contain an amide intermediate chain are metabolized by enzymes in the liver. The metabolic end product of the ester-type anesthetics is *para-aminobenzoic acid*—a compound that contributes to the development of allergic reactions in a small percentage of patients. Allergic reactions to the amide-type local anesthetics are extremely rare. Table 13.3 classifies local anesthetics by the type of their intermediate chains as well as by potency and duration of action. With the exception of tetracaine, the

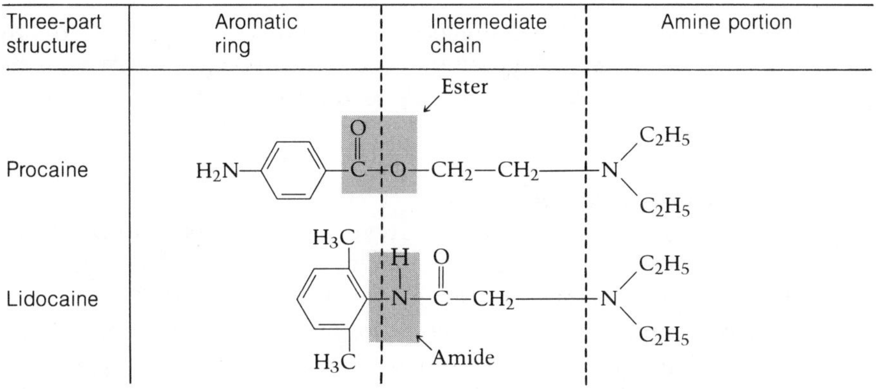

FIGURE 13.6

Structural formulas of procaine and lidocaine, illustrating the three-part structure of each. [Reproduced from R. M. Julien,[22] p. 121, with permission of the publisher.]

TABLE 13.3

Classification of local anesthetics.

Generic name	Trade name	Class	Onset	Potency	Toxicity	Duration (min)
Low potency, short duration of action						
Procaine	Novocain	Ester	Moderate	1	1	60
Chloroprocaine	Nesacaine	Ester	Fast	1	1	45
Intermediate potency and duration of action						
Lidocaine	Xylocaine	Amide	Fast	2	2	120
Mepivacaine	Carbocaine	Amide	Moderate	2	2	150
High potency, long duration of action						
Tetracaine	Pontocaine	Ester	Slow	10	10	180
Bupivacaine	Marcaine	Amide	Moderate	10	10	200+
Etidocaine	Duranest	Amide	Moderate	6	6	200+

Source: R. M. Julien,[22] p. 121.

ester-type local anesthetics are less potent and have a shorter duration of action than the amide type. Note that as their potency increases, their toxicities (discussed in the following section) also increase.

Uses of Local Anesthetics

Local anesthetics are used to block reversibly the conduction of nerve impulses through the nerve fibers that lie close to the point of injection. Therefore, they are used to (1) provide local anesthesia when they are injected into the skin, (2) to block major nerve trunks that are distal to the site of injection prior to surgery, (3) to produce complete sensory and motor blockade prior to surgery when they are injected into the spinal canal (as a spinal or epidural anesthetic), or (4) to relieve the pain that is associated with labor and delivery.

Side Effects and Toxicities

Following their injection near nerve fibers, local anesthetics are slowly absorbed into the bloodstream. If concentrations of the anesthetic reach sufficient levels in the plasma, effects can occur both in the brain and in the cardiovascular system.

In the brain, local anesthetics initially produce sedation, dizziness, and light-headedness. As levels in the brain increase, toxicities are associated with slurred speech, muscular twitching, and convulsions with loss of consciousness. This toxicity can be reduced by administering a benzodiazepine, such as diazepam, although in some cases mechanical support of ventilation also may be necessary.

Local anesthetics can produce significant effects on the cardiovascular system. At low doses, local anesthetics are mild cardiac depressants and are clinically useful in treating certain types of cardiac arrhythmias. Lidocaine, for example, suppresses ventricular arrhythmias, an effect that can be lifesaving in cardiac emergencies. At high doses, these depressant effects can lead to hypotension and cardiovascular collapse. The most cardiotoxic of the local anesthetics that are available currently are the long-acting amide anesthetics, bupivacaine and etidocaine.

All local anesthetics cross the placenta, which is a matter of concern when these drugs are used for the relief of pain during labor and delivery. However, no adverse effects appear to result from such placental transport. Indeed, local anesthetics are widely used (especially in epidural anesthesia) during labor and delivery to provide relief of pain for the mother without exerting adverse effects on the fetus.

STUDY QUESTIONS

1. What is a seizure? Through what mechanisms might a seizure be controlled?

2. Name the two newest antiepileptic drugs. For what use (other than seizures) were these drugs discussed? (See Chapter 8.)

3. Describe the etiology of Parkinson's disease.

4. Through what mechanisms might the symptoms of Parkinson's disease be alleviated? Give an example of a drug that might act by each mechanism.

5. Why is a dopa-decarboxylase inhibitor administered together with levodopa?

6. Discuss the enzyme subtypes MAO-A and MAO-B, and describe how they relate to the treatment of both depression and parkinsonism. (See Chapter 8.)

7. Selegeline is metabolized to by-products that include amphetamine. How does this occurrence affect parkinsonian therapy?

8. Differentiate between the actions of aspirin and of morphine.

9. Compare and contrast aspirin and acetaminophen.

10. How do local anesthetics work?

NOTES

1. American Medical Association, "Antiepileptic Drugs," in *Drug Evaluations Annual 1991* (Milwaukee, Wis.: American Medical Association, 1990), pp. 303–338.

2. M. A. Dichter and G. F. Ayala, "Cellular Mechanisms of Epilepsy: A Status Report," *Science* 237 (1987): 157–164.

3. K. Gale, "GABA in Epilepsy," *Epilepsia* 30, Supplement 3 (1989): S1–S11.

4. T. W. Rall and L. S. Schleifer, "Drugs Effective in the Therapy of the Epilepsies," in A. G. Gilman, T. W. Rall, A. S. Nies, and P. Taylor, eds., *Goodman and Gilman's The Pharmacological Basis of Therapeutics*, 8th ed. (New York: Pergamon, 1990), pp. 436–462.

5. D. M. Woodbury, J. K. Penry, and C. E. Pippenger, eds., *Antiepileptic Drugs*, 2d ed. (New York: Raven Press, 1982).

6. American Medical Association, "Drugs Used in Extrapyramidal Movement Disorders," in *Drug Evaluations Annual 1991* (Milwaukee, Wis.: American Medical Association, 1990), pp. 339–356.

7. J. M. Cedarbaum and L. S. Schleifer, "Drugs for Parkinson's Disease, Spasticity, and Acute Muscle Spasms," in A. G. Gilman, T. W. Rall, A. S. Nies, and P. Taylor, eds., *Goodman and Gilman's The Pharmacological Basis of Therapeutics*, 8th ed. (New York: Pergamon, 1990), pp. 463–484.

8. J. W. Tetrud and J. W. Langston, "The Effect of Deprenyl (Selegiline) on the Natural History of Parkinson's Disease," *Science* 245 (1989): 519–522.

9. B. Bishop, "Spasticity: Its Physiology and Management," *Physical Therapy* 57 (1977): 371–401.

10. R. R. Young and P. J. Delwaide, "Drug Therapy of Spasticity," *New England Journal of Medicine* 304 (1981): 28–33, 96–99.

11. J. M. Cedarbaum and L. S. Schleifer, "Drugs for Parkinson's Disease, Spasticity and Acute Muscle Spasms," in A. G. Gilman, T. W. Rall, A. S. Nies, and P. Taylor, eds., *Goodman and Gilman's The Pharmacological Basis of Therapeutics*, 8th ed. (New York: Pergamon, 1990), pp. 479–482.

12. American Medical Association, "Drugs Used for Spasticity and Muscle Spasm," in *Drug Evaluations Annual 1991* (Milwaukee, Wis.: American Medical Association, 1990), p. 368.

13. R. M. Pinder, et al. "Dantrolene Sodium: Review of Pharmacological Properties and Therapeutic Efficacy in Spasticity," *Drugs* 13 (1977): 323.

14. G. A. Gronert, "Malignant Hyperthermia," *Seminars in Anesthesia* 2 (1983): 197–204.

15. P. A. Insel, "Analgesic-Antipyretics and Anti-Inflammatory Agents: Drugs Employed in the Treatment of Rheumatoid Arthritis and Gout," in A. G. Gilman, T. W. Rall, A. S. Nies and P. Taylor, eds., *Goodman and Gilman's The Pharmacological Basis of Therapeutics*, 8th ed. (New York: Pergamon, 1990), pp. 638–681.

16. American Medical Association, "Analgesics," in *Drug Evaluations Annual 1991* (Milwaukee, Wis.: American Medical Association, 1990), pp. 101–119.

17. G. Weissmann, "Aspirin," *Scientific American* 264 (1991): 84–90.

18. P. Pinsky, E. S. Hurwitz, L. B. Schonberger, and W. J. Gunn, "Reye's Syndrome and Aspirin. Evidence for a Dose-Response Effect," *Journal of the American Medical Association* 260 (1988): 657–661.

19. L. B. Seeff, B. A. Cuccherini, H. J. Zimmerman, E. Adler, and S. B.

Benjamin, "Acetaminophen Hepatotoxicity in Alcoholics. A Therapeutic Misadventure," *Annals of Internal Medicine* 104 (1986): 399–404.

20. Medical Letter, Inc., "Ketorolac Tromethamine," in *The Medical Letter on Drugs and Therapeutics* 32 (1990): 79–81.

21. M. M.-T. Buckley and R. N. Brogden, "Ketorolac: Review of Its Pharmacodynamic and Pharmacokinetic Properties, and Therapeutic Potential," *Drugs* 39 (1990): 86–109.

22. R. M. Julien, *Understanding Anesthesia* (Stoneham, Mass.: Butterworth, 1984), pp. 119–124.

23. J. M. Ritchie and N. M. Green, "Local Anesthetics," in A. G. Gilman, T. W. Rall, A. S. Nies, and P. Taylor, eds., *Goodman and Gilman's The Pharmacological Basis of Therapeutics*, 8th ed. (New York: Pergamon, 1990), pp. 311–331.

24. American Medical Association, "Local Anesthetics," in *Drug Evaluations Annual 1991* (Milwaukee, Wis.: American Medical Association, 1990), pp. 141–155.

Birth Control and Fertility

How Drugs Modify Reproductive Systems

Neurons interact with one another through the liberation of chemical neurotransmitters. A neurotransmitter is secreted from the presynaptic terminal of one neuron; it diffuses across a narrow synaptic cleft; and then it acts on the postsynaptic membrane of the next neuron. These chemical transmitters are also appropriately called *neurohormones* because, by definition, a hormone is a substance that is released by one type of cell and then (after traveling some distance) exerts its effect on a different organ or structure. However, the neurotransmitters only travel a very short distance from their sites of release to their sites of action (across the synaptic cleft). The other normal hormones of the body (compounds such as estrogen, insulin, thyroid hormone, growth hormone, testosterone, and so on) are released by secretory cells into the bloodstream, and then they are transported to target organs that are a great distance away.

In addition to this physiological similarity between hormones and neurotransmitters, the brain exerts a regulatory role over the synthesis and release of both. For example, estrogen is the female hormone that is

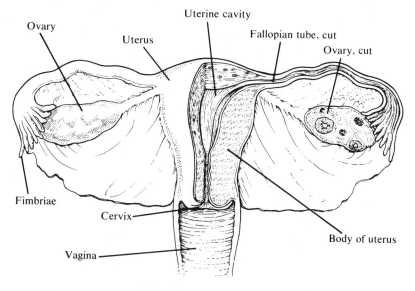

Ovary

Uterus

Uterine cavity

Fallopian tube, cut

Ovary, cut

Fimbriae

Cervix

Vagina

Body of uterus

FIGURE 14.1

Principal organs of the female reproductive system.

released from the ovaries, but it is regulated by another hormone that is released from the hypothalamus (which has a receptor for estrogen) and is, therefore, sensitive to the level of estrogen in the bloodstream. When the level of estrogen is low, the hypothalamus releases a hormone that causes stimulation of the ovaries, which, ultimately, results in the production and release of estrogen. Birth-control pills, which contain a form of estrogen that is synthetically produced and a form of progesterone (called a *progestin*) that is also synthetically produced, prevent conception largely through the actions of these two drugs on their receptors that are located in the hypothalamus. Thus, estrogen exerts prominent effects on the hypothalamus, and this "hormone feedback loop" is the mechanism through which the levels of estrogen are regulated in the body.

Regulation of the Menstrual Cycle

Figure 14.1 illustrates the principal organs of the human female reproductive system. These organs include the ovaries, the fallopian tubes, the uterus, and the vagina. The reproductive process involves the development of ova (eggs) in the ovaries. Once developed, a single ovum is released and is taken up (captured) by extensions of the fallopian tubes, called *fimbriae* (see Figure 14.1), which gather the ovum into the fallopian tube. The ovum is then transported down the tube into the uterus. If the ovum becomes fertilized by a sperm (usually during its passage down the fallopian tube), it implants itself in the body of the uterus, where it develops into a fetus and a placenta.

The Monthly Ovarian Cycle

After puberty and the development of ovarian function, the normal sex life of a woman is characterized by monthly rhythmic changes in the secretion of various sex hormones, together with corresponding changes in the activity of the female sexual organs themselves. The duration of this cycle averages 28 days, but it may vary from 20 days to as long as 45 days.

In order to accomplish the two most important aims of this cycle—the development and release of a single ovum and the proliferation of a uterine endometrium that is prepared for the implantation of a fertilized ovum—a coordinated sequence of hormonal events must occur. This sequence of events is illustrated in Figure 14.2. At the beginning of the cycle, the levels of both estrogen and progesterone in the bloodstream are low, the endometrium that was built up during the preceding cycle begins to slough, and a several-day period of menstruation occurs. Because the levels of estrogen and progesterone are low, the cells in the hypothalamus begin to release the gonadotropin-releasing factor (GRF) hormone. GRF is a 10 amino acid peptide (a small protein), which, on release, is transported in the bloodstream from the hypothalamus to the pituitary gland, where it induces release of the follicle-stimulating hormone (FSH) and the luteinizing hormone (LH) from the pituitary gland.[1] In response to FSH in the bloodstream, a variable number of ovarian follicles (each one containing an ovum) begin to enlarge. Then, after 5 or 6 days, one of these ovarian follicles begins to develop more rapidly than the others, and the ovum begins to mature.

The maturing ovum then begins to release small quantities of estrogen into the circulating blood. The estrogen inhibits further secretion of GRF from the hypothalamus and, therefore, inhibits further release of FSH from the pituitary gland. This inhibition results in the regression of the other follicles that had also started to develop. The secretion of estrogen by the one maturing ovum and the follicle in which it is contained reaches a peak just before midcycle (day 14). Near the end of this preovulatory phase, LH release peaks and prepares the ovarian follicle for ovulation by stimulating it to grow rapidly. The

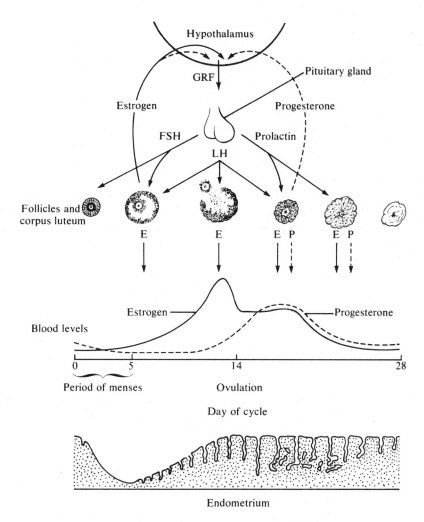

FIGURE 14.2

Sequence of events in brain, ovaries, and uterus during the monthly ovarian cycle in females. GRF, gonadotropin-releasing factor; FSH, follicle-stimulating hormone; LH, luteinizing hormone; E, estrogen; P, progesterone. *Solid arrows*, stimulation. *Dashed arrows*, inhibition.

follicle swells to the point at which it eventually ruptures, and the developed ovum is released. This occurrence is referred to as the time of *ovulation*. Because LH is necessary for the final preovulatory development of the follicle and subsequent ovulation, the follicle will not rupture and ovulation will be inhibited if LH is not present (even with large quantities of FSH).

After ovulation, the ovum is gathered by the fimbriae into one of the fallopian tubes, where fertilization by a sperm may occur. The ovum (whether it is fertilized or not) then enters the uterus. The follicle from which the ovum was released changes to become a structure (called the *corpus luteum*) that secretes both estrogen and progesterone. These hormones released from the corpus luteum maintain the uterus in a state that is conducive to receiving a fertilized ovum. This state is established by the maintenance of a highly vascular endometrial lining (or endometrium) on the wall of the uterus. In addition, the estrogen and progesterone that are released from the corpus luteum act on the hypothalamus to inhibit the release of GRF. During the next 10 days, the corpus luteum regresses and, within about 12 days, it ceases to function. Estrogen and progesterone are no longer released by the corpus luteum, menstruation begins, and a new cycle follows if fertilization does not occur. If the ovum is fertilized and implanted, the endometrium begins to secrete large quantities of hormones that act to maintain pregnancy and prevent menstrual sloughing.

Oral Contraceptives

Oral contraceptives are the most effective technique for preventing pregnancy. Preparations that are available can be classified according to their steroid content (Table 14.1):

1. Fixed combinations that contain constant amounts of an estrogen (usually ethinyl estradiol) and progestin (for example, norethindrone).[*]
2. Multiphasic combinations that contain constant amounts of estrogen that are combined with variable amounts of progestin (the dose of progestin changes from 1 week to the next).
3. "Minipills" that contain constant amounts of progestin only.[2]

During the early 1960s, the availability of orally absorbed estrogen and progestin fueled the technology to develop pharmacological control of ovulation as a means of preventing pregnancy. The problem was to find an appropriate combination of estrogen and progestin that

---

[*]Naturally occurring estrogen and progesterone cannot be utilized, since neither of them is absorbed following oral administration. Thus, synthetically produced derivatives that are effectively absorbed from the gastrointestinal tract are used. Two estrogens and four progestins are available in currently marketed products (Table 14.1).

TABLE 14.1

Oral contraceptives that are available in the United States.

| Trade name | Manufacturer | Steroid composition | | | |
		Progestin	mg	Estrogen	µg
Brevicon	Syntex	Norethindrone	0.5	Ethinyl estradiol	35
Demulen 1/35	Searle	Ethynodiol	1.0	Ethinyl estradiol	35
Demulen 1/50	Searle	Ethynodiol	1.0	Ethinyl estradiol	50
Loestrin-1/20	Parke-Davis	Norethindrone	1.0	Ethinyl estradiol	20
Loestrin-1.5/30	Parke-Davis	Norethindrone	1.5	Ethinyl estradiol	30
Lo/Ovral	Wyeth	Norgestrel	0.3	Ethinyl estradiol	30
Micronor	Ortho	Norethindrone	0.35	—	—
Modicon	Ortho	Norethindrone	0.50	Ethinyl estradiol	35
Nordette	Wyeth	Levonorgestrel	0.15	Ethinyl estradiol	30
Norinyl 1 & 35	Syntex	Norethindrone	1.0	Ethinyl estradiol	35
Norinyl 1 & 50	Syntex	Norethindrone	1.0	Mestranol	50
Norlestrin -1/50	Parke-Davis	Norethindrone	1.0	Ethinyl estradiol	50
Norlestrin-2.5/50	Parke-Davis	Norethindrone	2.5	Ethinyl estradiol	50
Nor-Q.D.	Syntex	Norethindrone	0.35	—	—
Ortho-Novum 7/7/7	Ortho	Norethindrone	0.5, 0.75, 1	Ethinyl estradiol	35
Ortho-Novum 10/11	Ortho	Norethindrone	0.5, 1.0	Ethinyl estradiol	35
Ortho-Novum 1/35	Ortho	Norethindrone	1.0	Ethinyl estradiol	35
Ortho-Novum-1/50	Ortho	Norethindrone	1.0	Mestranol	50
Ortho-Novum-1/80	Ortho	Norethindrone	1.0	Mestranol	80
Ortho-Novum-2	Ortho	Norethindrone	2.0	Mestranol	100
Ovcon-35	Mead Johnson	Norethindrone	0.4	Ethinyl estradiol	35
Ovcon-50	Mead Johnson	Norethindrone	1.0	Ethinyl estradiol	50
Ovral	Wyeth	Norgestrel	0.5	Ethinyl estradiol	50
Ovrette	Wyeth	Norgestrel	0.075	—	—
Tri-Norinyl	Syntex	Norethindrone	0.5, 1, 0.5	Ethinyl estradiol	35
Tri-Levlen	Berlex	Levonorgestrel	0.5, 0.075, 0.125	Ethinyl estradiol	30, 40, 30
Triphasil	Wyeth	Levonorgestrel	0.5, 0.075, 0.125	Ethinyl estradiol	30
Levlen	Berlex	Levonorgestrel	0.15	Ethinyl estradiol	30
Nelova 1/35	Warner-Chilcott	Norethindrone	1.0	Ethinyl estradiol	35
Nelova 10/11	Warner-Chilcott	Norethindrone	0.5, 1.0	Ethinyl estradiol	35
Nelova 1/50	Warner-Chilcott	Norethindrone	1.0	Ethinyl estradiol	50
Norethin 1/35	Searle	Norethindrone	1.0	Ethinyl estradiol	35
Norethin 1/50	Searle	Norethindrone	1.0	Ethinyl estradiol	50

would effectively suppress ovulation but limit the number and the intensity of side effects that occur as a result of its use. Excessive amounts of estrogen and progestin produce abnormal menstrual bleeding, whereas insufficient amounts might not completely inhibit the release of GRF, which might result in an unwanted pregnancy. Today, four decades after the introduction of these agents, it can truly be said that close-to-optimal balances have been achieved. The new oral contraceptives are extremely safe and very effective at blocking conception.[3] Indeed, we are likely at, or near, the lowest dose levels that can be achieved without sacrificing efficacy.

All but three of the oral contraceptive products that are currently available are combination products, which are in the form of low-dose, regular, or variable-dose preparations. The low-dose combination pills contain 30 to 35 micrograms of ethinyl estradiol and afford a reasonable compromise between the toxicities that are produced by too much estrogen and the bothersome breakthrough bleeding that results from too little estrogen. Because the regular-dose products contain 50 micrograms of ethinyl estradiol, use of them is diminishing rapidly in favor of the lower-dose products (which appear to be equally effective in preventing pregnancy, while causing only modest increases in breakthrough bleeding). A small number of products contain more than 50 micrograms of estrogen (usually mestranol), and these products are used even less frequently (most are among the earliest products marketed). The variable-dose products are either *biphasic* or *triphasic*, depending on the number of dosage variations that are possible for administration within a given month's cycle. These products are designed to reduce the total hormone content that is administered to the body throughout the menstrual cycle and, at the same time, to provide contraception that is comparable to that obtained from products that contain higher doses.

The three progestin-only pills are occasionally termed "minipills," and the rationale for their use is discussed later.

The combination oral contraceptives are taken for 21 days of the menstrual cycle (usually days 5 to 24, counting day 1 as the first day of menstruation). This is followed by 1 week without medication, toward the end of which withdrawal bleeding (menstruation) occurs. The progestin-only pills are taken daily and continuously.

Combination of Estrogen and Progestin

By combining estrogen and progestin, release of both FSH and LH is blocked (by means of negative feedback effects on both the pituitary gland and the hypothalamus); ovarian follicles do not develop; and no ovulation occurs. The estrogen primarily inhibits the release of FSH. The progestin suppresses the release of LH and acts directly on the uterus to produce an endometrium that will not accept the implantation of a fertilized ovum. The progestin thickens the normal mucus discharge of the cervix so that sperm cannot gain access to the uterus and fallopian tubes (where fertilization occurs). In addition to suppressing FSH release, the estrogen also stabilizes the uterine lining (the endometrium) so that irregular shedding and unwanted breakthrough bleeding will not occur. The estrogen also potentiates the action of the progestin.[3] All these actions minimize the likelihood of conception and implantation as long as the pills are taken faithfully.

Progestational Contraceptives

During the early 1980s, there was concern that long-term use of the estrogen that is contained in the combination estrogen–progestin contraceptives might be harmful. These fears prompted the use of continuous progestational therapy without concomitant administration of estrogen.

If a progestational agent is given alone (in which case an ovarian follicle might still mature), an endometrium that is not receptive to an ovum and a thick cervical mucus that is impervious to sperm transport are produced. Thus, even if fertilization does occur, the progestin will tend to prevent implantation of the fertilized ovum in the endometrium.

This discussion of *tendencies,* however, illustrates that the administration of a product that consists only of progestin (of which three are currently available) is not quite as reliable as the administration of a combination product (statistics indicate an approximately threefold increase in the incidence of unwanted pregnancies). However, for women who experience significant side effects as a result of using combination products, the administration of products that contain progestin only affords better contraceptive protection than do foams, creams, jellies, or rhythm; and it is certainly far better than no contraception at all. Table 14.2 offers a comparison of pregnancy rates for women who take oral contraceptives with rates for those who use other nonsurgical forms of contraception.[3]

Undesirable Effects

The frequent, mild side effects that are induced by the contraceptive pill resemble those that are experienced during early pregnancy and are generally attributed to the estrogen that is contained in the combination

TABLE 14.2

Pregnancies per 100 woman-years.

Contraception method	Range
Oral contraceptive pills, combination	1
Oral contraceptive pills, progestin only	2–3
Intrauterine device (IUD)	1–6
Diaphragm with spermicidal cream or gel	2–20
Condom	3–36
Spermicidal aerosol foams	2–29
Spermicidal gels and creams	4–36
Periodic abstinence ("rhythm")	
All types	1–47
Calendar method	14–47
Temperature method	1–20
Mucus method	1–25
No contraception	60–80

products. These side effects are usually related to the dose, and products that have less estrogen generally have milder side effects. These effects include nausea, occasional vomiting, headache, dizziness, weight gain, and breast discomfort.

All these side effects may be alleviated if a product is taken that has low doses of estrogen (30 micrograms) or progestin only. The incidence of breakthrough bleeding decreases with increasing doses of estrogen.

Other side effects are generally not too bothersome; they include weight gain and psychological changes that may result in depression in some women. These side effects are most frequently seen when progestin-only pills are taken or when Depo-Medrol (a long-acting, injectable progestin) is injected every three months (quarterly). Vaginal infections appear to be more common and more resistant to treatment in women who take oral contraceptives than in women who do not.

When administration of these agents is stopped, normal cyclic periods are usually resumed, but often not immediately reestablished. It may take several months or, possibly, even longer to reestablish a normal cycle, presumably because the hypothalamus, pituitary gland, and ovaries have been suppressed for a prolonged period of time. Approximately 95 percent of women whose menstrual periods were normal before taking oral contraceptives resume normal periods within a few months after they stop taking the drug. Indeed, in those women who discontinue oral contraceptives to become pregnant, 50 percent conceive within 3 months and, more important, after 2 years, only 7 to 15 percent have failed to conceive. Thus, infertility does not seem to occur often, if at all, in women who discontinue the use of oral contraceptives.

Serious Side Effects

The possibility that oral contraceptives will cause serious side effects has been a source of concern. However, with the advent of the newer, low-dose oral contraceptives, such concerns have largely dissipated. Concerns that we will address include: (1) cardiovascular risks (arteriosclerosis, venous thromboembolism, heart attacks, stroke, hypertension, and lipoprotein and cholesterol imbalance), (2) cancer risks (especially uterine, cervical, liver, or breast), (3) diabetes mellitus (sugar diabetes), and (4) postpill effects on reproduction.

No group of pharmacological agents has been studied more than the oral contraceptives.[4] All efforts have been directed at maximizing the benefits of drug use while minimizing potential risks, especially those involving the cardiovascular system. Decreasing the amount of estrogen from 100–150 micrograms per tablet (levels in the pills of the 1960s) to 30–35 micrograms per tablet (levels of today) has been accompanied by drastic reductions in the *cardiovascular risks*. In healthy women who are not predisposed to these conditions, the risks of thromboembolism, stroke, heart attack, hypertension, and arteriosclerosis are minimal.[3,5–10] All reports state that women who use oral contraceptives can reduce their risk of cardiovascular disease by reducing or eliminating cigarette smoking.[11]

The risks of cancer have been a great concern. Such concern follows from the fact that high doses of various types of estrogen (doses that are much higher than those used for birth control) have been associated with vaginal, uterine, and, perhaps, breast cancers as well as noncancerous liver tumors.[12] Indeed, in older studies of high-dose products that were used during the 1960s, a slightly increased risk of cervical cancer may have occurred. Today, such a risk is no longer considered significant. Investigators today are near unanimous in their conclusion that no increased risk of breast or cervical cancer results from the use of low-dose oral contraceptives.[13–15] Indeed, the use of oral contraceptive products *reduces* a woman's risk of uterine and ovarian cancer by 40 to 50 percent,[15,16] and no cases of liver tumors have been identified.[3]

Other risks that may be associated with the use of oral contraceptives are altered metabolism of glucose, altered utilization of insulin, and the possible production of diabetes mellitus (sugar diabetes).[17] Drug-induced production of diabetes is probably not a cause for great concern. In their text, Speroff, Glass, and Kase summarize:

> Insulin and glucose changes with the low dose monophasic and multiphasic pills are so minimal that it is now believed that they are of no clinical significance. . . . It can be stated definitively that birth control pill use does not produce an increase in diabetes mellitus. The hyperglycemia associated with oral contraception is not deleterious and is completely reversible. Even women who have risk factors for diabetes in their history do not seem to be affected.[3]

Mishell[16] concurs with this assessment that the current risk of adverse metabolic (diabetogenic) potential is minimal.

Postpill reproductive toxicities have been a concern, but they have not been substantiated. After cessation of oral contraceptive use, there is no increase in the occurrence of spontaneous abortions, pregnancy complications, or congenital malformations.[18]

Conclusions and Contraindications

Stolley, Strom, and Sartwell[11] offer reasonable guidelines for the use of oral contraceptives:

1. Women over 35 years of age should avoid the use of these products.
2. Women who smoke cigarettes should avoid the use of these products and users should not smoke.
3. The product that is effective at the lowest dose of estrogen that does not cause unacceptable breakthrough bleeding should be chosen.
4. Women who experience high blood pressure, migraine headaches, or diabetes should be carefully educated and monitored.

Oral contraceptives are contraindicated in women who experience

1. Venous thrombophlebitis, thromboembolic disorders, cerebral vascular disease, or coronary artery disease.
2. Impaired liver function or jaundice.

3. Known or suspected cancer of the breast or uterus.
4. Abnormal genital bleeding.
5. Known or suspected pregnancy.
6. Congenitally elevated blood cholesterol or lipid levels.
7. An addiction to cigarettes (who are over the age of 35 years).

Alternatives to Oral Contraceptives

Unfortunately, only a few *effective* alternatives to birth-control pills presently exist for women who want to avoid pregnancy. The most effective contraceptive practices include the use of (1) oral contraceptives, (2) an implanted, long-acting, progestin-releasing contraceptive (Norplant), (3) a long-acting, injected (depot) progestin (Depo-Provera), (4) male or female sterilization, or (5) abstention.

Diaphragms, condoms, or intrauterine devices (IUDs) are only approximately 90- to 95-percent effective (Table 14.2). Even less effective are vaginal spermicides, the rhythm method, *coitus interruptus*, or douching. The most effective practices for *temporary and effective* prevention of unwanted pregnancy are the use of oral contraceptives and abstention. Sterilization of men or women (although 100 percent effective) is *permanent* and should not be considered reversible.

Depo-Provera

Certain long-acting, injectable preparations can be used as contraceptive agents. Medroxyprogesterone acetate (Depo-Provera), which is a long-acting injectable progestin, is used worldwide as an effective contraceptive. Approximately 3.5 million women use this method of contraception. A single dose of 100 to 400 milligrams, which is injected intramuscularly every 3 to 6 months, has proved to be effective. The advantages of using this form of contraception include freedom from taking daily tablets, freedom from the side effects of estrogen (this is a progestin-only product, containing no estrogen), and the maintenance of normal FSH activity. Depo-Provera inhibits ovulation by blocking the midcycle surge of LH. It induces thickening of the cervical mucus and inhibits the development of the lush uterine endometrium that is necessary for the fertilized ovum to survive. Follicular development is not suppressed, because the normal estrogen cycle is not prevented. The contraceptive protection that Depo-Provera provides is approximately equal to that afforded by the combination-type oral con-

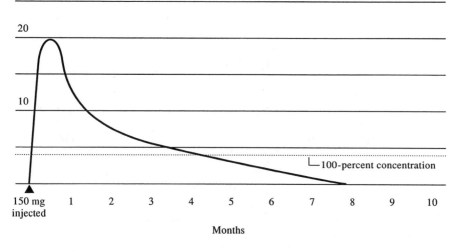

Provera blood level
ng/ml

20

10

└─100-percent concentration

150 mg   1   2   3   4   5   6   7   8   9   10
injected

Months

FIGURE 14.3

Blood levels of Depo-Provera following intramuscular injection. [From L. Speroff, R. H. Glass, and N. G. Kase,[3] p. 489.]

traceptives. Disadvantages of this mode of therapy include break-through bleeding, weight gain, depression, headaches, and abdominal bloating. Irregular menstrual cycles and spotting are quite common. Use of this technique has not been associated with an increased risk of cancer. However, two observations are important: first, it requires 6 to 8 months for the drug to clear totally from the average woman, and second, the effective level of contraception is maintained for 4 months (Figure 14.3). Therefore, 150 milligrams of Depo-Provera, given intramuscularly every 3 months, assures 100-percent contraception.[3]

Depo-Provera is being used currently in more than 70 countries. In the United States, the drug has not been approved for use in contraception, but it is used for other purposes. Its use is particularly appropriate for patients who cannot tolerate other forms of contraception or those who live in geographical areas where other contraceptive agents are not available. Uneducated or noncompliant patients have been the best candidates for its use. Depo-Provera has also been used for patients who are impaired intellectually or psychologically and in whom pregnancy might be unwise. Norplant (discussed next), however, may be even more appropriate for such uses.

Norplant

Recently approved and available is a new hormonal contraceptive device that delivers pregnancy-preventing progestin (levonorgestrel) for a maximum of five years following subcutaneous implantation (under a woman's skin). The device consists of six flexible silicone rubber tubes, each of which is filled with progestin and is about the size of a matchstick. It is inserted in a fan-like manner through a small skin incision on the inside of a woman's upper arm. This implant has the advantage that it can be discontinued at will (by removing the product from under the skin). Sufficient drug is released over a five-year period to protect against pregnancy. A failure rate of 4 to 5 per 1000 users every year has occurred.[19-21] Side effects are usually minimal and resemble those observed in women who take progestin-only oral contraceptives (that is, irregular periods and breakthrough bleeding).

Postcoital Contraception

When intercourse has occurred without contraceptive protection and pregnancy is not desired, certain pharmacological measures may be used to thwart an unwanted pregnancy. *Postcoital* techniques include high doses of estrogen in preparations that are often referred to as "morning after" pills. One such preparation contains large doses of diethylstilbestrol (about 25 milligrams) administered twice daily for 5 days. This type of drug apparently shortens the time that is required for a fertilized ovum to pass down the fallopian tube into the uterus, which impairs its ability to implant and survive in the endometrium. In other regimens, high doses of either ethinyl estradiol (the oral contraceptive Ovral) or conjugated estrogens (Premarin) are prescribed.

One should note that such regimens may be effective for contraception, but *routine* use of them may be dangerous. However, when there is a great desire to avoid pregnancy, such as for women who have been subjected to rape or incest, they can be very useful. Severe nausea, vomiting, and breast tenderness are noted frequently following treatment.

Mefepristone as an Abortifacient

Progesterone is a hormone that is required to maintain the uterine lining (endometrium). Pharmacological blockade of progesterone receptors will provoke endometrial necrosis and shedding (menstruation). Thus, if a woman is in the early stages of pregnancy, the growing fetus will be aborted if she takes a progesterone antagonist. Mefepristone (RU-486) is the first clinically available progesterone antagonist. It is used widely in Europe (especially in France) and in the Far East.[22] When a pharmacological abortion is desired, the drug is administered to the pregnant woman, and 2 days later an injection of prostaglandin is given (to stimulate uterine contractions). After a delay of 2 to 3 hours, vaginal bleeding and cramping will ensue. About one week later a physical examination is done and, if necessary, a surgical abortion is performed. Aside from its use as an abortifacient, mefepristone has been used to induce menstruation, to serve as a postcoital contraceptive, and to induce labor after intrauterine fetal demise.[23-25] The outcomes of moral controversies regarding pharmacological abortion ("contragestion"[22]) as a method of birth control will likely determine whether this method is used.

Agents That Increase Fertility

Women who are having difficulty becoming pregnant may respond to a drug that can *increase* fertility. Infertility may be caused by many factors (physical or psychological) in either the man or the woman. Certain types of physical infertility in women are susceptible to pharmacological manipulation. One such pharmacological approach is a direct extension of the scheme that is illustrated in Figure 14.2.

When estrogen acts on the hypothalamus, the release of GRF is inhibited, the release of FSH and LH by the pituitary gland is decreased, and follicular development is inhibited. If the action of estrogen on the hypothalamus were blocked, GRF would be released, which would stimulate the release of FSH and LH from the pituitary gland. Subsequently, one or more ovarian follicles would develop and, eventually, at least one ovum would be released. For a drug to block the inhibitory action of estrogen on the hypothalamus, it would need the ability to attach to normal estrogen receptors (thus blocking the normal access of estrogen to the receptor) without causing any changes in cellular behavior.

Clomiphene (Clomid), a compound that is frequently referred to as a "fertility pill," is such a drug. Clomiphene has enabled many women who were previously unable to conceive to become pregnant. The drug has also been responsible for causing multiple births; sometimes four or five ova are released and fertilized in women who take clomiphene. However, the possibility of bearing more than one child is usually not considered a problem for couples who have not been able to conceive by other methods. Because the action of clomiphene occurs in the hypothalamus, the pituitary gland and ovaries must be functional if the drug is to improve a woman's chances of conception. Thus, the drug is ineffective when infertility is caused by a deficit in the man or when the woman's infertility is caused by pituitary or ovarian dysfunction.

Ordinarily, the administration of clomiphene is started on day 5 of the menstrual period (day 1 being the first day of menses), and then it is taken daily for 5 days. The drug is stopped until the next menstrual cycle if the woman does not become pregnant. The procedure is then repeated, often with slowly increasing doses. A recent study indicates that approximately 35 percent of formerly infertile women become pregnant when they take clomiphene. Side effects of clomiphene include ovarian cysts (14 percent), multiple pregnancies (8 percent), and birth defects (2.4 percent). The incidence of birth defects in nontreated women is approximately 1 percent.

If a woman does not become pregnant after several trials on clomiphene, Pergonal (human postmenopausal hormone), Follutein (chorionic gonadotropin), or bromocriptine can be tried. Pergonal contains FSH and LH, which are extracted from the urine of postmenopausal women. Follutein is a hormone that is produced by human placenta, which is extracted from the urine of pregnant women. It exerts actions that are virtually identical to those of pituitary LH. Thus, sequential injections of Pergonal and then Follutein can, in anovulatory women, simulate normal FSH and LH release in the same manner that it occurs in fertile women. Pergonal is injected daily for 9 to 12 days, and then, after a day of rest, the woman is given a single injection of Follutein. Approximately 75 percent of women who are treated by this method will ovulate, and approximately 25 percent of them will become pregnant.

Bromocriptine is an agonist of dopamine receptors (Chapter 13) that inhibits the pituitary secretion of prolactin, restoring gonadotropin function and ovarian responsiveness. It seems to increase a woman's responsiveness to clomiphene.[3]

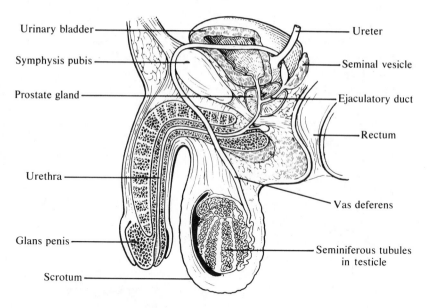

Urinary bladder

Symphysis pubis

Prostate gland

Urethra

Glans penis

Scrotum

Ureter

Seminal vesicle

Ejaculatory duct

Rectum

Vas deferens

Seminiferous tubules
in testicle

FIGURE 14.4

Principal organs of the male reproductive system.

The Male Reproductive System

Figure 14.4 illustrates some of the important structures of the male reproductive system. The testes are situated within the scrotal sac and are composed of great numbers of seminiferous tubules, in which sperm cells are formed. Once they are formed, the sperm cells empty into the epididymis, where they are stored until they mature. The epididymis leads into a long duct (the vas deferens), and the sperm cells are transported through that duct into the seminal vesicles and the prostate gland. In the upper vas deferens, they are mixed with fluids from both the prostate gland and the seminal vesicles. During ejaculation, the prostate gland, the vas deferens, and the seminal vesicles all contract simultaneously, so that the fluids and sperm cells are mixed and expelled through the ejaculatory duct and penis.

The actual neural control of erection and completion of the male sexual act is extremely complicated, involving sensory input to the spinal cord and the brain and final coordination of motor activity to cause erection with eventual ejaculation. This discussion, however, is focused not so much on the act itself as on the hormonal regulation of the male reproductive system as a possible site of action for a male contraceptive.

If a drug could be developed to serve as a contraceptive for men, it would probably have to affect testicular sperm production, sperm storage and maturation in the epididymis, sperm transport in the vas deferens, or the chemical constitution of the seminal fluid. All four processes are theoretically susceptible to modification by drugs.

Hormonal Regulation of Male Fertility

The production of male sex hormones is closely controlled by hormones that are released by the hypothalamus and the pituitary gland (Figure 14.5). The most important male hormone is testosterone, which is formed in the testes by cells that are near the seminiferous tubules. The hormone is released into the bloodstream and distributed throughout the body. In general, testosterone is responsible for the distinguishing characteristics of men, that is, the development of male features, including distribution of body hair, a low voice, muscular development, bone growth, and so on.

The production of testosterone is controlled by the hypothalamus. When testosterone levels decrease in the bloodstream, GRF is secreted from the hypothalamus. It is carried in the bloodstream to the pituitary gland, where it induces the release of LH, which then acts to promote the synthesis of testosterone in the testes. Testosterone, in turn, acts on the hypothalamus to slow the rate of its own synthesis by blocking the release of GRF.

The formation of sperm cells is controlled by FSH in conjunction with testosterone. The eventual formation of spermatozoa (a very complicated process) takes 74 days. After the spermatozoa leave the testes, an additional 12 to 26 days are required before they appear in the ejaculate.

Male Contraceptives

An effective male contraceptive would have to interfere with sperm production consistently and reversibly to produce temporary infertility.

> The development of safe, effective, and reversible contraceptive methods for men is an important goal in expanding the choices available for couples to regulate family size. The shortcomings of

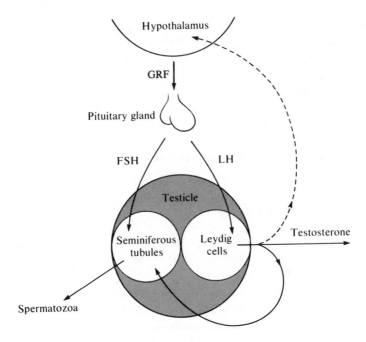

FIGURE 14.5

Hormonal regulation of male fertility. *Solid arrows*, stimulation. *Dashed arrows*, inhibition. (See legend for Figure 14.2 for explanation of abbreviations.) Note that the brain (hypothalamus and pituitary gland) is involved in the control of male fertility, just as it is in the control of female fertility. Note also, however, that fertility in the male is not subject to periodic cycling as it is in the female.

the currently available methods are a major barrier to the greater involvement of men in family planning. Nonetheless, that nearly 60 million men have had a vasectomy and nearly 40 million use condoms, indicates that men already have a wide involvement in family planning.[26]

To date, no satisfactory product has been developed for male contraception. Products that inhibit sperm production by suppressing sex hormones have been produced. However, the side effects and the inconvenient schedules for injection that are required have limited their usefulness.

Sperm production is, ultimately, controlled by pituitary FSH and LH, so it can be suppressed by the end product, testosterone. However, suppressing the pituitary hormones would decrease the production of the androgens that are necessary for the development of male characteristics. Early attempts to reduce sperm production involved injection of testosterone and estrogens.[27] More recently, a World Health Organization Task Force[26] has reported effective blockade of sperm production following weekly injection of a testosterone ester (testosterone enanthate) for a period of 12 months. The average time from the start of injections to the disappearance of sperm from ejaculate was 120 days. Recovery time following cessation of injections was about 100 days (these data correlate well with the normal 86 to 100 days that are required for sperm production and transport). Major limitations to the effectiveness of testosterone enanthate were the reluctance of male subjects to receive weekly injections, the delay in the onset of sterility, the long delay in recovery of fertility, and the inability of the injection to block sperm formation completely in all subjects. The results demonstrate, however, that male fertility can be temporarily, effectively, and reversibly controlled.

The only currently effective contraceptive methods for men are vasectomy (an irreversible method) and condoms (the only reversible method that is available).[28] Thus, much more study of the pharmacological limitation of male fertility is indicated.

Regarding vasectomy, it can be seen from Figure 14.4 that cutting the vas deferens would interfere only with the *transport* of sperm cells from the epididymis to the ejaculatory duct. Vasectomy does not interfere with masculinity, with sexual activity, with sperm production, or with the production of testosterone. Therefore, it does not interfere with male virility, libido, or function. Fluids are still secreted from the prostate gland and seminal vesicles into the ejaculatory duct and, during the sexual act, fluid is still expelled on ejaculation. The only difference in function is that this fluid does not contain sperm cells.

STUDY QUESTIONS

1. Differentiate between a neurotransmitter and a neurohormone. Give examples of each.
2. Where does fertilization occur?
3. Classify the various types of oral contraceptives. How do the newer contraceptives differ from those that were available during the 1960s?

4. What is the major trade-off that prevents further reductions in the amount of estrogen that is contained in oral contraceptives?

5. How do the steroid hormones in oral contraceptives work to block fertility?

6. Over the past 30 years, there has been much discussion about long-term harmful effects of oral contraceptives. Discuss the areas of concern and the current impression of such potential toxicity.

7. Differentiate among precoital contraception, postcoital contraception, and pharmacological abortifacients. Give examples of each.

8. What drugs are available to increase fertility in women?

9. Describe current techniques that are available to limit fertility in men. List advantages and disadvantages of each.

10. How might male fertility be hormonally regulated or limited?

NOTES

1. L. Speroff, R. H. Glass, and N. G. Kase, *Clinical Gynecologic Endocrinology and Infertility*, 4th ed. (Baltimore: Williams & Wilkins, 1989), pp. 51–61.

2. D. B. Bartosik, "Female Sex Hormones, Oral Contraceptives, and Fertility Agents," in J. R. DiPalma and G. J. DiGregorio, eds., *Basic Pharmacology in Medicine*, 3d ed. (New York: McGraw-Hill, 1990), p. 521.

3. L. Speroff, R. H. Glass, and N. G. Kase, *Clinical Gynecologic Endocrinology and Infertility*, 4th ed. (Baltimore: Williams & Wilkins, 1989), pp. 461–481.

4. B. Hedon, "The Evolution of Oral Contraceptives. Maximizing Efficacy, Minimizing Risks," *Acta Obstetricia et Gynecologica Scandinavica* 152, Supplement (1990): 7–12.

5. D. R. Mishell, Jr., "The Pharmacologic and Metabolic Effects of Oral Contraceptives," *International Journal of Fertility* 34, Supplement (1989): 21–26.

6. P. G. Stubblefield, "Cardiovascular Effects of Oral Contraceptives: A Review," *International Journal of Fertility* 34, Supplement (1989): 40–49.

7. M. Thorogood and M. P. Vessey, "An Epidemiologic Survey of Cardiovascular Disease in Women Taking Oral Contraceptives," *American Journal of Obstetrics and Gynecology* 163 (1990): 274–281.

8. G. Samsioe and L. A. Mattsson, "Some Aspects of the Relationship Between Oral Contraceptives, Lipid Abnormalities, and Cardiovascular Disease," *American Journal of Obstetrics and Gynecology* 163 (1990): 354–358.

9. E. P. Frohlich, "Vascular Complications in Women Using the Low Steroid Content Combined Oral Contraceptive Pills: Case Reports and Review of the Literature," *Obstetrical and Gynecological Survey* 45 (1990): 578–584.

10. R. J. Derman, "Oral Contraceptives and Cardiovascular Risk. Taking a Safe Course of Action," *Postgraduate Medicine* 88 (1990): 119–122.

11. P. D. Stolley, B. L. Strom, and P. E. Sartwell, "Oral Contraceptives and Vascular Disease," *Epidemiologic Reviews* 11 (1989): 241–243.

12. F. Murad and J. A. Kuret, "Estrogens and Progestins," in A. G. Gilman, T. W. Rall, A. S. Nies, and P. Taylor, eds., *Goodman and Gilman's The Pharmacological Basis of Therapeutics*, 8th ed. (New York: Pergamon, 1990), p. 1407.

13. D. A. Grimes, "Results of Oral Contraceptive Epidemiologic Studies Regarding Neoplastic and Cardiovascular Effects," *International Journal of Fertility* 34, Supplement (1989): 27–33.

14. H. Olsson, "Oral Contraceptives and Breast Cancer. A Review," *Acta Oncologica* 28 (1989): 849–863.

15. K. Gast and T. Snyder, "Combination Oral Contraceptives and Cancer Risk," *Kansas Medicine* 91 (1990): 201–208.

16. D. R. Mishell, Jr., "Correcting Misconceptions About Oral Contraceptives," *American Journal of Obstetrics and Gynecology* 161 (1989): 1385–1389.

17. I. F. Godsland, D. Crook, and V. Wynn, "Low-Dose Oral Contraceptives and Carbohydrate Metabolism," *American Journal of Obstetrics and Gynecology* 163 (1990): 348–353.

18. L. Speroff, "The Effects of Oral Contraceptives on Reproduction," *International Journal of Fertility* 34, Supplement (1989): 34–39.

19. D. Shoupe and D. R. Mishell, "Norplant: Subdermal Implant System for Long-term Contraception," *American Journal of Obstetrics and Gynecology* 160 (1989): 1286–1292.

20. C. W. Bardin, "Long-Acting Steroidal Contraception: An Update," *International Journal of Fertility* 34, Supplement (1989): 88–95.

21. K. Singh, O. A. Viegas, and S. S. Ratnam, "A Three-year Evaluation of Metabolic Changes in Singaporean Norplant Acceptors," *Advances in Contraception* 6 (1990): 11–21.

22. E. E. Baulieu, "Contragestion by the Progesterone Antagonist RU 486:

A Novel Approach to Human Fertility Control," *Contraception* 36, Supplement (1987): 1–5.

23. I. M. Spitz, D. Shoupe, R. Sitruk-Ware, and D. R. Mishell, Jr., "Response to the Antiprogestogen RU 486 (Mefepristone) During Early Pregnancy and the Menstrual Cycle in Women," *Journal of Reproduction and Fertility* 37, Supplement (1989): 253–260.

24. A. Ulmann and C. Dubois, "Clinical Trials with RU 486 (Mefepristone): An Update," *Acta Obstetricia et Gynecologica Scandinavica* 149, Supplement (1989): 9–11.

25. O. Heininheimo, O. Ylikorkala, and P. Lahteenmaki, "Antiprogesterone RU 486: A Drug for Non-surgical Abortion," *Annals of Medicine* 22 (1990): 75–84.

26. World Health Organization Task Force on Methods for the Regulation of Male Fertility, "Contraceptive Efficacy of Testosterone-Induced Azoospermia in Normal Men," *Lancet* 336 (1990): 955–959.

27. U. A. Knuth and E. Nieschlag, "Endocrine Approaches to Male Fertility Control," *Baillieres Clinical Endocrinology and Metabolism* 1 (1987): 113–131.

28. American Medical Association, *Drug Evaluations Annual 1991* (Milwaukee, Wis.: American Medical Association, 1990), pp. 973–974.

Drugs and Society

Priorities and Alternatives

PSYCHOACTIVE DRUGS AS BEHAVIORAL REINFORCERS

As far back as recorded history, every society has used drugs that produce effects on mood, thought, and feeling. Moreover, there were always a few individuals who digressed from custom with respect to the time, the amount, and the situation in which these drugs were to be used. Thus, both the nonmedical use of drugs and the problem of drug abuse are as old as civilization itself.[1]

Lessons From the Laboratory

If we accept the above statement as true, we can begin an analysis of drug abuse by examining the factors that contribute to the user's attraction to drugs. Use of drugs can progress from experimentation to casual use, intensive use, compulsive abuse, and, finally, dependence. Perhaps we should begin by extending our discussion of pharmacology to an examination of the *reinforcing properties* of psychoactive drugs. Socially, we tend to focus on the nonmedical use and abuse of drugs, together with all the social disruptions that can result from both the direct pharmacological effects (for example, automobile accidents) and the extended consequences (for example, crime) that accompany the procurement and use of illicit drugs. However, we can step back from human use of these drugs and examine how these drugs are used by animals under experimental conditions, thus separating the inherent attractiveness of drugs from human social and cultural issues.

Laboratory animals will self-administer many psychoactive drugs in varying degrees. Indeed, the patterns by which an animal will self-administer a particular drug closely parallel the patterns of abuse that are exhibited by human users of the same drug.[2]

For example, cocaine is self-administered to excess by every species of animal that has been tested, including rats, squirrel monkeys, rhesus monkeys, pigtail macaques, baboons, dogs, and humans.[3] Certainly, the same behavior in a variety of species is evidence of the impressive behavioral reinforcing property of cocaine. Indeed, with cocaine:

> Animals will press a lever more than 4,000 times to get a single injection of cocaine, and when given free access, they generally self-administer high daily doses that may produce severe toxic effects and induce self-mutilating behavior. . . . Generally the animals die of toxic effects and inanition [starvation] after a period of several weeks of continuous use.[2]

The self-administration of strongly reinforcing drugs by several species dispels the notion that the drug abuser (compared to a casual user or a nonuser) may have some kind of inherent, specific pathological condition (for example, preexisting psychopathology) that *creates* a propensity for abusing drugs. Rather, the drugs themselves are powerful behavioral reinforcers. Thus, we must examine briefly the reinforcing properties of the major psychoactive drugs.

Cocaine and the *amphetamines* are likely the most powerful reinforcing drugs.[4] Animals will self-administer cocaine or any of the amphetamines in preference to food or water; and they will eventually die from weight loss, dehydration, and drug toxicity. Likely, this reinforcing property is the most important factor in the development of compulsive abuse by humans, and it plays a major role in establishing the drug's attractiveness to users.

Morphine, heroin, and other opioids are readily self-administered by animals, but this self-administration has different characteristics from the self-administration of cocaine and the amphetamines.

> Animals self-administering morphine gradually raise the daily dose over a period of weeks, then self-administer the drug at a steady rate that avoids gross toxicity and withdrawal symptoms.[2]

The initial increase in dose probably reflects the development of drug tolerance. The subsequent dose stabilization probably reflects a reduction in the pleasurable effect of the drug over time, with drug use being continued primarily to avoid the unpleasant withdrawal symptoms.

Nicotine is not initially self-administered by animals. However, over time, the rate of self-administration increases, and self-administration decreases rapidly when saline is substituted for the drug.[5]

Caffeine has been thougl.t to be relatively weak as a behavioral reinforcer. Recent evidence, however, indicates that the behavioral reinforcing properties of caffeine may be much greater than previously thought.[6,7]

Ethanol (ethyl alcohol) is not particularly effective as a behavioral reinforcer, because animals usually will not self-administer ethanol without prior exposure; they will use ethanol primarily to avoid withdrawal symptoms.

Chlorpromazine and other neuroleptic drugs are never self-administered, and, in fact, animals learn to avoid behaviors that result in the receipt of an injection of a neuroleptic drug.

Cannabinols, psychedelics (such as LSD), and *clinical antidepressants* are not strong behavioral reinforcers.[8] The latter compounds, in fact, reduce the frequency of self-administration of cocaine and the amphetamines by animals.

Mechanism of Reinforcement Action

There is now a general consensus that the behavioral reinforcing properties of many psychoactive drugs involve a potentiation of dopamine neurotransmission within specific pathways in the CNS (particularly the limbic system).[2,9] Indeed, the limbic dopaminergic systems must be intact for the user to experience the behavioral reinforcing properties of drugs.*

---

*Jaffe[2] describes these systems as originating "in the ventral tegmental area of the brain and making connections with the nucleus accumbens and either directly or indirectly with the limbic cortex, ventral pallidum, and frontal cortex. Activation of these pathways releases dopamine in the nucleus accumbens and is associated with rewarding or reinforcing events." Opioids inhibit neurons that, in turn, inhibit dopaminergic neurons in the ventral tegmental area, while cocaine and amphetamines act directly on dopamine neurons, as described in Chapter 6. Drugs that block dopamine receptors (such as the antipsychotic agents) raise the threshold for activation of this system. Clinical antidepressants that exert little effect on dopamine neurons (acting primarily on serotonin reuptake) are, as would be predicted by this model, not considered to be behaviorally reinforcing drugs.

From the previous discussion it appears that

1. Behavioral reinforcement follows from the inherent ability of a drug directly or indirectly to augment dopamine neurotransmission in the limbic system of the brain.
2. A psychopathological process is probably not involved in the reinforcing response of a human drug abuser.
3. A drug's potential for abuse can be evaluated readily in nonhuman species to evaluate both its propensity to exert behavioral reinforcement and the degree to which self-administration may dominate behavior and control health.[5]
4. This knowledge can be extended (with limitations) to legal, social, medical, and treatment approaches for dealing with human drug-abuse problems.

DRUG USE AND ABUSE

If we decide that we wish to reduce the level of drug abuse that exists in our society, we will find that our choice of methods is limited. Over the years, we have attempted to pass laws that are designed to limit the availability of drugs and to punish those users whom we determine to be dangerous to themselves or to society because of their drug use. Brecher,[10] in a classic text, describes the successes and failures that have resulted from this approach. When these laws are strictly enforced, such an approach can reduce drug use by persons who fear reprisal. However, it can create problems of its own. Although history has shown that aggressive legislation will not effectively control a person's desire for mind-altering drugs (driven by the reinforcing properties already discussed), even today such an approach continues. As stated in the 1989 White House report *National Drug Control Strategy*:

> In short, legalizing drugs would be an unqualified national disaster. In fact, *any* significant relaxation of drug enforcement—for whatever reason, however well-intentioned—would promise more use, more crime, and more trouble for desperately needed treatment and education efforts.[11]

Such statements are made despite a 1990 federal antidrug budget that totaled almost $8 billion—the largest dollar increase in history.[11] Furthermore, for the 1991–1992 federal budget, the White House increased its request to $11.7 billion, which includes $5.2 billion for law enforcement.

Other traditional techniques that are used in attempts to reduce drug abuse usually involve education, combined with efforts to develop negative attitudes toward drugs in both users and potential users. Today, we are realizing that such efforts have brought limited results, perhaps because the problem was rooted in our basic approach; that is, maybe our goals were misguided and our efforts were uncoordinated. Perhaps it is time to determine the degree to which we, as a society, want to discourage the misuse or abuse of legal or illicit drugs. Do we focus solely on drugs as being "evil," as deleterious to the physical or psychological health of the user, as potentially dangerous to ourselves as a consequence of someone else's use of drugs, or, more generally, as a means by which the degradation of society has occurred because of widespread use? Perhaps all these considerations are valid. However, the reality may go deeper, involving the core of each person's sense of self-worth, self-respect, and dignity. Perhaps it is time to acknowledge the following statements:

1. Drugs are potent behavioral reinforcers, and that fact alone will always lead to misuse that is proportionate to the degree of a particular drug's inherent reinforcing properties.
2. There will always be a segment of a society that will abuse behavioral reinforcing drugs.
3. Given a market, there will always be an available supply of drugs.
4. Potential drug users, suppliers, and drugs themselves will never disappear entirely.
5. A drug-free society should not be a goal of government policymakers.
6. Ultimately, we must learn to coexist with the presence of drugs, that is, teach potential users to make conscious decisions about drugs.
7. Harmful drugs (for example, alcohol and nicotine) have been accepted and legalized.
8. It is necessary to teach people how to coexist with potentially harmful drugs and yet not be harmed by them.

One of the most excitingly heartening developments today is the widening effort to restore the teaching of moral values in our nation's schools. The direness of the drug epidemic has provided immense, immediate impetus. Further, more Americans now realize that the best way to prevent drug addiction is to inculcate a sense of personal worth and personal integrity. No other task is more vital as a priority in our students' curricula.[12]

When we look at this emphasis on moral values, it is clear that both the family and the extended community are vital in the quest to prevent drug abuse. Parental example, concern, influence, clarification of values, open communication, and teaching of individual responsibility are essential. Parental example should certainly include abstinence from cigarettes, moderation in the use of alcohol, and avoidance of driving after drinking. Parents can be positive educators if they provide good role models, an accurate education, and examples of alternatives to the drug experience. Similarly, peer programs and peer influence can be effective in building a person's sense of self-worth and, it is to be hoped, in reducing drug attractiveness.

As a society, we can undertake educational and legislative goals that seek both short-term and long-term objectives, remembering the ultimate goal of improving the perception of self-worth, integrity, and dignity of the individual. To this end, education has been a classic and continuing effort.

Shedler and Block[13] have expanded on this concept of values and upbringing as a determinant of proneness for drug abuse. They reported that significant behavioral maladjustments occurring in adolescents who are frequent abusers of drugs precede (to the earliest years of childhood) the initiation of drug use. Drug use is therefore a symptom, not a cause, of personal and social maladjustment. These authors emphasize that the meaning of drug use and abuse can be understood only in the context of an individual's personality structure and developmental history. Drug abuse is only part of a broad psychological syndrome that is not adequately explained in terms of peer influences. Social policy, they emphasize, should not be aimed at eliminating drug experimentation by adolescents. Indeed, adolescents with a history of drug experimentation (but who are not frequent users of drugs) can be quite stable and well adjusted. Societal efforts should be aimed at encouraging sensitive and empathic parenting, building self-esteem, fostering interpersonal relationships, and promoting involvement and commitment to meaningful goals.

The classic approach to teaching people about the actions of psychoactive drugs is to describe (1) how the body absorbs, distributes, metabolizes, and excretes them; (2) how the brain is organized and operates; (3) how neuronal function is related to behavior; and (4) how these functions are altered when drugs are ingested. Such a scheme avoids many of the complications that are inherent in an emotion-laden approach to drug education. The facts that are provided leave no room for mystery.

Of course, such an approach provides explicit directions for people who are seeking to satisfy existing needs with drugs. This result has been amply demonstrated in comprehensive education programs that *increased* the extent of drug use rather than decreased it, contrary to our original expectations.[14] However, the goal of drug education is not only to decrease drug use. Education provides accurate information for people who need to make informed decisions about their own use of, and attitudes toward, drugs. With such information, they can examine and modify their own risk-taking behavior, and they can be prepared to make the active, conscious decisions that are necessary for leading a healthy life in the wider community, where even relatively inexpensive psychoactive drugs are available.

The Objectives of Drug Education

No program of drug education can be designed that will guarantee the elimination of, or even a drastic reduction in, the use of psychoactive drugs. However, society will eventually learn about all the beneficial and harmful effects of a given drug (both licit and illicit). Education serves only to hasten the process of increasing people's knowledge about the risk-to-benefit ratio that accompanies all drug use. This knowledge will, more or less rapidly, be disseminated into the community, and as people learn about the risks and benefits of taking a particular drug, a level of drug use (and/or abuse) will be established that relates to this knowledge. In short, it is hoped that, as a result of education, society will be able to view drugs in proper perspective. Education can function only to present the truth as far as it is known. Indeed, although solid facts *can* be misinterpreted, they will serve society best in the long run.

This factual approach is also taken in the hope of countering much of the magic, mysticism, and emotionalism that surrounds the use of psychoactive drugs. In many social circles, discussion of psychoactive drugs evokes a very emotional response. It is hoped that by using this method of presentation, discussion of the actions of psychoactive drugs will be concentrated on the drugs themselves—as chemical entities and as compounds that alter existing processes in the brain.

Now that the pharmacology of these drugs has been presented, one should be able to compare and contrast the pharmacological effects that are induced by the different compounds. For example, there is controversy about the different effects that are induced by drinking alcohol or smoking marijuana. Chapters 4 and 12 should provide enough information to compare the divergence of attitudes toward the use of these drugs—a divergence that demonstrates the fact that some people will defend stoutly their own use of certain drugs while condemning others' use of different drugs. For example, an adult might attempt to justify his or her own alcohol use while attacking the use of marijuana by young adults. That same adult might even be relieved if the youth abandons marijuana and adopts the adult pattern of alcohol use. The pharmacology of these two drugs suggests that we should question the wisdom of such a shift.

Practical and Immediate Efforts

Practical and immediate efforts to deter the use of drugs that cause the *most* harm to society (and extract a multibillion-dollar toll in loss of lives, health, and productivity) must focus on *cigarettes* and *alcohol*. These substances should now—and in the future—be the major focus of educational, regulatory, and enforcement efforts.

In addition, we must meet the challenge of the sudden and episodic emergence of fashionable, potent, and dangerous drugs, such as crack cocaine, methamphetamine, or "designer" derivatives of fentanyl and other narcotics. Such drugs are undoubtedly potent behavioral reinforcers—usually behavioral stimulants (euphoriants) or narcotics. Those persons who are most resistant to educational and legislative efforts are the long-term abusers of such agents, especially when the drugs are administered intravenously, although potent reinforcing drugs that are inhaled (smoked) do produce nearly identical problems.

Cigarettes

The extent of people's addiction to cigarettes, which is clearly illustrated by many persons' inability to abstain from smoking, is clear. The more serious toxicities that are associated with smoking (bronchial irritation, wheezing, chest pain, lung congestion, and lung cancer) have

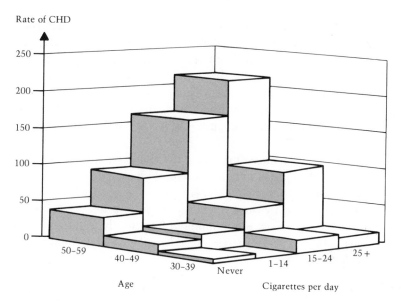

Rate of CHD

FIGURE 15.1

Rates of total coronary heart disease (CHD) per 100,000 person-years (vertical scale) among women according to cigarette use and age. [From W. C. Willett et al.,[16] p. 1306.]

been examined. The toxic effects of smoking on the cardiovascular system—coronary artery disease, peripheral vascular arteriosclerosis, increases in heart rate and blood pressure, and, possibly, an increased predisposition to the formation of blood clots—have been shown as well. The effects on the developing fetus, including increased rates of spontaneous abortion, stillbirths, and early postpartum death in infants who are born of mothers who smoked during pregnancy, have been especially emphasized.

Cigarette smoking by *younger women* is reaching crisis proportions.[15] Lung cancer is now the greatest cause of cancer-induced deaths in women. In addition, the risk of fatal or nonfatal heart attacks in those who smoke more than one pack of cigarettes per day is more than 500 percent of the risk in nonsmokers.[16] Even in light smokers (one to four cigarettes per day), the risk of heart attacks is more than doubled. Among heavy smokers, more than 80 percent of heart attacks are caused by smoking (Figure 15.1).

Finally, the worst consequences of smoking by women are the effects on reproduction and children. Some of these consequences have been discussed already. Less appreciated is the fact that maternal smoking during pregnancy has long-term effects on children, affecting growth, intellectual and emotional development, and behavior. Cigarette smoking during pregnancy is incompatible with giving an unborn child the best chance of being normal both at birth and during later development. The increase in cigarette smoking by women has been largely attributed to cigarette advertisements:

> Over the past half century and with remarkable consistency, tobacco advertising has linked smoking with women's emancipation and achievement of equality with men. Themes like "You've come a long way, baby" and the introduction of a new cigarette "For women who know the meaning of free" testify to the continuing marketing appeal of stressing independence and equal right to enjoyment.[17]

Marketing to women includes special packaging for feminine appeal and the introduction of "designer" cigarettes, promising sophistication, attractiveness, a slender body, and sex appeal. Sponsorship of sporting events, coupled with sports themes in cigarette advertisements, deceptively associates smoking with enhanced physical capacity.[17]

Cigarette smoking is clearly the most widespread example of drug dependence and the most preventable cause of disease and disability in this country. Fifty-six million Americans still smoke, and cigarettes cause more illness and death than do any of the other drugs. The major problem that most people have with recognizing and accepting this fact is that most of the toxicities are delayed in onset—often until someone has smoked for 20 years or more, at which time much of the damage is irreversible. Smoking and dependence develop early (even in 15- to 30-year-olds)—at an age when the feeling of personal invulnerability is maximal. The inevitable toxicity is not appreciated until the smoker reaches middle age.

The latest data (1988) show that *annual* health-related costs of cigarette smoking in the United States are greater than $60 billion. This estimate includes direct medical costs and salary losses for smokers who suffer from lung cancer, heart attacks, emphysema, and other respiratory illnesses. More than 450,000 deaths occur yearly as a result of smoking, which result in more than 4 million person-years lost.

If 56 million American smokers are responsible for $60 billion in yearly medical and social costs, each smoker is responsible for a yearly expense of $1070 ($60 billion divided by 56 million smokers). Thus, a person who smokes two packs of cigarettes daily (730 packs per year) incurs an average health-related cost of $1.46 for each pack of cigarettes that he or she smokes—an estimate that is probably conservative.

Given these facts and statistics, what should be our educational, legislative, and enforcement response? The following suggestions might constitute a starting point:

1. Continue educational efforts to warn people about the dangers of smoking, and depict smoking as dangerous.
2. Encourage health-care providers (such as pharmacies) not to sell cigarettes, even to cigarette-addicted adults.
3. Designate all health-care facilities as smoke-free areas.
4. Discontinue direct or indirect cigarette promotion to youths (those under 21 years old). This effort should include cigarette sponsorship of athletic events, automobile races, youth-oriented music concerts, and so on. (Blum[18] recently documented the finding that sponsorship of motor racing has become one of the major promotional activities that is used by the tobacco industry. During a recent 1.5-hour televised auto race, the Marlboro logotype was shown 5933 times and was visible for 46 minutes during the 93-minute race.)
5. Eliminate cigarette-containing vending machines.
6. Enforce laws that discourage sales and promotion of cigarettes to persons who are less than 21 years of age.
7. Eliminate free sampling of cigarettes.
8. Eliminate cigarette advertising and promotion on college campuses.
9. Continue to create smoke-free zones.
10. Regulate advertising to separate smoking from the youthful, macho, and avant-garde image that is currently portrayed.
11. Remove all government subsidies for tobacco growing.
12. Create a national cigarette health-care fund to contribute to the health-care expenses of smokers. Based on current cost estimates, a surcharge of $1.50 per pack of cigarettes would help to fund the health-care costs that are incurred by cigarette-induced toxicities.

These suggestions are intended to highlight the health dangers of cigarettes, to prevent the development of dependence in youths, to provide for future payment of medical costs that are incurred by smokers, to remove the attractions of smoking, and to discredit the concept that cigarette smoking is compatible with a youthful, active, healthy lifestyle. Although they do not suggest that we remove cigarettes from our culture, they might prepare adults to live cigarette-free in a society where cigarettes are freely available to them. If these suggestions could be implemented successfully, they could then be applied to alcohol and marijuana—two sedative-like drugs that are also freely available.

Alcohol

In addition to the dangers of cigarettes, we should become equally concerned about the use of alcohol. As illustrated in Chapter 4, alcohol predisposes one to various states of behavioral disinhibition, which can be manifested by a variety of behavioral patterns, including euphoria, aggression, hostility, and altered driving ability.

Alcohol is the direct pathological cause of death for more than 31,000 Americans each year and an indirect cause of more than 37,000 deaths by accident or violence. Fifty percent of our highway deaths involve alcohol, and the drug is a factor in 70 percent of homicides. Every year, the average American consumes 3 gallons of absolute alcohol. This amount of alcohol is equivalent to a yearly personal consumption of 591 (12-ounce) cans of beer, 115 fifths of table wine, or 35 fifths of 80-proof whiskey, gin, or vodka. We pay about $90 billion per year for alcohol-related problems. These problems include medical treatment of alcoholism; alcohol-related illness; fetal alcohol syndrome; loss of life, productivity, and property (including fire losses); crime; motor vehicle accidents; and social responses. One out of four families is troubled by family members who drink alcohol—the highest incidence of problem drinking in 37 years. An estimated 10 million adults in the United States are alcoholics, and 7 million adults are problem drinkers. Alcohol-associated deaths account for at least 25 times more deaths than those caused by all the illegal drugs combined.

Especially devastating are the injuries and fatalities to youths. A few statistics follow:

1. More than 40 percent of teenage deaths result from automobile accidents, and more than half of them involve alcohol.
2. Approximately 10 youths that are between 15 and 19 years old die each day from alcohol-related traffic accidents.
3. Youths that are between 15 and 24 years old account for 37 percent of all alcohol-related traffic deaths.

4. A yearly cost that is greater than $6 billion is incurred by teenage drivers who cause automobile accidents while they are under the influence of alcohol.
5. By the time a teenager is 18 years old, he or she has seen more than 100,000 beer commercials.[19]

An appropriate social goal might be to limit the numbers of persons who are harmed by alcohol by promoting some general policies:

1. Eliminate alcohol promotion to minors, for example, on college campuses.
2. Strictly enforce drinking laws in places where minors are present.
3. Teach people responsible methods of drinking for those occasions when they feel it is necessary, or socially appropriate, to drink.
4. Enforce drunk driving laws more strictly. Reduce the "legal" blood alcohol limit to 0.08 grams-percent for adults and to 0.00 (zero) grams-percent for those who are under 18 years of age.
5. Educate judges so that they understand the need for harsh penalties and rehabilitation when they are sentencing intoxicated drivers.[20] This should include immediate suspension of the driver's license of any driver found with a blood-alcohol level above the legal limit.
6. Increase education in such a way that people will learn to dissociate the drinking of alcoholic beverages from the smoking of cigarettes. Relatively few long-term drinkers are nonsmokers, and some toxicities are additive.
7. Discourage all advertising that associates the use of alcohol with socializing. In this manner, advertising would become primarily institutional in form.[19]

Comments on CNS Depressants

First, all CNS depressants are virtually identical pharmacologically. They are nonselective depressants of the central nervous system (Chapter 3). They are not magic bullets, love drugs, magic potions, or elixirs; nor do they possess any other magical or mystical qualities. Each of these drugs has a potential for harm as well as a potential for certain inherent psychosocial benefits.

Second, the extent to which these compounds are used and the negative health and economic consequences that follow their use must be emphasized. The statistics on alcohol, benzodiazepines, and marijuana have been emphasized throughout this text. Many persons have not recognized that these compounds are psychoactive drugs— they have all the positive behavioral reinforcing properties and all the negative health consequences that are associated with illegal drugs. We seem to have become desensitized to the deaths, illnesses, traffic accidents, family traumas, social havoc, and dollar costs that are associated with their use.

Third, the use and abuse of sedative-hypnotic compounds is not a fad. It will not go away; it cannot be legislated away; and it will remain a very widespread and serious problem.

Fourth, as stated previously, we must teach people to make active, conscious decisions about the use of CNS depressants. Certainly, the time has come to teach people how to drink alcoholic beverages. For example, we all know that alcohol interferes with a person's ability to drive an automobile, yet people who drink alcohol continue to drive. Few people seem to understand the relationship between drinking alcohol, the blood levels of alcohol that result, and the impairment of driving ability that follows.

In many states, a blood alcohol concentration (BAC) of 0.10 percent indicates "intoxication," and a person who drives with a BAC of 0.10 percent or greater may be charged with "driving while under the influence of alcohol." Thus, many people assume that a level of 0.09 percent is "O.K." but that a level of 0.11 percent is "bad." However, the behavioral effects of alcohol are not all or none; alcohol (like *all* sedatives) exerts a *graded, progressive* impairment of a person's ability to function. Thus, the 0.10-percent blood level is only a *legally established, arbitrary* value. Driving ability is minimally impaired at a BAC of 0.01 to 0.04 percent. However, at 0.05 to 0.09 percent, the driver's judgment and reactions become progressively impaired, a state of disinhibition occurs, and his or her risk of having an accident quadruples. The deterioration of a person's driving ability continues at a BAC of 0.10 to 0.14 percent, leading to a sixfold to sevenfold increase in the risk of having an accident. At 0.15 percent and higher, a person is 25 times more likely to become involved in a serious accident.

Figure 15.2 illustrates the correlation between the amount of alcohol that a person ingests, his or her resultant BAC, and the impairment of driving performance that occurs. To use this chart, first glance at the left margin and find the number that is closest to your body weight (in pounds). Then, look across the columns to the right and find

Blood Alcohol Concentration—a guide

Drinks: One drink equals 1 ounce of 80 proof alcohol; 12 ounce bottle of beer; 2 ounces of 20% wine; 3 ounces of 12% wine.

Weight (lb)	1	2	3	4	5	6	7	8	9	10
100	.029	.058	.088	.117	.146	.175	.204	.233	.262	.290
120	.024	.048	.073	.097	.121	.145	.170	.194	.219	.243
140	.021	.042	.063	.083	.104	.125	.146	.166	.187	.208
160	.019	.037	.055	.073	.091	.109	.128	.146	.164	.182
180	.017	.033	.049	.065	.081	.097	.113	.130	.146	.162
200	.015	.029	.044	.058	.073	.087	.102	.117	.131	.146
220	.014	.027	.040	.053	.067	.080	.093	.106	.119	.133
240	.012	.024	.037	.048	.061	.073	.085	.097	.109	.122

CAUTION   DRIVING IMPAIRED   LEGALLY DRUNK

Alcohol is "burned up" by your body at .015% per hour, as follows:

No. hours since starting first drink	1	2	3	4	5	6
Percent alcohol burned up	.015	.030	.045	.060	.075	.090

Calculate your BAC

Example: 180 lb man—8 drinks in 4 hours is .130% on chart.
Subtract .060% burned up in 4 hours. BAC equals .070%—DRIVING IMPAIRED.

FIGURE 15.2

Relation between blood alcohol concentration, body weight, and the number of drinks ingested. See text for details. Wallet-sized copies of this table are available from the Washington State Liquor Control Board, Capitol Plaza Building, Olympia, Washington 98504. [Data developed by Richard Zylman, Center for Alcohol Studies, Rutgers University, New Brunswick, N.J.]

the column that shows the number of drinks that you have consumed. By matching your body weight with the number of drinks that you have ingested, you can find your BAC. From this number, subtract the amount of alcohol that is metabolized per hour (remember from Chapter 4 that approximately 1 ounce of "hard" liquor is metabolized in 1 hour). The final figure is your approximate BAC. By calculating this number, you can predict the degree to which your driving ability would be impaired.

The following examples illustrate how these data can be used. Consider a 140-pound man who takes six drinks in 2 hours. The chart value for the blood alcohol concentration is 0.125 percent. Subtract 0.030 percent for metabolism (0.015 percent × 2 hours). His resulting BAC is 0.095 percent, which is not legally intoxicating (in most states) but is enough to impair his driving ability. Next, consider a 120-pound woman who also takes six drinks in 2 hours. The chart value is 0.145 percent. Subtract the same 0.030 percent for metabolism. Her resulting BAC is 0.115 percent, which is a legally intoxicating value. And, finally, consider a 160-pound man who takes four drinks in 4 hours. The chart value is 0.073 percent. Subtract 0.060 percent for metabolism. His resulting BAC is only 0.013 percent. At this level, the man's driving ability is only minimally impaired. Although caution is advised for this man, one can state that if he chooses to drive, his behavior is reasonably responsible.

Another point concerning alcohol and driving is that the presence of another sedative in the body will potentiate the effects of alcohol. Such drug potentiation is not included in Figure 15.2. Thus, although the BAC that is illustrated in Figure 15.2 remains true, a person who has ingested other sedatives as well as alcohol will experience an impairment that is magnified greatly.

Fifth, people should understand the circumstances that are appropriate for seeking or accepting tranquilizers that are prescribed by a physician or otherwise obtained. The benzodiazepines (Chapter 5), for example, were never intended to be made available to patients for the long-term "coping" management of problems that are associated with day-to-day living. They are intended only for the short-term, symptomatic alleviation of extreme anxiety or tension.

Sixth, I feel that we should recognize the legal inequities that are associated with the use of sedative drugs. We should work to equate the legal penalties for using certain drugs with the personal and societal costs that accompany the misuse of each agent. Certainly, there has been a movement in recent years to reduce the legal consequences of possessing marijuana, to bring penalties more in line with possible dangers to society. On the other hand, sedatives, such as alcohol, which cause greater risks and costs to society, should be dealt with more seriously. This assertion is not intended to advocate the reinstitution of prohibition (because such prohibition failed) but to urge stricter enforcement of the laws that are relevant to the use of alcohol and other sedatives when such use might endanger others.

The Nosology of Drug Abuse

The term *drug abuse* is difficult to define.[21] In general, it seems to imply the use of any drug for reasons other than its assigned purposes. However, the concept of *assigned purposes* is vague. Does it refer to use only in medical treatment or to use that is limited to a doctor's prescription? Does this mean that all use of drugs for reasons other than the treatment of medically diagnosed disorders is abuse of drugs? Are there no

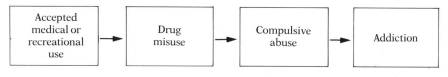

FIGURE 15.3

A continuum of the use and abuse of psychoactive drugs.

legitimate uses of drugs for recreational pursuits, for relaxation, for experience, or for temporary escape from reality? The history of human use of psychoactive drugs (including alcohol) clearly indicates that psychoactive drugs may become an acceptable form of recreation, relaxation, or escape when one feels that there are no better alternatives. Thus, the alternatives should be developed now—before psychoactive drugs *do* become the only recourse.

Figure 15.3 presents a continuum of use and abuse of psychoactive drugs. This continuum progresses from accepted drug use (both medical and recreational) to drug misuse, compulsive abuse, and drug addiction. Legitimate uses of psychoactive drugs are not all necessarily medical and cannot be dictated by law. Thus, we accept the notion that drugs can be used legitimately for recreation and as a means of experiencing altered states of consciousness.

Compulsive abuse is an extension of misuse. It refers to a state that is experienced by a person who is no longer flexible in his or her drug behavior, who uses the drug despite adverse social or medical consequences. The user has developed an intense reliance on the effects of self-administered drugs.

Addiction is a further extension of drug use. It refers to a state that is experienced by a person who is overwhelmingly involved with using a drug (compulsive abuse) and securing its supply. The addicted person has a high tendency to relapse after the drug has been withdrawn. Drug use thus pervades the total life activity of the user and controls his or her behavior.

The vagueness of the terms *misuse* and *abuse* recently led the World Health Organization to recommend abandonment of these terms and replacement with the following definitions:

(1) Unsanctioned Use—Use of a drug that is not approved by a society or a group within that society. Who disapproves should be made clear when the term is used. The term implies the acceptance

of disapproval as a fact in its own right, without having to determine or justify its basis, e.g., certain psychedelics.

(2) Hazardous Use—Use of a drug that will probably lead to harmful consequences for the user—either to dysfunction or to harm. This category essentially includes the idea of risky behavior, e.g., smoking 1 pack of cigarettes a day.

(3) Dysfunctional Use—Use of a drug that is leading to impaired psychological or social functioning (e.g., loss of job or marital problems).

(4) Harmful Use—Use of a drug that is known to have caused the particular person tissue damage or mental illness.[21]

Because exposure to strongly reinforcing drugs will inevitably lead to problems in significant numbers of people, drug education and treatment must include consideration of the extent of a person's behavioral and physiological involvement with psychoactive drugs. Although educational programs and drug alternatives may be useful, formal treatment programs are necessary for those persons who experience patterns of compulsive abuse or addiction. As stated by Jaffe:

> The indications for treatment vary with the drugs being used as well as with the social and cultural factors determining the particular pattern of drug use. Some patterns of drug use, such as weekly use of [less reinforcing drugs such as] marihuana, do not require treatment any more than does the occasional smoking of tobacco or the social use of alcohol. Such casual use is not without hazard, and it may jeopardize vocational status. . . . However, such patterns of use do not necessarily constitute a treatable disorder. It is likely that changing views about drug use will continue to create gray areas where the indications for treatment are unclear. However, there is general agreement that treatment is appropriate for the adverse consequences of drug use and for the compulsive drug user who voluntarily seeks help.[22]

Legitimate use of psychoactive drugs is recognized (Table 15.1), subject to social and legal restrictions. *Medically* legitimate uses of drugs include the treatment or prevention of diagnosed diseases or the alleviation of physical or mental discomfort. *Recreationally* legitimate uses of drugs generally include the achievement of altered states of mood or of consciousness, relief from anxiety, induction of euphoria, or escape from uncomfortable or oppressive circumstances.

Drug misuse (step two in Figure 15.3) can, therefore, be described as the use of any drug (legal or illegal) for a medical or recreational

TABLE 15.1

The medical and recreational uses of psychoactive drugs.

Medical
1. Treatment or prevention of diagnosed disease
2. Alleviation of physical or mental discomfort

Recreational
1. Relief from anxiety
2. Achievement of a state of disinhibition or euphoria
3. Achievement of altered states of consciousness
4. Expansion of creative abilities
5. Attempt to gain interpersonal or external insight
6. Escape from uncomfortable or oppressive surroundings
7. Experience of altered states of mood

purpose *when other alternatives are available, practical, or warranted or when drug use endangers either the users or others who are around them.* In medicine, drug misuse applies to the seeking, prescribing, or using of any drug for any purpose other than the prevention or treatment of diagnosed disease or the alleviation of physical or mental discomfort. A physician who prescribes a mild sedative (such as a benzodiazepine) for a patient merely because the patient requested it, or to terminate the interview with a patient, may be allowing the patient to misuse a drug. This situation would be an example of unsanctioned or hazardous use. A drug that may be used properly for recreational purposes is misused when it impedes the user's development beyond his or her use of drugs (dysfunctional use), when it results in a preoccupation with drug use, or when it endangers the physical or mental health of the user or others (harmful use).

Alternatives to Drugs

The concept of drug use that is presented in Table 15.1 leads to the final point of discussion in this book—namely, recognition of the fact that society must not only teach cognitive–behavioral decision-making skills to combat drug misuse, but it must also provide suitable alternatives. Consider the following:

Interviewer: Why do you use drugs?
User: Why not?
Interviewer: How could someone convince you to stop?
User: Show me something better.[23]

This terse dialogue is most significant. The recreational use of drugs will never disappear. Thus, an important aspect of teaching people to live in a world where drugs are available is to provide suitable alternatives to the reliance on recreational pharmacology as a diversion.

Recognizing the potent reinforcing properties of psychoactive drugs, recognizing the motives of persons who use drugs, and recognizing that it is basic human nature periodically to seek alterations in mood and altered states of consciousness, we can proceed to an active search for alternatives to drug use. As Cohen states:

> Alternative is not just a synonym for "substitute" since it implies an orientation which is *more effective* than drugs for giving the person real satisfaction.[24]

Numerous alternatives to using drugs must be made available, but only after matching them with an analysis of the types of experiences that drug users are seeking, their motives for seeking that experience, and possible alternatives that might help them (or potential users) to attain that experience without drugs. Provision of nondrug, natural highs, for example, might replace drug-induced altered states of consciousness. New experiences might be achieved by high-energy activities (athletics, dance, and so on), creative endeavors (photography or business training), interpersonal activities (for example, Outward Bound), or spiritual and self-worth training (religious study or experiences), to name only a few.

The implementation of these alternatives should be a high priority of the family, the community, and our society. Brecher remarked that

> . . . these and other "alternatives to the drug experience" are gaining favor among young people because they are superior to drugs, not because they are safer than drugs. An experienced drug user . . . often finds that some form of meditation more effectively satisfies his desire to get high. One sees a great many drug takers give up drugs for meditation, but one does not see any meditators giving up meditation for drugs. Once you have learned from a drug what being high really is, you can begin to reproduce it without the drug; all persons who accomplish this feat testify that the non-drug high is superior.[24]

Note, however, that provision of alternatives for drug-dependent or formerly drug-dependent persons requires a reduction in the "craving" for drugs. Here the use of opioid or dopamine antagonists may prove invaluable.[25]

STUDY QUESTIONS

1. What is meant when a particular psychoactive drug is called a *behavioral reinforcer*?
2. Why might the evaluation of drug reinforcing properties in animals be valuable in the assessment of human experiences?
3. Is a propensity to abusing drugs caused by a psychopathological process in the user or is it a property of the drug in particular? Defend your position.
4. On a mechanistic level, what might explain the lack of self-reinforcing action of phenothiazines or tricyclic antidepressants?
5. What is the mechanism that underlies the behavioral reinforcing properties of certain psychoactive drugs?
6. List several key principles that underlie a positive approach toward drug-abuse education.
7. Where has drug education failed? How might it be used successfully?
8. List, in descending order, the most harmful to the least harmful classes of psychoactive drugs that have been presented in this text. Defend your choices.
9. Reconcile the entries in the list you just made in terms of social acceptance and legal status.
10. Should certain drugs be more readily available? In what direction should our legislative efforts be focused?

NOTES

1. J. H. Jaffe, "Drug Addiction and Drug Abuse," in A. G. Gilman, T. W. Rall, A. S. Nies, and P. Taylor, eds., *Goodman and Gilman's The Pharmacological Basis of Therapeutics,* 8th ed. (New York: Pergamon, 1990), p. 522.
2. J. H. Jaffe, "Drug Addiction and Drug Abuse," in A. G. Gilman, T. W. Rall, A. S. Nies, and P. Taylor, eds., *Goodman and Gilman's The Pharmacological Basis of Therapeutics,* 8th ed. (New York: Pergamon, 1990), pp. 523–524.

3. C.-E. Johanson, "Behavioral Studies of the Reinforcing Properties of Cocaine," in D. Clouet, K. Asqhar, and R. Brown, eds., *Mechanisms of Cocaine Abuse and Toxicity*, NIDA Research Monograph 88, U.S. Department of Health and Human Services (Rockville, Md.: National Institute on Drug Abuse, 1988), pp. 107–124.

4. R. L. Balster, "Pharmacological Effects of Cocaine Relevant to Its Abuse," in *Mechanism of Cocaine Abuse and Toxicity*, NIDA Research Monograph 88, U.S. Department of Health and Human Services (Rockville, Md.: National Institute on Drug Abuse, 1988), pp. 1–13.

5. C.-E. Johanson, "Assessing the Reinforcing Properties of Drugs," in L. S. Harris, ed., *Problems of Drug Dependence, 1989*, NIDA Research Monograph 95, U.S. Department of Health and Human Services (Rockville, Md.: National Institute on Drug Abuse, 1990), pp. 135–145.

6. R. R. Griffiths, G. E. Bigelow, and I. A. Liebson, "Reinforcing Effects of Caffeine in Coffee and Capsules," *Journal of the Experimental Analysis of Behavior* 52 (1989): 127–140.

7. R. R. Griffiths and P. P. Woodson, "Reinforcing Effects of Caffeine in Humans," *Journal of Pharmacology and Experimental Therapeutics* 246 (1988): 21–29.

8. J. H. Jaffe, "Drug Addiction and Drug Abuse," in A. G. Gilman, T. W. Rall, A. S. Nies, and P. Taylor, eds., *Goodman and Gilman's The Pharmacological Basis of Therapeutics*, 8th ed. (New York: Pergamon, 1990), p. 567.

9. D. Clouet, K. Asqhar, and R. Brown, eds., *Mechanisms of Cocaine Abuse and Toxicity*, NIDA Research Monograph 88, U.S. Department of Health and Human Services (Rockville, Md.: National Institute on Drug Abuse, 1988).

10. E. M. Brecher and Consumer Reports editors, *Licit and Illicit Drugs* (Mt. Vernon, N.Y.: Consumers Union, 1972).

11. Office of National Drug Control Policy, *National Drug Control Strategy*, The White House, September 1989 (Washington, D.C.: U.S. Government Printing Office, 1989), p. 13.

12. M. S. Forbes, "Fact and Comment," *Forbes* (December 1, 1986), p. 25.

13. J. Shedler and J. Block, "Adolescent Drug Use and Psychological Health," *American Psychologist* 45 (1990): 612–630.

14. T. J. Glynn, ed., *Drug Abuse Prevention Research*, National Institute on Drug Abuse (Washington, D.C.: U.S. Government Printing Office, 1983).

15. J. E. Fielding, "Smoking and Women: Tragedy of the Majority," *New England Journal of Medicine* 317 (1987): 1343–1345.

16. W. C. Willett, A. Green, M. J. Stampfer, F. E. Speizer, G. A. Colditz, B. Rosner, R. R. Monson, W. Stason, and C. H. Hennekens, "Relative and Absolute Excess Risks of Coronary Heart Disease Among Women Who Smoke Cigarettes," *New England Journal of Medicine* 317 (1987): 1303–1309.

17. R. M. Davis, "Current Trends in Cigarette Advertising and Marketing," *New England Journal of Medicine* 316 (March 19, 1987): 725–732.

18. A. Blum, "The Marlboro Grand Prix. Circumvention of the Television Ban on Tobacco Advertising," *New England Journal of Medicine* 324 (1991): 913–917.

19. N. Postman, C. Nystrom, L. Strate, and C. Weingartner, *Myths, Men and Beer: An Analysis of Beer Commercials on Broadcast Television, 1987* (Falls Church, Va.: AAA Foundation for Traffic Safety, 1988).

20. M. Colquitt, P. Fielding, and J. F. Cronan, "Drunk Drivers and Medical and Social Injury," *New England Journal of Medicine* 317 (November 12, 1987): 1262–1266.

21. H. D. Kleber, "The Nosology of Abuse and Dependence," *Journal of Psychiatric Research* 24, Supplement 2 (1990): 57–64.

22. J. H. Jaffe, "Drug Addiction and Drug Abuse," in A. G. Gilman, T. W. Rall, A. S. Nies, and P. Taylor, eds., *Goodman and Gilman's The Pharmacological Basis of Therapeutics*, 8th ed. (New York: Pergamon, 1990), pp. 559–561.

23. A. Y. Cohen, "The Journey Beyond Trips: Alternatives to Drugs," in D. E. Smith and G. R. Gay, eds., *It's So Good Don't Even Try It Once: Heroin in Perspective* (Englewood Cliffs, N.J.: Prentice-Hall, 1972), p. 186.

24. E. M. Brecher and Consumer Reports editors, *Licit and Illicit Drugs* (Mt. Vernon, N.Y.: Consumers Union, 1972), p. 510.

25. M. Holloway, "Rx for Addicition," *Scientific American* 264 (March, 1991): 94–103.

Appendixes I–III

Introduction to
Neuropsychopharmacology

Basic Anatomy of the Nervous System

Because the brain is the most complex of all biological structures, any discussion about its anatomy and function is necessarily complicated. Still, a number of introductory and straightforward principles can be described that may lead to a relatively uncomplicated outline of the anatomy and physiology of the brain and help explain the actions of psychoactive drugs in terms of their discrete effects on brain function as well as on behavior.

Introductory Terminology

For ease in understanding, the nervous system can be divided into two major functional systems: the *central nervous system (CNS)* and the *peripheral nervous system*. The CNS consists of all the neurons that are situated inside the skull and the spinal cord. The peripheral nervous system consists of all the neurons that are located outside the skull and spinal cord, including all sensory and motor nerves that innervate the muscles, glands, and organs of the body.

The CNS may be sudivided conveniently into two major parts: the brain and the spinal cord. The brain is a collection of some 20 billion

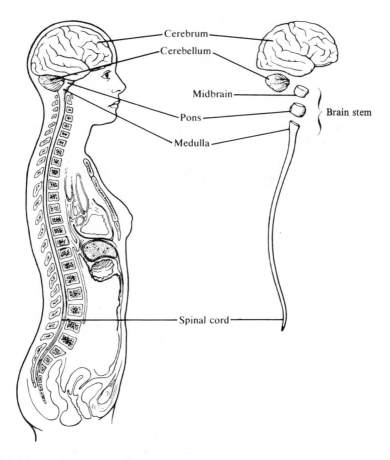

FIGURE I.1

The central nervous system. The location of the brain and spinal cord within the body (*left*) and the principal components of the central nervous system (*right*).

neurons, along with their dendrites and axons, that are contained entirely within the skull (Figure I.1). The lower part of the brain, which is attached to the upper part of the spinal cord, is referred to as the *brain stem*. The brain stem is situated entirely within the skull. All the impulses that are conducted (in either direction) between the spinal cord and the brain must, of necessity, be conducted through the brain stem, which is also important in the regulation of vital body functions. The brain stem is a site of action for many psychoactive drugs (discussed in Appendix III).

If we divide the brain into its component parts (Figure I.1), we see that the top, or front end, of the CNS (the *cerebrum*) is considerably larger than the brain stem and the spinal cord. As the upper part of the spinal cord enlarges, it separates into three distinct, yet completely interconnected segments, which are referred to as the *medulla*, the *pons* (or bridge), and the *midbrain*. These three segments form the brain stem. The area immediately above the brain stem, which is referred to as the *diencephalon*, is covered by the cerebrum. This area includes the hypothalamus, the pituitary gland, the fiber tracts from the eyes (optic tracts), and the thalamus. The region below the thalamus is referred to as the *subthalamus*. Finally, almost completely covering the brain stem and the diencephalon are the two *cerebral hemispheres*, which extend to the left and the right.

The Spinal Cord

The spinal cord extends from the lower end of the medulla to the upper levels of the sacral vertebrae (Figure I.1). It consists of a mass of neurons and fiber tracts (bundles of axons that travel as a group from one area to another). The spinal cord is involved in (1) carrying sensory information (from skin, muscles, joints, and internal body organs) to the brain, (2) organizing and modulating the motor out-flow to the muscles (to produce coordinated muscle responses), (3) modulating sensory input, such as limiting nociceptive (painful) information (Chapter 9), and (4) providing autonomic (involuntary) control of vital body functions.

The neurons of the spinal cord both communicate with higher centers in the brain and exert local control over spinal reflexes. An example that is relevant to analgesia is that both local endorphin neurons and the long, descending, inhibitory fiber tracts from the brain stem modulate the intensity of nociceptive input as substance P–releasing afferent neurons enter the spinal cord (Chapter 9).

Thus, neurons that are located in the spinal cord are strongly influenced by information that is received from the brain. For example, drugs that cause behavioral sedation decrease the flow of information from the brain to the spinal cord. Such drugs are used as muscle relaxants, because they decrease the spinal cord's control over muscle tone by decreasing indirectly the activity of the motor neurons (Chapter 13).

The Brain Stem and Midbrain

The brain stem and the midbrain lie inside the skull and connect the spinal cord with the cerebral hemispheres and the thalamic–hypothalamic areas. The major subdivisions of the brain stem are the *medulla, pons,* and *midbrain* (Figure I.1). Behind the midbrain is a large bulbous structure, which is called the *cerebellum.*

The brain stem is the direct continuation of the spinal cord in the skull. All ascending and descending fiber tracts that connect the brain and the spinal cord pass through the various structures of the brain stem. Also present are centers that are largely responsible for the control of respiration (breathing), blood pressure, pulse, heart function, gastrointestinal functioning, and sleeping and wakefulness. The brain stem is also involved in behavioral alerting, attention, and arousal responses. Depressant drugs (such as the barbiturates, Chapter 3) depress these centers; and such neuronal depression probably underlies the hypnotic action of those drugs. Other agents that are used clinically for the treatment of high blood pressure exert at least part of their hypotensive effect by depressing brain-stem centers that control vascular tone.

The major biological amine–containing neurons that project to the cerebrum are also found within the brain stem. These brain-stem regions are also the primary relay areas for sensory information that enters the CNS from the face, head, and most visceral organs (through the cranial nerves).

Cerebellum

The cerebellum is a large, highly convoluted structure that is situated immediately behind the brain stem and is connected to it by large fiber tracts. The cerebellum is necessary for the proper integration of movement and posture. Some drugs exert noticeable effects on cerebellar activity. Drunkenness, which is characterized by loss of coordination, staggering, loss of balance, and other deficits, appears to be caused largely by an alcohol-induced depression of cerebellar function.

The Diencephalon

The diencephalon is a portion of the brain that is situated above the brain stem, below the cerebral cortex, and buried between the right and left cerebral hemispheres. The diencephalon may be subdivided further into several areas, three of which will be discussed: the *thalamus,* the *hypothalamus,* and the *subthalamus.*

Thalamus

The thalamus is the largest structure of the diencephalon, and it is actually a group of many smaller structures. It lies in the center of the brain, beneath the cerebral hemispheres and basal ganglia, and just above the hypothalamus. Physiologically, the thalamus is often referred to as a way station, where incoming sensory pathways, which are traveling up the spinal cord and through the brain stem, synapse before they pass into the various areas of the cerebral cortex. Thus, the thalamus may be thought of as one of the primary relay stations of the brain.

Various subdivisions of the thalamus receive projections from specific sensory organs and, in turn, the neurons in these subdivisions relay information to specific areas of the cerebral cortex. Inputs from vision, hearing, touch, pressure, position, pain, and so on, feed into specific regions of the thalamus before they are relayed to the areas of the cerebral cortex that are specifically associated with the senses. Other areas of the thalamus, which are not well defined, are referred to as *association areas.* These areas integrate incoming information and relay it to the association areas of the cerebral cortex. Other areas of the thalamus connect caudally with the reticular formation, the hypothalamus, and the limbic system. These areas form the diffuse thalamic projection system, which has been implicated as a site of action for several psychoactive drugs. Electrical stimulation of the diffuse thalamic projection system yields behavioral alerting reactions that are similar to those that follow stimulation of the reticular activating system. This diffuse thalamic projection system may, therefore, be an extension of the brain-stem activating areas.

Subthalamus

The subthalamus is a small area that is underneath the thalamus and above the midbrain; it contains a variety of small structures which, together with the basal ganglia, constitute one of our motor systems: the *extrapyramidal system.* Patients who have Parkinson's disease—a disorder that is characterized by exaggerated motor movements—have a deficiency of the neurotransmitter dopamine in the terminals of their nerve axons, which originate from cell bodies in the substantia nigra (one of the subthalamic structures). Administration of levodopa to these patients replaces the dopamine and ameliorates the symptoms (Chapter 13). Thus, in humans, as well as in lower mammals and birds, the subthalamic structures, together with the cerebellum, seem to be important in the coordination of motor activity.

Hypothalamus

The hypothalamus consists of a collection of nuclei in the lower portion of the brain that is near the junction of the midbrain and the thalamus. It is located near the base of the skull, just above the pituitary gland (the function of which it largely modulates). The hypothalamus is the principal center in the brain that is responsible for the integration of our entire autonomic (involuntary, or vegetative) nervous system. It contains important centers for the control of such vegetative functions as eating, drinking, sleeping, the regulation of body temperature, sexual behavior, blood pressure, emotion, and water balance. In addition, hormonal output of the pituitary gland (Chapter 14) is controlled closely by the hypothalamus. Neurons in the hypothalamus produce and secrete substances that are called *releasing factors*, which travel to the nearby pituitary gland (Figure I.2). There, they induce the production and secretion of hormones that act on both female and male sex organs to cause sexual development, menstrual cycling, ovulation, and sperm formation.

The hypothalamus is a site of action for many psychoactive drugs—either as a site for the primary action of a drug or as a site that is responsible for side effects that are associated with the use of a drug. Finally, it is pertinent to mention the hypothalamic reward centers (the self-stimulation and behavioral reinforcing centers) that involve the median forebrain bundle and the limbic system. These centers contain norepinephrine-secreting neurons which modulate specific types of reward and avoidance behaviors.

Limbic System

Closely associated with the hypothalamus is the limbic system, the major components of which are the *amygdala*, the *hippocampus*, the *mammillary bodies*, and a variety of other smaller structures. These structures exert primitive types of behavioral control; they integrate emotion and behavior with motor and autonomic functions. Because the limbic system and the hypothalamus interact in the regulation of emotion and emotional expression, these structures are logical sites for the study of psychoactive drugs that alter mood, affect, emotion, or responses to emotional experiences. The classical notion that the limbic system is

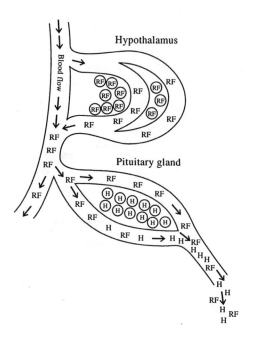

FIGURE I.2

Blood flow enters the hypothalamus, carrying hypothalamic releasing factors (RF) as it leaves the structure. The releasing factor induces the release of pituitary hormones (H: FSH, LH, and others), which are released into the blood that leaves the gland.

important in the functions of learning and memory has prompted investigations of both this structure and the hypothalamus as sites of action for compounds that affect these functions. For example, scopolamine (Chapter 11) impairs learning and memory, producing amnesia with a loss of short-term memory (which somewhat resembles the amnesia that is observed in patients who experience dementia of the Alzheimer's type; Appendix III).

The Cerebral Cortex

In humans, the cerebral cortex constitutes the largest portion of the brain. It is separated into two distinct hemispheres: the left and the right. Numerous fiber tracts interconnect the two hemispheres both at a level above the thalamus and through the multisynaptic pathways in

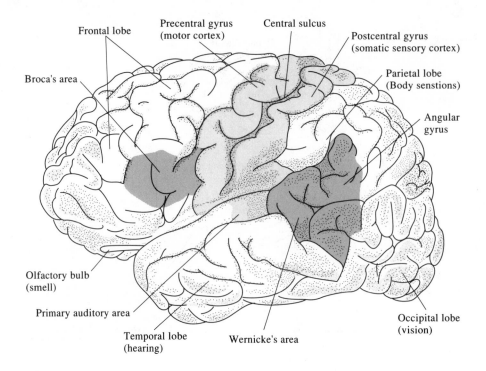

Frontal lobe

Precentral gyrus
(motor cortex)

Central sulcus

Postcentral gyrus
(somatic sensory cortex)

Broca's area

Parietal lobe
(Body senstions)

Angular
gyrus

Olfactory bulb
(smell)

Primary auditory area

Occipital lobe
(vision)

Temporal lobe
(hearing)

Wernicke's area

FIGURE I.3

(*Above*) Surface structure of the brain, showing major areas of the cerebral cortex. (*Facing page*) Cross section of the brain, showing major structures. [Panel above modified from N. Geschwind, "Specializations of the Human Brain," in *The Brain*, a *Scientific American* book (San Francisco: W. H. Freeman and Company, 1979), p. 111.]

the brain stem. In humans, the skull size is limited and the cerebral cortex is so large, so the cortex is deeply convoluted and fissured. Like other portions of the brain, the cerebral cortex is divided functionally— that is, it contains distinct centers for vision, hearing, speech, sensory perception, emotion, and so on.

The various regions of the cerebral cortex can be classified in several different ways. The most useful classification for this discussion is a subdivision by the type of function or sensation that is processed (Figure I.3). The anterior (front) and posterior (back) portions of the cerebral cortex can be divided by a lateral longitudinal groove, which is called the *central sulcus*. The area of cortex that is immediately in front of the central sulcus is called the *precentral gyrus*. The precentral gyrus is involved in the control of motor movement (the *pyramidal system*, as opposed to the extrapyramidal system, which involves the basal ganglia). The area that is

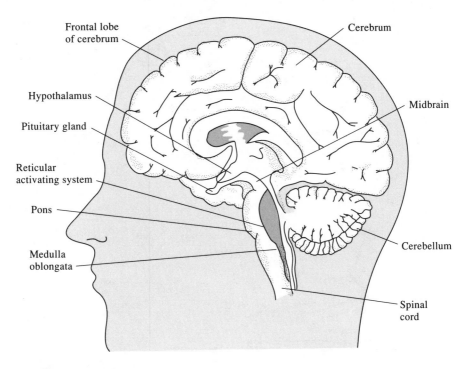

Frontal lobe
of cerebrum

Cerebrum

Hypothalamus

Midbrain

Pituitary gland

Reticular
activating system

Pons

Cerebellum

Medulla
oblongata

Spinal
cord

FIGURE I.3 (continued)

behind the central sulcus is the *postcentral gyrus*, which is the major
processing center for the sensation of touch (Figure I.4). Posterior to the
postcentral gyrus lies the *parietal* and *occipital* lobes, which process body
sensation and vision, respectively. In front of the precentral gyrus lies the
frontal lobe, which is involved in behavior, learning, memory, visceral sensations, abstract thought, and other specialized functions. Finally, below
the central sulcus lies the *temporal lobe* (Figure I.3), which is involved in,
primarily, hearing and the integration of hearing with speech in nearby
areas (Brocha's and Wernicke's areas).

The nervous system is extremely complex in structure and function,
and the cerebral cortex represents the ultimate development of this
complexity. Only now are we beginning to understand something of the
brain's precise functioning and how it relates to the actions of psychoactive drugs.

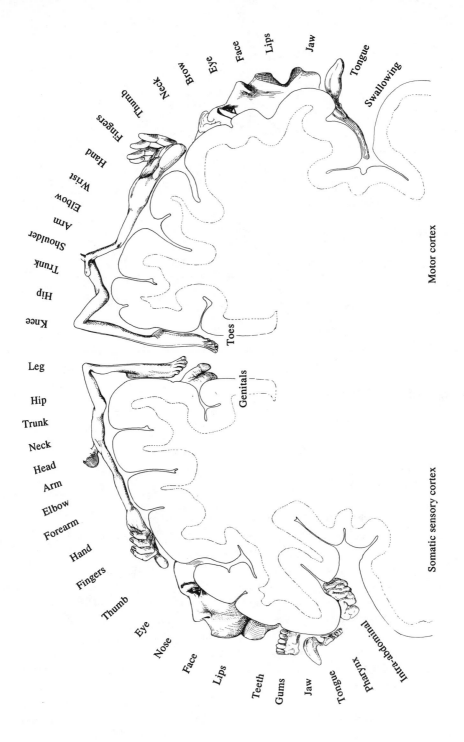

Motor cortex

Somatic sensory cortex

FIGURE 1.4

Somatic sensory and motor regions of the cerebral cortex are specialized in the sense that every site in these regions can be associated with some part of the body. In other words, most of the body can be mapped onto the cortex, yielding two distorted homunculi. The distortions come about because the area of the cortex dedicated to a part of the body is proportional not to that part's actual size but to the precision with which it must be controlled. In humans, the motor and somatic sensory regions given over to the face and the hands are greatly exaggerated. Only half of each cortical region is shown: the left somatic sensory area (which receives sensations primarily from the right side of the body) and the right motor cortex (which exercises control over movement in the left half of the body). [From N. Geschwind, "Specializations of the Human Brain," in *The Brain*, a *Scientific American* book (San Francisco: W. H. Freeman and Company, 1979), p. 110.]

The Physiology
of the Neuron

The Neuron as the Basic Component of the Brain

In a study of the nervous system, structure and function must be considered together, because they are intimately related. Further, to understand the effects of drugs on the nervous system, the principles of the structure and function of the *nerve cell* (the *neuron*), which is the basic component of the nervous system, must be described.

Neurons exhibit two special properties that distinguish them from all other cells in the body. The first property is their ability to conduct electrical impulses over long distances. The second property is their ability to carry out specific input and output relations with both other nerve cells and other tissues of the body, the functions of which the neurons may control. These input–output connections determine the function of a particular neuron and, in turn, the patterns of behavioral response that neuronal activity may elicit.[1]

The human brain contains about 100 billion neurons.[2] Most of these neurons share common structural and functional characteristics (Figure

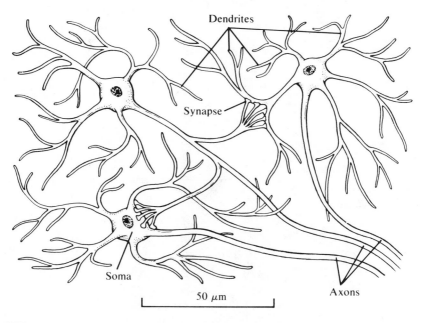

FIGURE II.1

Schematic representation of three nerve cells, showing the major subdivisions of such cells and the interactions between them.

II.1). Structurally, a typical neuron consists of a cell body (the *soma*), which contains the nucleus of the cell. Extending from the soma, many short fibers, called *dendrites* (consisting of hundreds or thousands of widely branched extensions), connect with the axons of other neurons to receive impulses through receptor sites, which are located on the dendritic membrane.[2] An electrical current is then generated and travels down the dendrite to the soma. Extending from the soma is an elongated process, called an *axon,* which varies in length from as short as a few millimeters to as long as 1 meter (for example, the axons that project down the spinal cord or that run from the motor neurons of the spinal cord out to the muscles that they innervate). The axon, in essence, transmits activity from the soma to other neurons or to muscles, organs, or glands of the body. Normally, the axon conducts impulses in one direction only: from the soma, down the axon, to a specialized structure, which, together with one or more dendrites from another neuron, forms a complex microspace, called a *synapse* (Figure II.2).

A synapse is a minute space that exists between the presynaptic membrane (which is the axon terminal) of one neuron and the

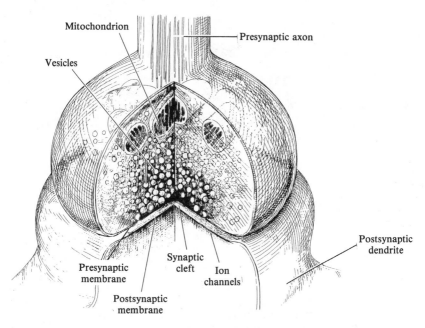

Mitochondrion

Presynaptic axon

Vesicles

Postsynaptic
dendrite

Presynaptic
membrane

Synaptic
cleft

Ion
channels

Postsynaptic
membrane

FIGURE II.2

A synapse is the relay point at which information is conveyed by chemical transmitters from one neuron to another. A synapse consists of two parts: the knob-like tip of an axon terminal at the presynaptic side and the receptor region on the dendritic surface of another neuron at the postsynaptic side. The membranes are separated by a synaptic cleft some 200 nanometers across. Molecules of chemical transmitter, stored in vesicles in the axon terminal, are released into the cleft by arriving nerve impulses. The transmitter changes the electrical state of the receiving neuron, making it either more likely or less likely to fire an impulse. [From C. F. Stevens, "The Neuron," in *The Brain*, a *Scientific American* book (San Francisco: W. H. Freeman and Company, 1979), p. 11.]

postsynaptic membrane (which is usually located on a dendrite)[*] of the receiving neuron.[2] The presynaptic terminal contains numerous structural elements, the most important of which (for the purposes of this discussion) are the small synaptic vesicles, each of which contains several thousand molecules of neurotransmitter chemical. These vesicles, therefore, store the transmitter, which is available for release (Figure II.3). Through a process of exocytosis, molecules of transmitter are released into the synaptic cleft itself. The transmitter substance diffuses across the synaptic cleft and attaches to receptors on the dendrite of the next neuron, thereby transmitting information chemically from one neuron to another. The neurons do not physically touch each other; thus, synaptic transmission is a chemical (rather than an electrical) process.

Usually, only one axon will arise from the soma, but, in its projection, the axon may give off many side branches, sending impulses to hundreds or thousands of other neurons (causing a *divergence of information*). Several dendrites can arise from one soma. The dendrites branch profusely and receive several thousand contacts from other cells (which results in the *convergence of information*). The dendrites then process the impulses and passively transmit electrical activity to the soma. The soma, in turn, actively transmits the impulses down the axon to as many as 10,000 other neurons. Thus, thousands of neurons converge on a single neuron, which, in turn, spreads its own impulses to thousands of other neurons.

As a consequence of this convergence and divergence of electrical activity, neurons tend to group together and form circuits. The properties of these circuits determine the way in which information is handled in the nervous system. The neural circuits form the discrete brain structures that were discussed in Appendix I. Thus, one can distinguish those areas of the brain where cell bodies and their dendrites are concentrated (these areas are referred to as *nuclei*) from those regions that consist mainly of axons that project from one group of neurons to another (these regions are referred to as *fiber tracts*). Thus, axons are

---

[*]In this introductory discussion, we discuss most synapses as occurring between axon terminals of one neuron and postsynaptic receptors located on the dendrites of a second neuron. Axon terminals are also located on the soma of the second neuron, in which instance the transmitter substance is most often inhibitory in nature, exerting a profound inhibitory effect on neuronal function. In addition, some axons synapse directly on the axon terminals of a second neuron. Again, these are usually inhibitory in nature. In this instance, the process is termed "presynaptic inhibition". Such synapses are thought to function in a type of negative feedback inhibition, since the discharge of the second neuron causes the release of inhibitory neurotransmitter directly on the presynaptic terminal of the first neuron, limiting its ability to release further amounts of transmitter.

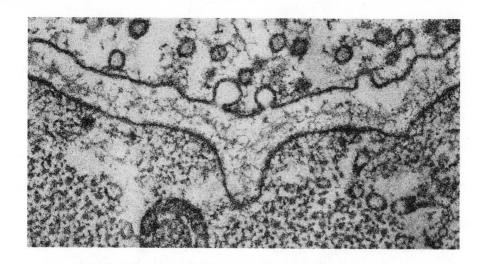

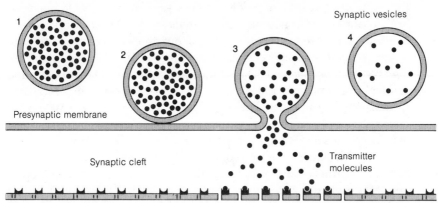

FIGURE II.3

Transmitter is discharged into the synaptic cleft at the synaptic junction between neurons by vesicles that open up after they fuse with the axon's presynaptic membrane, a process called *exocytosis*. This electron micrograph, made by Heuser, has caught the vesicles in the terminal of an axon in the act of discharging acetylcholine into the neuromuscular junction of a frog. The structures that appear in the micrograph are enlarged some 115,000 diameters. Synaptic vesicles are clustered near the presynaptic membrane. The diagram shows the probable steps in exocytosis. Filled vesicles move up to the synaptic cleft, fuse with the membrane, discharge their contents, and are reclaimed, re-formed, and refilled with transmitter. [From C. F. Stevens, "The Neuron," in *The Brain*, a *Scientific American* book (San Francisco: W. H. Freeman and Company, 1979), p. 24.]

sometimes called *fibers* or *nerve fibers*. In the peripheral nervous system (that is, outside the brain and spinal cord), bundles of axons are commonly referred to as *nerves*.

In the brain, the somas of several thousand individual neurons group together to form structures (nuclei). Further, those nuclei tend to congregate to form yet larger structures (such as the *thalamus, hypothalamus, amygdala,* and *hippocampus*). Each nucleus consists of tens of thousands of individual nerve-cell bodies (somas). The fiber tracts of the brain are often given names that indicate the areas of the brain that are connected by the tracts. For example, the bundle of sensory axons that runs from the spinal cord to the thalamus is referred to as the *spinothalamic tract.*

In addition to neurons, other types of cells are also found in the brain. The most conspicuous of these are the *glial cells* (which make up more than half the volume of the brain). One type of glial cell (the *astrocyte*) surrounds blood capillaries in the brain to form part of the blood-brain barrier (Chapter 1). Other glial cells provide structural support for the brain and metabolic support for the neurons in a fashion that has not yet been well identified.

In summary:

> The brain, then, is an immense number of spidery nerve cells, interconnected in a complex net, and embedded in a supporting and protecting meshwork of neuroglia. Dendrites spring from the neuron cell body, branch profusely, and along with the soma receive myriads of axon terminals, making it possible for a single nerve cell to gather information from hundreds of others. Furthermore, cell bodies are collected into groups, the nuclei, and these, in turn, into clusters. Running back and forth between nuclei, or between collections of nuclei, are fiber tracts, the main channels of communications between one part of the brain and another. Altogether, these structures are arranged in an orderly way to form the brain of the animal and to provide the anatomical basis for neural function.[1]

Further,

> It is reasonable to think of the brain as a symphony of almost infinite orchestration with assemblies of instrumentations evoking an infinite ensemble of informational responses. The brain, vast and adaptable, is capable of providing for all the subtleties of sensing, integrating and responding. . . . The neuron is the basic information processor and transmitter.[2]

Relevant to this anatomy and critical to the study of neuro-psychopharmacology is the fact that psychoactive drugs exert their behavioral effects secondary to their production of very specific altera-tions in the synaptic function of neurons that are located within specific areas of the brain.

The Axon

As discussed previously, the neuron consists of three main elements: the dendrites, the soma, and the axon. In brief, electrical impulses originate in the dendrites; they are integrated in the soma (where the action potentials are formed); and they are transmitted down the axon to the synapse. Unlike the dendrites and the soma, the axon is specialized solely for the reliable conduction of electrical activity, which occurs in the form of electri-cal impulses, called *action potentials*. All action potentials are conducted down a given axon rapidly and without alteration. The only way to change the content of information that is relayed by an axon is to alter the number of action potentials that are conducted each second.

The axon is, in general, not a major site of action for psychoactive drugs, but it is the site of action for local anesthetics (Chapter 13). Lidocaine (Xylocaine), for example, is a local anesthetic that, if it is injected into the tissues that surround the axons that carry sensory stimuli from a tooth, effectively blocks the transmission of pain im-pulses from the tooth to the brain. The anesthetic does not affect the generation of pain impulses in the tooth directly; rather, it blocks the axonal conduction of the nociceptive stimuli to the brain.

The Dendrites

How do action potentials (which are conducted down the axon) in-fluence the activity of other neurons? Information is transferred be-tween neurons in the following manner. As discussed previously, the terminal boutons of an axon align themselves at the synapse in close approximation to one or more of the dendrites of the next neuron.

Dendrites are specialized structures that receive chemical transmitter released from other neurons. When action potentials have been conducted down the axon of a neuron and transmitter has been released from that neuron, the dendrites of the postsynaptic neuron will exhibit an electrical change, the magnitude of which is proportional to the degree of postsynaptic receptor stimulation by transmitter (Figure II.4). Thus, when action potientials reach the synapse, a chemical transmitter is released, which diffuses across a small, fluid-filled gap (the synaptic cleft) and attaches to receptors on the postsynaptic (dendritic) membrane (Figure II.3). If the transmitter chemical affects the membrane in such a way that the membrane is depolarized, the neuron becomes more excitable (Figure II.4). This depolarization is referred to as an *excitatory postsynaptic potential* (EPSP). Note from Figure II.4 that a slight delay (approximately 0.5 millisecond) occurs between the arrival of an action potential at a nerve terminal and the EPSP in the postsynaptic (dendritic) membrane. This time lag is called the *synaptic delay*. It is explained by the time that is required for the transmitter substance, which is released by the axon, to reach the dendrite of the next cell.

In the CNS, all neurons are held in a balance between excitation and inhibition. If all synapses were excitatory, every cell in the brain would discharge at an uncontrolled rate. Thus, to balance excitation, a process of inhibition must also occur. Indeed, some transmitter chemicals (Appendix III), instead of depolarizing the dendrites, induce a *hyperpolarization* of the dendritic membrane. This hyperpolarizing potential is referred to as an *inhibitory postsynaptic potential* (IPSP). This IPSP opposes the action of the EPSP; it stabilizes the neuron and tends to prevent the generation of action potentials.

All the neurons in the CNS receive impulses from both excitatory and inhibitory synapses. Indeed, the exquisite beauty of the nervous system is maintained by this delicate balance between excitation and inhibition. Psychoactive drugs, because they affect synaptic transmission, tend to upset this balance. It is the result of this alteration of excitability within specific areas of the nervous system that leads to drug-induced alterations in behavior.

The Soma

The dendrites and soma (Figure II.5) receive input from other neurons through synapses and respond by becoming either depolarized (increased excitability) or hyperpolarized (decreased excitability). All the impulses that are received by the dendrites and the soma affect the level of excitability of the soma (the cell body), which gives rise to a single axon and, therefore, to a single channel through which these impulses are transmitted to other neurons. The soma integrates (or averages) the impulses that are gathered by the dendrites and the soma. If the influence of ex-

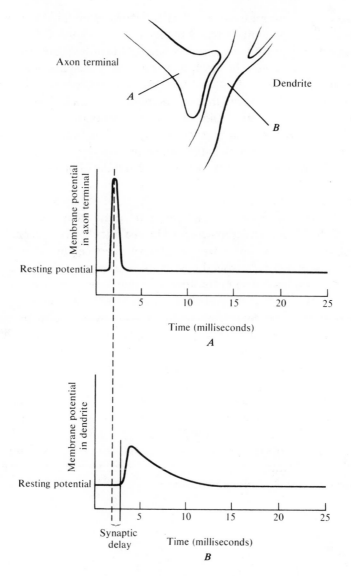

FIGURE II.4

Transmission of impulses from one neuron to another at a synapse. Graph A is a recording of electrical activity in the axon terminal as an action potential arrives at the synapse. Graph B is a recording of electrical activity in the dendrite of the next neuron, showing the postsynaptic activity resulting from the transmission of impulses across the synapse. [Modified from C. F. Stevens, *Neurophysiology: A Primer* (New York: Wiley, 1966), Figure 3.2, p. 35.]

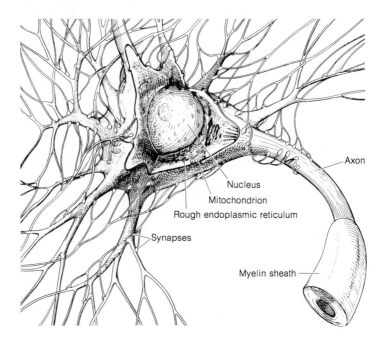

FIGURE II.5

The cell body of a neuron contains the genetic material and complex metabolic apparatus common to all cells. Unlike most other cells, however, neurons do not divide after embryonic development; an organism's original supply must serve a lifetime. Projecting from the cell body are several dendrites and a single axon. The cell body and dendrites are covered by synapses—knob-like structures where information is received from other neurons. Mitochondria provide the cell with energy. Proteins are synthesized on the endoplasmic reticulum. A transport system moves proteins and other substances from the cell body to sites where they are needed. [From C. F. Stevens, "The Neuron," in *The Brain*, a *Scientific American* book (San Francisco: W. H. Freeman and Company, 1979), p. 17.]

citatory synapses is greater than the influence of inhibitory synapses, the soma will respond by producing an action potential. The action potential spreads into the axon, and then it is conducted to the next synapse. If, instead, the influence of inhibitory synapses predominates, the soma will hyperpolarize, and the neuron will become less excitable. The soma, therefore, expresses the integration of synaptic input.

Properties of Excitable Membranes

All body fluid that is outside the bloodstream is either inside cellular membranes (*intracellular fluid*) or outside the cells, surrounding them but remaining outside the bloodstream (*extracellular fluid*). An impor-

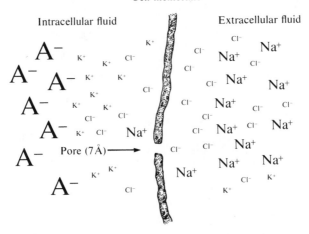

FIGURE II.6

Distribution of ions across a cell membrane. The cell membrane is a protein–fat barrier (see Figure 1.4) that apparently contains small pores, approximately 7 Å in diameter, and allows the passage of water and of certain small ions: Na+, sodium ions; Cl–, chloride ions; K+, potassium ions; A–, large protein molecules that contain negative charges. As their relative sizes indicate, potassium and chloride ions are able to diffuse freely through the pores; sodium ions are less able to do so; and protein molecules are largely not able to diffuse.

tant difference between extracellular and intracellular fluid is in their concentrations of certain ions (small, electrically charged molecules). This imbalance between extracellular and intracellular fluids results largely from the varying permeability of the cell membrane to water-soluble, fat-insoluble substances. The cell membranes (Chapter 1) are structures of protein and fat that contain small, water-filled pores, which are about 7 angstroms in diameter. The membrane is freely permeable to potassium ions and chloride ions (which are smaller than 7 angstroms); it is relatively impermeable to sodium ions; and it is quite impermeable to large protein molecules. The concentrations of sodium and chloride are much higher in extracellular fluid; and the concentration of potassium is much higher in intracellular fluid (Figure II.6).

As a consequence of this ionic imbalance on either side of the cell membrane, an electrical potential (difference in voltage) occurs across the membrane. This electrical potential may reach minus 50 to minus 90 millivolts; the inner side of the membrane is negative in relation to the outer side. Such a difference in potential exists in every cell of the body (not only neurons), and it is referred to as the *resting potential* of the cell

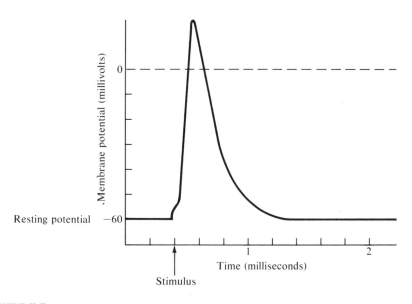

FIGURE II.7

Graph of an action potential. A stimulus was applied at the time indicated by the arrow. [From C. F. Stevens, *Neurophysiology: A Primer* (New York: Wiley, 1966), Figure 2.3, p. 14.]

The magnitude of the resting potential varies from one cell type to another.

Assuming that all cells of the body exhibit this resting potential, what distinguishes nerve cells (which are excitable structures that are capable of generating action potentials) from all other cells of the body? When the neuron (the intracellular fluid) becomes less negatively charged (in relation to the extracellular fluid), the axon is said to be depolarized (Figure II.7). When the axon is depolarized by a few millivolts, a "threshold" is reached and the permeability of the membrane is uniquely altered so that the membrane rapidly becomes more permeable to sodium. Indeed, within a fraction of a millisecond, sodium channels open in the membrane, resulting in a flow of sodium (along its concentration gradient) from the outside to the inside of the cell, neutralizing the electrical potential that was formerly maintained across the membrane. At this point, the entry of sodium into the neuron during depolarization produces a flow of potassium (along its concentration gradient) out of the neuron[2] (all of which takes about 1 millisecond to happen!), restoring the resting potential. Then, through a "pump," the membrane redistributes the

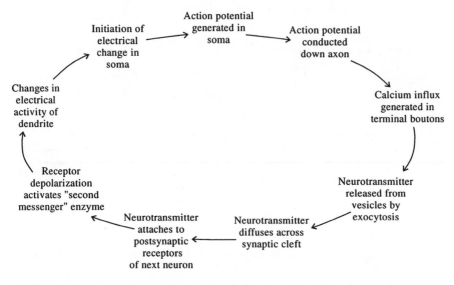

FIGURE II.8

Sequence of the transmission of information between neurons.

ions and restores the original distribution of sodium and potassium. When the action potential arrives near the axon terminal, calcium channels in the membrane open and calcium crosses the neuronal membrane into the cell. This influx of calcium triggers the release of transmitter chemical (through exocytosis) for 1 to 2 milliseconds.[3] This entire sequence of information transfer is diagrammed in Figure II.8.

Appendix III continues this discussion by focusing on the process of synaptic transmission, the chemical substances that are involved, and some general concepts that relate to drug-induced alterations of synaptic transmission.

NOTES

1. C. F. Stevens, "The Neuron," in *The Brain*, a *Scientific American* book (San Francisco: W. H. Freeman and Company, 1979), pp. 15–25.
2. S. Cohen, *The Chemical Brain* (Irvine, Calif.: Care Institute, 1988), pp. 1–10.
3. J. R. Cooper, F. E. Bloom, and R. H. Roth, *The Biochemical Basis of Neuropharmacology*, 5th ed. (New York: Oxford, 1986).

Synaptic Transmission and Transmitters

In Appendix II, we discussed the electrical phenomena that characterize neurons as unique entities and that are the basis of nervous system function. We introduced the concept that all information transfer in the brain occurs through the interaction of one neuron with another, which is accomplished through a process that involves the liberation of chemical transmitters into a synaptic junction between two neurons. Although today we universally accept chemical transmission as a fact, this concept developed slowly over the past 50 to 70 years. Today, this theory is so well accepted that the actions of most psychoactive drugs can be interpreted in terms of the alterations that occur in the identifiable steps of synaptic transmission.

This appendix begins with a discussion of the steps that are involved in synaptic transmission and the criteria that a chemical must meet to be called a *transmitter substance*. Next, we present specific substances that are known to function in the CNS as synaptic transmitters. Finally, the role of these transmitters both in neuropsychological disorders and in the action of psychoactive drugs is discussed as an introduction to the extensive presentation that is provided in the chapters of this text.

Historical Background

The first suggestion that chemical substances might be involved in the transmission of information between neurons was probably made in 1877. Subsequent work by such physiologists as Langley (1901), Elliot (1904), Dixon (1907), Dale (1914) and Loewi (1921) established the foundation for the concept that neuronal excitation results in the local release of a chemical substance, which causes specific activity by combination with some constituent of the end-organ, muscle, or gland. The work of these early physiologists led to the identification of acetylcholine and epinephrine as transmitter substances in the peripheral nervous system (nerves that lie outside the brain and spinal cord). Indeed, numerous studies from the 1920s through the 1940s established quite conclusively that a chemical mediator is instrumental in the transmission of impulses across synapses.

The second phase of neurochemical research extended from 1946 through the early 1970s, when a flood of research delineated the neurochemical pathways and prototype neurotransmitters (primarily acetylcholine, serotonin, norepinephrine, and dopamine), while numerous amino acids and peptides were considered to be possible candidates. Studies focused on psychedelic drug action considered it a secondary occurrence to either stimulation or blockade of the steps in the process of synaptic transmission.

During the past decade, a third phase of research has refined our understanding of the relation between neurotransmitters and drug action (at least until the next phase of research, which will continue through the 1990s and the 21st century). We now recognize that many more neurotransmitters exist than we previously thought (our estimate had been approximately six to eight "classic" substances). In reality, 40 or more neurotransmitters exist; some serve as primary transmitters, while many others function as modulators (for example, they modulate, presynaptically, the release of a primary transmitter) or as neurohormones (autacoids) that alter postsynaptic neuronal responsiveness (see the discussion of caffeine; Chapter 7). However, it is not clear whether a single neuron liberates one or several transmitter substances. (We formerly thought that one neuron was capable only of manufacturing and releasing a single neurotransmitter, neuromodulator, or neurohormone.) As stated by Cohen:

> It may be that most neurons contain multiple transmitters, for example, an amine or amino acid [as a primary transmitter], along with a neuropeptide to modulate the transmission and sometimes

a neurohormone to prolong the transmission. All neurochemical information circuits are widely dispersed and are almost never localized in discrete brain areas. As a corollary, many neurotransmitting systems converge on single brain regions. These features of transmitter function make simple statements about the effects of various transmitters incomplete. Furthermore, the receptors exhibit a considerable self-regulatory capability, changing their sensitivity during excessive or infrequent use.

Many of the important transmitters are amines and are called biogenic [biological] amines as a group. Most are monoamines; that is, they have a single ammonium (NH_2) radical in their structure. The biogenic amines derived from catechol (dihydrobenzene) are named catecholamines and include dopamine, norepinephrine, and epinephrine. Another monoamine is serotonin, 5-hydroxytryptamine. Acetylcholine is not an amine. It does not contain an NH_2 group. It can be classified as a choline ester.[1]

Thus, the past decade has yielded much new (and often confusing) information about an increasing number of neurotransmitters and neuromodulators as well as the diversity of effects that are attributed to them. This information greatly increases (and confuses) the possible sites of action for psychoactive drugs, making our initial biological amine hypotheses (of the 1950s through the 1970s) often appear simplistic. The older concepts, however, provided a framework for experimentation and interpretation, which can now be modified to fit our new concepts. Indeed, the concepts of mechanisms that underlie both neuropsychological disorders and the actions of psychoactive drugs have been modified in this text to reflect this new phase of neuropsychopharmacology.

Steps in Synaptic Transmission

The synapse is centrally important to the functioning of the nervous system and to the action of psychoactive drugs. Thus, it is useful to examine, in more detail, the structural features of the synapse and its process of transferring information from one cell to another. Figure III.1 shows a schematic representation of an idealized synapse. The axon terminal is located in close approximation to the dendrite, with a narrow space of about 200 angstroms between them. This space (the *synaptic cleft*) separates the presynaptic membrane (the *axon terminal*) from the postsynaptic membrane of the dendrite. Mitochondria (which are

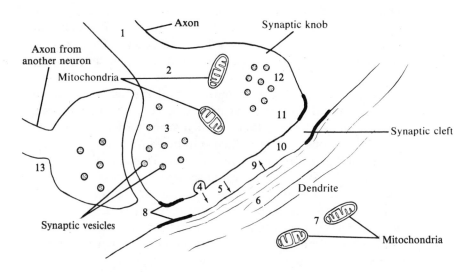

FIGURE III.1

Schematic diagram of an idealized synapse within the central nervous system. The steps in the transmission of information across such a synapse are numbered in this diagram:

1. Conduction of the action potential down the presynaptic axon.
2. Arrival of the action potential at the nerve terminal.
3. Synthesis and storage of transmitter in the synaptic vesicles (this may occur before steps 1 and 2).
4. Release of transmitter from synaptic vesicles (by a process of exocytosis) into the synaptic cleft when an action potential arrives.
5. Diffusion of transmitter across the synaptic cleft.
6. Stimulation of the postsynaptic receptors by transmitter.
7. Postsynaptic cellular response to receptor activation.
8. "Adaptive" or "plastic" processes on presynaptic and postsynaptic membranes in response to excess or deficient amounts of transmitter.
9. Release of transmitter from postsynaptic receptors back into the synaptic cleft.
10. Metabolism of some of the transmitter in the synaptic cleft by extracellular enzymes.
11. Reuptake of some of the transmitter back into the presynaptic nerve terminal.
12. Uptake of transmitter that is free in the intracellular fluid of the presynaptic nerve terminal into the synaptic vesicles, where it is protected from destruction by enzymes located in the cytoplasm.
13. Axon exerting presynaptic inhibition.

the metabolic "factories" of the cell) and numerous small synaptic vesicles are located in the *presynaptic terminal*. These vesicles are approximately 300 to 600 angstroms in diameter. In the nervous system, they are almost universally found intracellularly adjacent to the presynaptic membrane. In fact, the presence of these synaptic vesicles is considered to be proof of the presence of a synapse. The transmitter chemical is stored in these vesicles before it is released. The postsynaptic membrane is similar to membranes found elsewhere in the nervous system.

This, then, is the general organization of the synapse. Structure alone, however, does not explain the sequence of events that occurs between the arrival of an action potential at the terminal of one axon and the alterations that are then produced in the postsynaptic membrane of the dendrite of the next neuron. There are about a dozen steps to consider in the synaptic transmission process (numbered in Figure III.1), and each one constitutes a possible site of drug action. The steps include those that occur within the presynaptic terminal, on the presynaptic membrane, within the synaptic cleft, on the postsynaptic membrane, or within the postsynaptic neuron. Presynaptically and within the synaptic cleft itself, some events can involve long-term cellular adaptive mechanisms (possibly involved in drug tolerance and/or dependence); or they can involve presynaptic modulation which may control or otherwise determine the transmitter release response to the calcium influx which follows arrival of an action potential.

Of increasing interest are events that occur within the postsynaptic membrane. The postsynaptic receptor for transmitter consists of specific recognition sites (located on the outer layer of the membrane) for transmitter. The remainder of the receptor complex serves as a sort of transducer that relays the signal (the fact that the receptor has been activated) to the inner part of the dendrite (or soma). This signal, in turn, generates either the excitatory postsynaptic potential (EPSP) or the inhibitory postsynaptic potential (IPSP) by opening or closing the ion channels of the postsynaptic neuron. In addition, it may activate a "second messenger" system (the presynaptically released transmitter was the first messenger) that can have several possible effects: activation of enzymes that manufacture certain neuronal proteins, alteration of membrane conductance, or change in the rate of protein synthesis.

Criteria for a Transmitter Substance

There is an ongoing search for specific neurotransmitters in the CNS—a search that has greatly increased the number of defined or highly likely compounds identified. A number of criteria must be satisfied to prove that a chemical is, in fact, a neurotransmitter (Table III.1).

TABLE III.1

Criteria for a chemical neurotransmitter.

1. The proposed compound must be contained within the presynaptic nerve terminal
2. The proposed compound must be released from nerve endings on stimulation of the nerve
3. Injection of the proposed neurotransmitter must mimic the synaptic action that normally occurs after transmitter is released
4. There must be some mechanism (enzymatic or otherwise) by which transmitter action can be terminated and that fits the time course of transmitter action
5. Drugs that interfere with the actions of the proposed transmitter must exert an identical interfering action on the effects of nerve stimulation at the synapse in question

Certainly, the first criterion is that the transmitter chemical must be contained within a presynaptic terminal, or, at least, an immediate precursor (a substance that will eventually become the transmitter) must be present. Second, this transmitter substance in the presynaptic terminal must be released from the synaptic nerve ending in response to the arrival of an action potential. In the peripheral nervous system, performing assays to satisfy this second criterion is relatively easy, but in the CNS, it is more difficult, because it is almost impossible to stimulate one axon selectively and then to collect any substance that is released from the terminals of that axon. The third criterion is that an injection of a suspected synaptic transmitter must exert an effect on the postsynaptic membrane that is identical to the effect that normally follows the release of transmitter. The same technical difficulties that hinder satisfaction of the second criterion also hinder satisfaction of the third criterion. The fourth criterion is the existence of a mechanism (enzymatic or otherwise) that can terminate the action of the transmitter and that fits the time course of action of the transmitter substance. This criterion can be satisfied more easily, but it is difficult to pinpoint precisely the exact mechanisms that are involved. The fifth criterion is that drugs that are known to alter the synthesis, release, action, reuptake, or degradation of a supposed transmitter substance must exert an identical action at the synapse in question.

To date, there are few sites in the brain where a postulated transmitter substance has been shown to meet all these criteria, primarily because of the enormous technical difficulties that are involved in isolating and studying single synapses in the brain. However, several substances have shown physiological and pharmacological evidence that is strong enough to identify them as putative neurotransmitters.

Specific Transmitter Substances

In this section, we discuss the major neurotransmitter substances: acetylcholine, norepinephrine, dopamine, serotonin, excitatory and inhibitory amino acids, the opioid peptides, and (briefly) other putative neurotransmitters.

Acetylcholine

Acetylcholine was first identified as a transmitter chemical in the peripheral nervous system. We now know that large amounts of acetylcholine are present in brain tissue. Thus, we shall discuss the evidence for and against the role of acetylcholine as a transmitter in the CNS.

The chemical reactions in the nerve terminal that lead to the synthesis of acetylcholine are illustrated in Figure III.2. The dynamics of the acetylcholine nerve terminal (that is, a nerve terminal that releases acetylcholine) are portrayed in Figure III.3. Following synthesis, acetylcholine is stored inside the nerve terminal within synaptic vesicles. It is released into the synaptic cleft when an action potential arrives from the axon. The acetylcholine then diffuses across the cleft and attaches itself to receptors that are located on the dendrite of the next neuron, which results in the transmission of information between the two neurons. Scopolamine is a psychedelic drug that blocks the postsynaptic receptors for acetylcholine. Thus, in Chapter 11, it is referred to as an anticholinergic psychedelic drug.

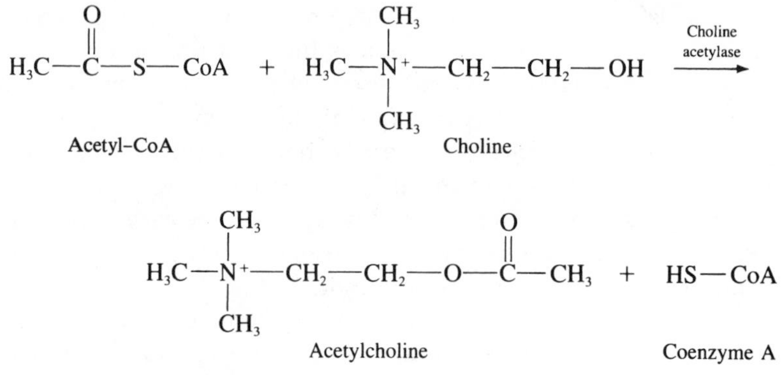

FIGURE III.2

Chemical reactions in the brain that are responsible for synthesis of acetylcholine (ACh). The acetylcholine is synthesized from acetyl-CoA and choline.

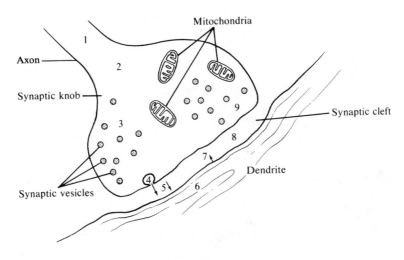

FIGURE III.3

Schematic diagram of an acetylcholine (ACh) synapse. The steps in transmission of information across such a synapse are numbered in this diagram:

1. Conduction of the action potential down the presynaptic axon.
2. Arrival of the action potential at the nerve terminal.
3. Synthesis of ACh (see Figure III.2) and storage of ACh in the synaptic vesicles (this may occur before steps 1 and 2).
4. Release of ACh from synaptic vesicles into the synaptic cleft when an action potential arrives.
5. Diffusion of ACh across the synaptic cleft.
6. Stimulation of the postsynaptic receptors by ACh.
7. Release of ACh from postsynaptic receptors back into the synaptic cleft.
8. Metabolism of ACh in the synaptic cleft by the enzyme AChE (see Figure III.4).
9. Uptake of choline that was produced by metabolism of ACh into the presynaptic nerve terminal for the resynthesis of ACh.

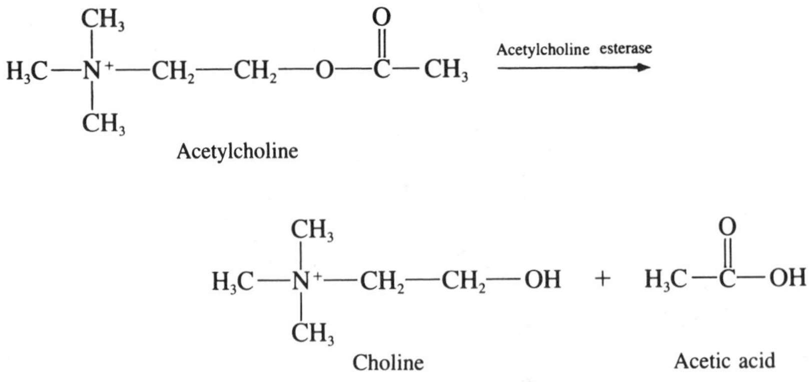

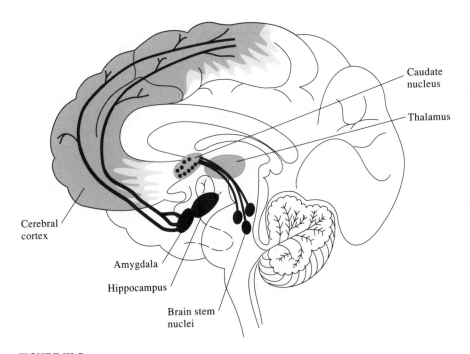

FIGURE III.4

Destruction of acetylcholine by the enzyme acetylcholine esterase (AChE).

FIGURE III.5

Cholinergic pathways in the human brain. Cell bodies and fiber tracts (axonal projections) are shown in black. Shaded areas show the locations of cholinergic terminals. [Modified from L. L. Iversen, "The Chemistry of the Brain," in *The Brain*, a *Scientific American* book (San Francisco: W. H. Freeman and Company, 1979), p. 77.]

Once acetylcholine has exerted its effect on the postsynaptic dendritic membrane, its action is terminated by the enzyme acetylcholine esterase (AChE). The process is illustrated in Figure III.4. The enzyme reaction that degrades acetylcholine is important, because many drugs (referred to as *AChE inhibitors*) will inhibit this enzyme. Such drugs are quite toxic. Commercially, this toxicity is exploited in agriculture, where AChE inhibitors are used as insecticides, and in the military where they are used as lethal nerve gases.

Acetylcholine is distributed widely in the brain (Figure III.5). The highest concentrations are found in the caudate nucleus, certain brain stem nuclei, and the cerebral cortex (especially the frontal cortex). High concentrations of acetylcholine are also found in the motor neurons that emerge from the spinal cord, which reflects the fact that acetylcholine is the transmitter at the neuromuscular junction.

In the basal ganglia, acetylcholine-containing neurons apparently persist after dopamine neurons degenerate in patients who have Parkinson's disease; and the relatively unopposed action of acetylcholine underlies the symptoms that are observed in patients who have that disorder. In patients who have died of Alzheimer's disease (presenile dementia), cerebral cortical acetylcholine receptors are conspicuously absent.[*2] Interestingly, scopolamine (Chapter 11) blocks acetylcholine receptors in the CNS. Scopolamine is a potent amnestic agent, and amnesia is a prominent symptom of Alzheimer's disease. Acetylcholine also appears to be important in mechanisms that are related to behavioral arousal, learning, memory, attention, energy conservation, mood, and REM activity during sleep. Acetylcholine neurons

---

[*]Cohen discusses the etiology of dementia of the Alzheimer's type (DAT): "In addition to the structural changes (senile plaques, neurofibrillary tangles, and cortical atrophy), some chemical alterations have been consistently documented in DAT. A decrease in choline acetyltransferase, the enzyme that makes ACh [acetylcholine], is found. ACh neuronal loss also occurs, so that cholinergic mechanisms tend to be severely reduced in DAT. Drugs that block muscarinic receptors (scopolamine, atropine), when given to normal young adults, reproduce a number of the cognitive defects of early DAT. Such agents will also worsen the disease. . . . No evidence exists that ingested choline increases ACh levels in the brain. Antipsychotic drugs, particularly haloperidol (Haldol), are used to provide dopamine blockade for the neurologic and the psychiatric aspects of these conditions and to reduce the ACh/DA imbalance.

"Mood changes caused by shifts in cholinergic activity have been reported: decreased activity evokes euphoria, and increased activity produces a depressive state.

"A nerve growth factor (NGF) previously found only in peripheral nerves has been recovered in brain neurons, particularly in cholinergic neurons. NGF is necessary for the development and maintenance of ACh mediated neurons, including those involved in memory."[3]

that are located in the hippocampus and cerebral cortex participate in learning, memory formation, and retrieval of memory.

Norepinephrine and Dopamine

The term *catecholamine* refers to three chemically related compounds: epinephrine, norepinephrine, and dopamine. Epinephrine is a neurohormone in the peripheral nervous system. It is important in the maintenance of such major body functions as blood pressure and heart rate. Epinephrine is not commonly found in the brain. During the last 10 years, a large body of evidence has accumulated which demonstrates that norepinephrine and dopamine are the primary catecholamine neurotransmitters in the brain. It has also become clear that many of the drugs that profoundly affect brain function and behavior exert their effects by altering the synaptic action of norepinephrine and dopamine in the brain. Thus, in many instances, the effects of new drugs on behavior have been predictable, because we know how they will affect the actions of catecholamine neurotransmitters.

Dopamine and norepinephrine are manufactured within catecholamine neurons by the steps shown in Figure III.6. Although we shall not discuss the details of this scheme, we will consider the step that involves the enzyme tyrosine hydroxylase as a catalyst. Inhibition of this enzyme by drugs, such as alpha-methyl-para-tyrosine, results in a reduction in brain catecholamines and induces sedation. This action apparently occurs secondary to the inhibition of norepinephrine synthesis by the inhibitiion of that enzyme, which would indicate that the levels and functioning of neurotransmitters within the brain underlie behavior. By similar reasoning, we might assume that drugs that alter behavior probably produce their effects secondary to alterations in chemical transmission between neurons. For example, patients who have Parkinson's disease exhibit a level of dopamine in the *caudate nucleus* of the brain that is lower than the amount that is normally present. Administration of dopamine into these patients' bodies is not useful therapeutically, because it does not cross the blood-brain barrier. However, the administration of dopa (the precursor to dopamine) *does* increase the level of dopamine in the caudate nucleus. Dopa can cross the blood-brain barrier, and it is converted into dopamine in the brain. This is an example of how knowledge of the chemical synthesis of a transmitter may be used to clinical benefit.

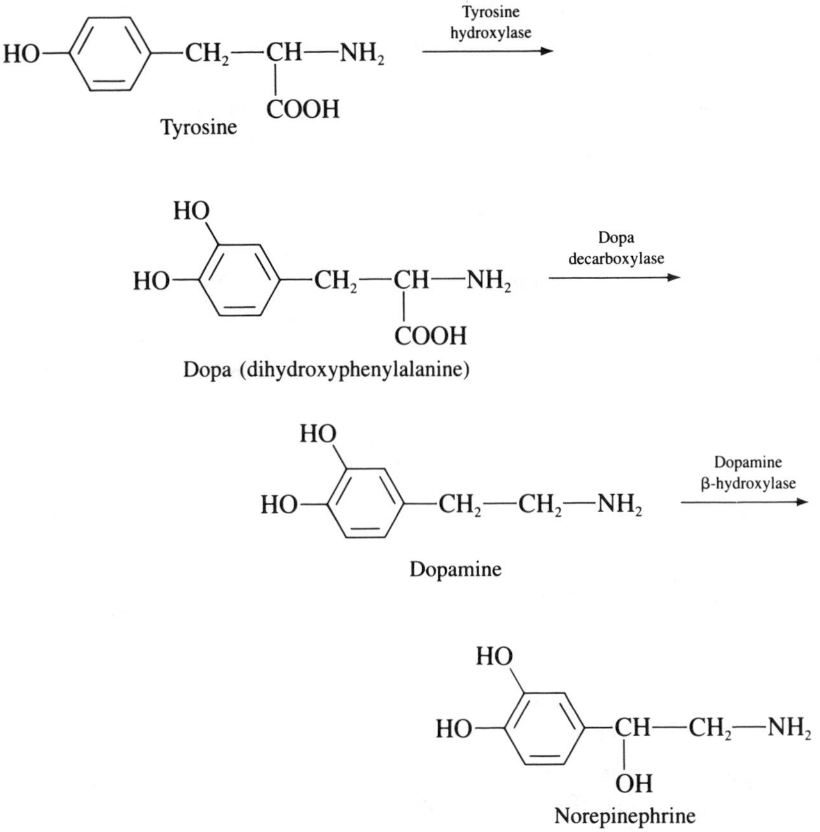

FIGURE III.6

Synthesis of norepinephrine (NE) from tyrosine. Note the intermediate compounds that are formed in this reaction: namely, dopa and dopamine.

METABOLIC FATE   A transmitter is synthesized, stored, and released; exerts a postsynaptic effect; and then is inactivated. Inactivation can occur by either, or both, of two processes: enzymatic destruction or reuptake of the transmitter from the synaptic cleft back into the presynaptic nerve terminal. Catecholamines are inactivated by the enzymes monoamine oxidase (MAO) and catechol *O*-methyltransferase (COMT) (Figure III.7). However, these enzymatic inactivations are much slower in the termination of dopamine or norepinephrine neurotransmission than is the destruction of acetylcholine by AChE in the termination of its neurotransmission. Thus, the postsynaptic effects of dopamine or norepinephrine are not terminated to any significant extent by enzymes. The actions of these transmitters are terminated

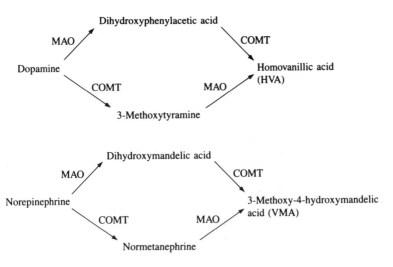

FIGURE III.7

Destruction of dopamine and norepinephrine. The inactivating enzymes are monamine oxidase (MAO) and catechol O-methyltransferase (COMT).

primarily by an active process of reuptake across the presynaptic nerve membrane back into the presynaptic nerve ending. When norepinephrine or dopamine is taken up in this way, it is then stored again in the synaptic vesicles to be reused later.

The principle of reuptake into the nerve terminal and then into the storage vesicles is crucially important, because certain drugs may block either (1) the active uptake process into the nerve terminal (thus prolonging the synaptic action of the transmitter) or (2) the uptake of the transmitter from the intracellular fluid in the nerve terminal back into the synaptic vesicles (thus decreasing the amount of stored transmitter available for release). Reserpine is an example of a drug that blocks the uptake of the transmitter back into the vesicle; cocaine is representative of drugs that block presynaptic reuptake of dopamine from the synaptic cleft into the nerve terminal; and the tricyclic antidepressants are drugs that block presynaptic reuptake into the nerve terminals of norepinephrine and serotonin neurons.

THE CATECHOLAMINE SYNAPSE   The dynamics of dopamine and norepinephrine resemble those of other CNS transmitters. A norepinephrine synapse is illustrated in Figure III.8. It is similar to the acetylcholine terminal that is presented in Figure III.3; that is, the presynaptic nerve terminal contains mitochondria and small vesicles that contain stored trans-

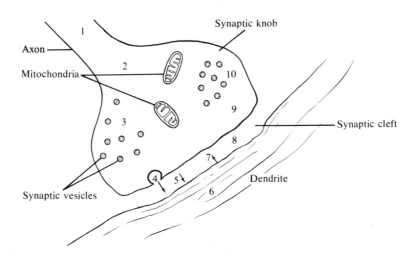

FIGURE III.8

Schematic diagram of a norepinephrine (NE) synapse within the central nervous system. The steps in the transmission of information across such a synapse are numbered in this diagram:

1. Conduction of the action potential down the presynaptic axon.
2. Arrival of the action potential at the nerve terminal.
3. Synthesis of NE (see Figure III.6) and storage of NE in the synaptic vesicles (this may occur before steps 1 and 2).
4. Release of NE from synaptic vesicles into the synaptic cleft when an action potential arrives.
5. Diffusion of NE across the synaptic cleft.
6. Stimulation of the postsynaptic receptors by NE.
7. Release of NE from postsynaptic receptors back into the synaptic cleft.
8. Metabolism of some of the NE in the synaptic cleft by extracellular enzymes.
9. Uptake of some of the NE back into the presynaptic nerve terminal.
10. Uptake of NE in the presynaptic nerve terminal into the presynaptic vesicles, where it is protected from destruction by the enzyme MAO.

mitter. Also, like the acetylcholine terminal, the catecholamine-containing presynaptic nerve terminal is separated from the postsynaptic dendritic membrane by a distance of approximately 200 angstroms. However, the dopamine and norepinephrine terminals contain chemical products entirely different from those in an acetylcholine terminal. The amino acid tyrosine (which is obtained from food) is actively taken up into the presynaptic terminal, where it is transformed to dopa, dopamine, and norepinephrine (Figure III.6). In those catecholamine nerve terminals in which the enzyme dopamine beta-hydroxylase is not present, dopamine is not converted to norepinephrine, and the dopamine itself serves as the transmitter substance.

After synthesis, the transmitter is stored in the synaptic vesicles. When an action potential arrives at the nerve terminal, a brief influx of calcium flows into the terminal, and the transmitter is released by exocytosis from the vesicles (which cluster close to the cleft) into the synaptic cleft. The transmitter then diffuses across the cleft and attaches to the postsynaptic membrane. The transmission process is terminated by the active reuptake of norepinephrine (or dopamine) back into the nerve terminal, where it is either metabolized by the intracellular enzyme MAO or else is taken up into, and stored by, the vesicles until it is released again.

NOREPINEPHRINE PATHWAYS AND FUNCTION   The cell bodies of norepinephrine neurons are located in the brain stem (Figure III.9). From there, axons project rostrally to nerve terminals that are located in the cerebral cortex, the limbic system, the hypothalamus, and the cerebellum. Caudally, axonal projections travel to the dorsal horns of the spinal cord, where they exert an analgesic action by limiting the release of substance P (Chapter 9).

The release of norepinephrine produces an alerting, focusing, orienting response (similar to the peripheral fight/flight/fright syndrome), positive feelings of reward, analgesia, and regulation of blood pressure. Basic instinctual behaviors such as hunger, thirst, emotion, and sex, may also be caused by a release of norepinephrine.

DOPAMINE PATHWAYS AND FUNCTION   The distribution of dopamine neurons and pathways in the CNS is more discrete than that of norepinephrine. Large amounts of dopamine are found in nerve terminals (synaptic boutons) that are located in the basal ganglia (a part of the *extrapyramidal motor system*), the frontal cortex, and the limbic system. The cell bodies of origin for these nerve terminals are largely found

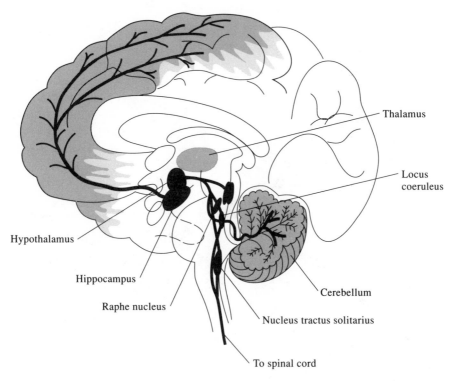

FIGURE III.9

Norepinephrine pathways in the human brain. Cell bodies and fiber tracts are shown in black. Norepinephrine terminals are represented by the shaded areas. [Modified from L. L. Iversen, "The Chemistry of the Brain," in *The Brain*, a *Scientific American* book (San Francisco: W. H. Freeman and Company, 1979), p. 77.]

in a brain-stem structure that is called the *substantia nigra* (Figure III.10) and in other discrete nuclei of the midbrain (that are associated with emotion and reward systems that involve the limbic system). Those axons that project to the frontal cortex seem to be involved with thought and the integration of emotions.

An alteration of dopamine function is important in at least two major disorders: schizophrenia and parkinsonism. In schizophrenics, an increased sensitivity of dopamine receptors occurs in the frontal cortex, which forms the rationale for treating schizophrenic patients with dopamine-receptor blockers (for example, phenothiazines; Chapter 10). The parkinsonism-like side effects of phenothiazines reflect a blockade of dopamine receptors in the basal ganglia (the drugs are not specific for dopamine receptors that are located in the frontal cortex).

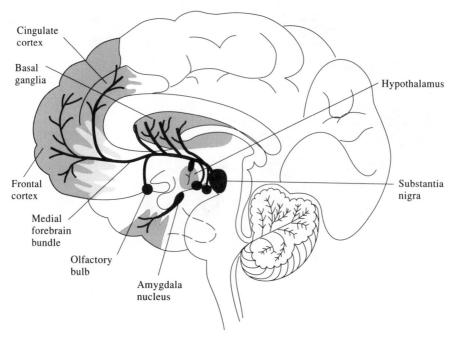

FIGURE III.10

Dopaminergic pathways in the rat brain. Cell bodies and fiber tracts (axonal projections) are shown in black. Dopaminergic terminals are represented by the shaded areas. [Modified from L. L. Iversen, "The Chemistry of the Brain," in *The Brain*, a *Scientific American* book (San Francisco: W. H. Freeman and Company, 1979), p. 77.]

Similarly, in patients who have Parkinson's disease (Chapter 13), the neurons in the basal ganglia are devoid of dopamine, so treatment that includes either replacement (with levodopa) or the administration of drugs that will stimulate dopamine receptors (agonists) can be useful. Finally, the behavioral stimulant and reinforcing properties of cocaine and amphetamine reflect the activation of dopamine receptors. Many drugs that affect dopamine neurons are discussed throughout this text.

Serotonin

Serotonin was first investigated as a CNS neurotransmitter when LSD was found to resemble serotonin structurally. At that time, a hypothesis

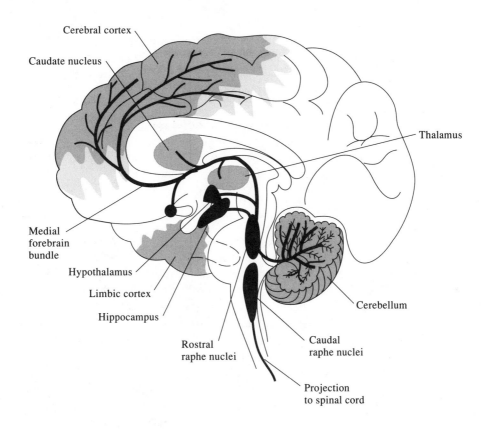

FIGURE III.11

Serotonin pathways in the rat brain. Cell bodies and fiber tracts (axonal projections) are shown in black. Serotonergic terminals are represented by the shaded areas. [Modified from L. L. Iversen, "The Chemistry of the Brain," in *The Brain*, a *Scientific American* book (San Francisco: W. H. Freeman and Company, 1979), p. 77.]

was advanced which asserted that drug-induced hallucinations might be caused by alterations in the functioning of serotonin neurons. In the brain, significant amounts of serotonin are found in the upper brain stem, with a large collection in the pons and the medulla (areas that are collectively called the *raphe nuclei*). Rostral projections from the brain stem terminate diffusely throughout the cerebral cortex, the hippocampus, the hypothalamus and the limbic system (Figure III.11). Because serotonin is an inhibitor of activity and behavior, these rostral projections are thought to function in sleep, wakefulness, mood, temperature regulation, feeding, and sexual activity. The serotonin projections largely parallel those of norepinephrine; and serotonin seems to have an effect that is opposite to that of norepinephrine (in a manner that is analogous to dopamine and acetylcholine opposing each other in the basal ganglia). Caudal projections of serotonin axons from the raphe nuclei inhibit the release of substance P in the spinal cord (Chapter 9) and control spinal reflexes.

Pharmacologically, the tricyclic antidepressants (especially the new serotonin-uptake blockers) relieve depression, improve mood, and improve eating and drinking behavior; all these actions likely occur through potentiation of serotonin neurotransmission.

Amino Acid Transmitters

Four amino acids function as CNS neurotransmitters: two (glutamic and aspartic acid) are excitatory to neuronal transmission, and two (gamma-aminobutyric acid, or GABA, and glycine) are inhibitory (Figure III.12).

GABA is a major inhibitor of neurotransmission in the brain. In drug studies, it has been shown that the antianxiety effects of benzodiazepines, such as diazepam (Valium), occur when the synaptic actions of GABA are facilitated. The benzodiazepines potentiate the actions of GABA in the brain by attaching to specific receptors, forming a complex of benzodiazepine, GABA, and the chloride channel (Chapter 5). The specific benzodiazepine antagonist (flumazenil) blocks this binding and reverses benzodiazepine overdoses. When it is marketed, it will be a significant advance in the management of patients who are suffering from benzodiazepine intoxication.

The identification both of the specific anxiolytic actions of the benzodiazepines and their specific action on GABA receptor complexes initiated a search for a "natural Valium." Although several candidate compounds have been postulated as an endogenous anxiolytic, none has yet emerged as a definitive winner. Recently, however, interest has focused on a stress-induced and stress-released neurohormone, *allopregnanolone*. This

---

*Cohen states: "The ability of various benzodiazepines to bind to the benzodiazepine receptor parallels their therapeutic potency. The highest concentration of these receptors is to be found in the limbic system, the hippocampus and the olfactory bulb, thus accounting for their antianxiety effects. Anxiety might be conceptualized as excessive firing in specfic brain areas, like the limbic system. The hyperexcitability feeds back to GABA neurons, after which GABA is released, opening the chloride channels and inhibiting neuronal firing. The presence of benzodiazepines enhances GABA binding and intensifies the antianxiety effect. Sudden withdrawal of the benzodiazepine after prolonged use may induce a rebound hyperexcitability with symptoms of sedative withdrawal. Eventually, GABA homeostasis is restored. Rather than a withdrawal syndrome, discontinuance of the benzodiazepine may permit the reemergence of preexisting anxiety that had been suppressed by the drug."[4]

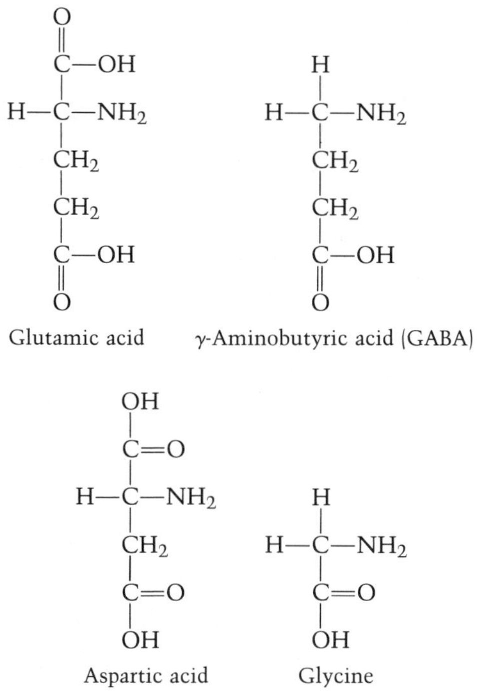

FIGURE III.12

Structures of four amino acid neurotransmitters within the CNS.

substance appears to exert a calming influence on patients. It binds to the GABA-chloride receptors (as do the benzodiazepines) and increases the activity of the neurotransmitter GABA. In turn, GABA inhibits the release of corticotropin-releasing hormone (which triggers normal stress responses) from the pituitary gland. Thus, stress-induced release of allopregnanolone may initiate a negative feedback response that limits the intensity of normal stress responses. Allopregnanolone is therefore a viable candidate for further study as an endogenous anxiolytic, the actions of which can be mimicked by the benzodiazepines.

Glycine is an inhibitory neurotransmitter in the spinal cord. When glycine receptors are blocked by *strychnine*, convulsions are produced.

Glutamate and *aspartate* are universally excitatory amino acids.[5] A synthetic derivative of aspartate (N-methyl-*d*-aspartate) is also excitatory. These agents appear to be involved in cellular metabolism by increasing ion conductance across membranes. Chapter 11 discusses the interaction between phencyclidine and N-methyl-*d*-aspartate.

Purines, expecially adenine, may function as CNS neurotransmitters and, posssibly, as neuromodulators. In Chapter 7, we described how the stimulant action of caffeine might result from the antagonism of inhibitory adenine neuromodulation.

Substance P is a peptide transmitter that is released by nociceptive afferent neurons that synapse in the dorsal horn of the spinal cord. Substance P is discussed at length in Chapter 9.

Opioid Peptides

In 1967, it was proposed that naturally occurring chemicals exist in the brain that provide analgesia by acting on their receptors and that the opioid narcotics might mimic these natural analgesic substances by binding to the same receptors. This proposal was based on three facts. First, opioids are highly specific; that is, certain very minor structural modifications convert an active drug into one that is almost totally inactive. Second, the extreme potency of some narcotics implies that only a specific receptor could account for this potency. For example, a narcotic named etorphine is 500 to 1000 times more potent than morphine. Thus, far fewer molecules of etorphine would be needed for the drug to exert its effects on the brain. Third, pure narcotic antagonists are available (see Chapter 9)—they displace pharmacologically active narcotics from their receptors.

In 1973, specific opioid receptors were identified in portions of the brain that contained a high concentration of nerve endings. It was then determined that only six areas of the brain have a high concentration of opioid receptors. First, high concentrations of opioid receptors are located in the brain stem, lining the wall of the fourth ventricle. In that area, either morphine or electrical stimulation produces analgesia, which can be blocked by naloxone. Second, the medial thalamus has a high concentration of opioid receptors. It is this area of the brain that appears to mediate deep pain that is poorly localized and is emotionally influenced—the kind of pain that is most strongly affected by narcotics. Third, opioid receptors are found in specific areas of the spinal cord that are involved with the receipt and integration of incoming sensory information. Here they function to reduce the intensity of painful stimuli. Fourth, receptors are also located in a specific nucleus of the brain stem that receives pain fibers from the face and the hands. Fifth, receptors are located in those centers of the brain stem that are involved in the mediation of cough, nausea and vomiting, maintenance of blood pressure, and control of stomach secretions. Finally, the greatest concentration of opioid receptors in the CNS is located in the limbic system—more specifically, in the amygdala. Although narcotics are not thought to exert analgesic actions through receptors in the limbic system, such receptors are probably associated with the influences of opioids on emotional behavior (see Chapter 9). Opioid receptors are only rarely found in the cerebral cortex, and none have been found in the cerebellum. Although opioid receptors have been found in all the vertebrates so far studied, they are not found in invertebrates.

In 1976, three types of opioid receptors were postulated: *mu, kappa,* and *sigma*. In 1981, a fourth type of receptor (the *delta* receptor) was added. More recent postulates focus on subtypes of these receptors.

Mu receptors are located primarily in the brain stem and medial thalamic areas. They appear to mediate morphine-induced analgesia and respiratory depression. Kappa receptors are located primarily in the spinal cord and mediate spinal analgesia (without respiratory depression). In the brain stem, these kappa receptors mediate the sedation and miosis (pupil constriction) that are induced by opioids. Sigma receptors are located primarily in the limbic system and mediate dysphoria and the psychotomimetic effects that are produced by certain of the opioids, especially pentazocine (Talwin) and butorphanol (Stadol). The newly described delta receptors are postulated to be involved in alterations of affective behavior and euphoria. These receptors appear to be specific target receptors for the enkephalin peptides.

Some opioid receptors are now divided further into subcategories. For example, a mu-1 receptor may be associated with analgesia, while a mu-2 receptor may be associated with respiratory depression. In the future, receptor-specific synthetic opioids might be developed so that specific mu-1 or kappa analgesia could be obtained in the absence of undesirable sigma, delta, or mu-2 side effects. Although this concept may seem far-fetched now, it should be remembered that this unfolding story only began during the late 1970s, and it is proceeding at breakneck speed.

Thus, although receptors for opioids have been found in specific areas of the brain, this discovery alone did not prove the existence of naturally occurring compounds in the brain that act on these receptors. However, in 1975, researchers isolated crude extracts from the brain that demonstrated actions that are similar to those of morphine in a preparation of small intestines from guinea pigs; that is, the brain extract inhibited intestinal contractions, and then that action was blocked by naloxone. Two proteins were isolated from this crude extract, each of which consisted of five amino acids. These two proteins were named *met-enkephalin* and *leu-enkephalin*. More recently, these proteins have been isolated from pig brain, beef brain, human cerebral spinal fluid, and the pituitary glands of several species. Also isolated from the pituitary gland was a longer protein (called *beta-lipotropin*), within which was found met-enkephalin and other peptides that have opioid activity (Figure III.13).

Beta-endorphin is the amino acid sequence 61–91 of the pituitary

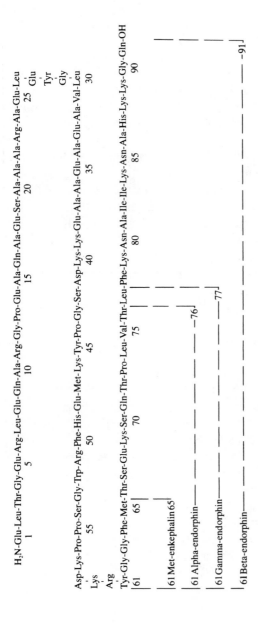

FIGURE III.13

The 91 amino acid sequence (primary structure) of beta-lipotropin. The four structures outlined below beta-lipotropin are fragments that are known to exert opioid-like activity.

peptide beta-lipotropin. Met-enkephalin is the amino acid sequence 61–65 of the same peptide (Figure III.13). Another pituitary peptide, designated *dynorphin,* is more potent than either beta-endorphin or met-enkephalin. Several possible functions, including neurotransmission and a role as "natural opioids," have been postulated for the endorphins, dynorphins, and enkephalins; however, their mechanism of analgesic action is not clear. The question then arises concerning the addictive potential of these compounds. Have we finally found a non-addicting opioid narcotic? Recent work indicates that the answer to this question is no. Physical dependence upon these proteins does develop, and both cross-tolerance and cross-dependence occur between these proteins and morphine. Therefore, these compounds probably have the same potential for addiction as the opioid narcotics, such as morphine.

A variety of evidence indicates that the enkephalins are physiological neurotransmitters that are located in specific neuronal systems in the brain. They mediate the integration of sensory inputs that are related to pain, perception, and emotional behavior. Probably, in animals, this system is relatively inactive; otherwise, pure narcotic antagonists, such as naloxone, would displace the proteins from their receptors and would initiate pain or an increased responsiveness to a painful stimulus. A limited investigation into the influence of enkephalins in acupuncture has suggested that these proteins may mediate acupuncture-induced analgesia.

The interesting possibility that enkephalins may play a role in stress responses and in mental illness has been raised. The narcotic antagonist, naloxone, seems to have some benefit in ameliorating the hallucinogenic episodes that are experienced by chronic schizophrenic patients. Also, in patients who experience chronic pain, enkephalin levels are altered by naloxone. Certainly, these reports will stimulate additional attempts to delineate more clearly the role of enkephalins in various emotional states.

Is it possible that enkephalins are involved in the tolerance and dependence that develop to opioid narcotics such as morphine? Administration of narcotic analgesics such as morphine produces intense stimulation of enkephalin receptors, and the activity of enkephalin neurons is suppressed through a negative-feedback mechanism. As the levels of enkephalins fall, increasing amounts of opioids must be administered to achieve the same effect (that is, *tolerance* develops). When the administration of morphine is stopped, neither morphine nor enkephalins are present at the receptor, and withdrawal symptoms appear (that is, *physical dependence*). Recovery from the withdrawal symptoms is achieved only when the activity of enkephalin neurons returns.

In conclusion, much research has identified endogenous compounds that exert opioid-like activity.[7-10] The receptors on which these compounds act appear to be the same receptors as those for the opioid narcotics. Whether opioid addiction can be explained on the basis of these endogenous substances—and the role of these substances in certain emotional states—remains to be delineated more clearly. Chapter 9 discusses the location of endorphin nuclei, their projections, and the influence of opioid agonists and antagonists on their function.

NOTES

1. S. Cohen, *The Chemical Brain: The Neurochemistry of Addictive Disorders* (Irvine, Calif.: Care Institute, 1988), p. 11.

2. P. J. Whitehouse, A. M. Martino, P. G. Antuono, P. R. Lowenstein, J. T. Coyle, D. L. Price, and K. J. Kellar, "Nicotinic Acetylcholine Binding Sites in Alzheimer's Disease," *Brain Research* 371 (1986): 146–151.

3. S. Cohen, *The Chemical Brain: The Neurochemistry of Addictive Disorders* (Irvine, Calif.: Care Institute, 1988), pp. 14–16.

4. S. Cohen, *The Chemical Brain: The Neurochemistry of Addictive Disorders* (Irvine, Calif.: Care Institute, 1988), p. 35.

5. D. T. Monaghan, R. J. Bridges, and C. W. Cotman, "The Excitatory Amino Acid Receptors: Their Classes, Pharmacology, and Distinct Properties in the Function of the Central Nervous System," *Annual Review of Pharmacology and Toxicology* 29 (1989): 365–402.

6. J. E. Shook, W. D. Watkins, and E. M. Camporesi, "Differential Roles of Opioid Receptors in Respiration, Respiratory Disease, and Opiate-Induced Respiratory Depression," *American Review of Respiratory Disease* 142 (1990): 895–909.

7. S. H. Snyder, "Drug and Neurotransmitter Receptors in the Brain," *Science* 224 (1984): 22–31.

8. E. L. Way, "Sites and Mechanisms of Basic Narcotic Receptor Function Based on Current Research," *Annals of Emergency Medicine* 15 (1986): 1021–1025.

9. M. L. Adams, D. A. Brase, S. P. Welch, and W. L. Dewey, "The Role of Endogenous Peptides in the Action of Opioid Analgesics," *Annals of Emergency Medicine* 15 (1986): 1030–1035.

10. F. E. Bloom, "Neurotransmitters: Past, Present, and Future Directions," *The FASEB Journal* 2 (1988): 32–41.

Glossary

Absorption, drug—mechanisms by which a drug reaches the bloodstream from the skin, lungs, stomach, intestinal tract, or muscle.

Abstinence syndrome—a state of altered behavior that is observed following cessation of drug administration.

Acetaminophen (Tylenol)—a nonnarcotic, nonsalicylate analgesic and antipyretic drug that is devoid of anti-inflammatory effects.

Acetylcholine (ACh)—a neurotransmitter in the central and peripheral nervous systems.

Additive effect—an increased effect that is observed when two drugs that have similar biological actions are administered. The net effect is the sum of the independent effects that are exerted by each drug.

Adenosine—a chemical neuromodulator in the CNS, primarily at inhibitory synapses.

Administration, drug—procedures through which a drug gains entrance into the body (oral administration of tablets or liquids, inhalation of powders, injection of sterile liquids, and so on).

Affective disorder—a type of mental disorder that is characterized by recurrent episodes of mania, depression, or both.

Agonist—a drug that attaches to a receptor and produces actions that mimic or potentiate those of an endogenous transmitter.

Alcohol (ethyl alcohol, ethanol)—a widely used sedative-hypnotic drug.

Aldehyde dehydrogenase—an enzyme that carries out a specific step in alcohol metabolism: the metabolism of acetaldehyde to acetate. This enzyme may be blocked by the drug disulfiram (Antabuse).

Alzheimer's disease—a progressive neurological disease that occurs primarily in the elderly. It is characterized by a loss of short-term memory and intellectual functioning. It is associated with a loss of function of acetylcholine neurons.

Amanita muscaria—the fly agaric mushroom, which is used for its psychedelic properties.

Amantadine (Symmetrel)—an antiviral drug that is useful in the treatment of Parkinson's disease.

Amphetamine—a behavioral stimulant.

Anesthetic drug—a sedative-hypnotic compound that is used primarily in doses that are capable of inducing a state of general anesthesia that involves both loss of sensation and loss of consciousness.

Antabuse—trade name for disulfiram, a drug that interferes with the breakdown of alcohol, resulting in the accumulation of acetaldehyde.

Antagonist—a drug that attaches to a receptor and blocks the action of either an endogenous transmitter or an agonist drug.

Antianxiety agent—a sedative-hypnotic compound that is used in subhypnotic doses.

Anticonvulsant—a drug that blocks or prevents epileptic convulsions.

Antidepressant—a drug that is useful in treating mental depression in depressed patients without producing stimulant effects in normal persons.

Antipsychotic drugs—a class of psychoactive drugs, all of which have the ability to calm psychotic states and make the psychotic patient more manageable.

Anxiolytic—a drug that is used to relieve the symptoms that are associated with anxiety and related disorders.

Ascending reticular activating system (ARAS)—a network of neurons in the brain stem that is thought to function in arousal mechanisms.

Aspirin—a nonnarcotic analgesic and anti-inflammatory drug.

Attention-deficit–hyperactivity disorder—a learning and behavioral disability that is characterized by reduced attention span and by hyperactivity. Formerly called **hyperkinetic syndrome, minimal brain disorder,** and **minimal brain dysfunction.**

Autonomic nervous system—the portion of the peripheral nervous system that controls or regulates the visceral, or automatic, functions of the body (such as heart rate and blood pressure).

Baclofen (Lioresal)—a GABA derivative that is useful in the treatment of spasticity.

Barbiturate—a class of chemically related sedative-hypnotic compounds, all of which share a characteristic six-membered ring structure.

Basal ganglia—that part of the brain that contains vast numbers of dopamine-containing synapses. Forms part of the **extrapyramidal system.** Parkinson's disease follows dopamine loss in this structure.

Benzodiazepine—a class of chemically related sedative-hypnotic agents, of which chlordiazepoxide (Librium) and diazepam (Valium) are examples.

Bipolar disorder—an affective disorder that is characterized by alternating bouts of mania and depression. Also referred to as **manic-depressive illness.**

Blackout—a period of time during which one may be awake, but memory is not imprinted. It is commonly seen in people who exhibit excessive alcohol consumption.

Brain syndrome, organic—a pattern of behavior that is induced when neurons are either reversibly depressed or irreversibly destroyed. Behavior is characterized by clouded sensorium; disorientation; shallow and labile affect; and impaired memory, intellectual function, insight, and judgment.

Brand name—a unique name that is given by license to one manufacturer to act as a marketer of a particular chemical entity. Contrasts with *generic name,* which is the name under which any manufacturer may sell a drug.

Bromocriptine (Parlodel)—a stimulant of dopamine receptors that is used occasionally in the treatment of Parkinson's disease.

Bufotenin—a psychoactive drug that is found in cohoba snuff, the skin and parotid gland of the toad, and in small amounts in the mushroom *Amanita muscaria.*

Caffeine—a behavioral and general cellular stimulant that is found in coffee, tea, cola drinks, and chocolate.

Caffeinism—habitual use of large amounts of caffeine.

Cannabis—the plant that contains marijuana.

Carbamazepine (Tegretol)—an antiepileptic drug.

Carbidopa (contained in Sinemet)—a drug that inhibits the enzyme dopadecarboxylase, allowing increased availability of dopa within the brain.

Central nervous system (CNS)—that portion of the body that contains the brain and spinal cord.

"China White"—a street term for illicit derivatives of fentanyl-type narcotics.

Chlordiazepoxide (Librium)—a benzodiazepine; sedative-hypnotic drug.

Chlorpromazine (Thorazine)—a phenothiazine; antipsychotic drug.

Cirrhosis—a serious, usually irreversible liver disease. Usually associated with chronic, excessive alcohol consumption.

Citalopram—a drug that selectively blocks the active reuptake of serotonin into presynaptic nerve terminals.

Clomiphene (Clomid)—an ovulation-inducing agent that is thought to act by blocking the inhibitory (negative-feedback) effect that estrogens exert on the hypothalamus.

Clonidine (Catapres)—an antihypertensive drug that is useful in ameliorating the symptoms of narcotic withdrawal.

Cocaine—a behavioral stimulant.

Codeine—a sedative and pain-relieving agent that is found in opium; it is structurally related to morphine, but less potent, and constitutes approximately 0.5 percent of the opium extract.

Convulsant—a drug that produces convulsions by blocking inhibitory neurotransmission.

Crack—a street name for a smokable form of potent, concentrated cocaine.

Cross–dependence—a condition in which one drug can prevent the withdrawal symptoms that are associated with physical dependence on a different drug.

Cross-tolerance—a condition in which tolerance of one drug results in a lessened response to another drug.

Dantrolene (Dantrium)—a drug that acts to limit the release of calcium ions in muscle, thereby reducing muscle spasticity.

Delirium tremens (DTs, "rum fits")—a syndrome of tremulousness, with hallucinations, psychomotor agitation, confusion and disorientation, sleep disorders, and other associated discomforts, lasting several days after alcohol withdrawal.

Dementia—a general designation for nonspecific mental deterioration.

Dependence, drug—a state in which the use of a drug is necessary for either physical or psychological well-being.

Depo-Provera—a long-acting, injectable preparation of progesterone, which is useful as a long-acting female contraceptive.

"Designer drug"—a street term for illicit derivatives of fentanyl-type narcotics.

Detoxification—the process of allowing time for the body to metabolize and/or excrete accumulations of drug. Usually a first step in drug evaluation and treatment.

Diazepam (Valium)—a benzodiazepine; antianxiety drug.

Diethylstilbestrol—a synthetically produced estrogen that is used occasionally in high doses as a postcoital contraceptive.

Dimethyltryptamine (DMT)—a psychedelic drug that is found in many South American snuffs.

Disinhibition—a physiological state within the central nervous system that is characterized by decreased activity of inhibitory synapses, which results in a net excess of excitatory activity.

Dose-response relation—a graph that illustrates the relation between drug doses and the response that was elicited at each dose level.

Droperidol (Inapsine)—an antipsychotic drug that is classified chemically as a butyrophenone.

Drug—any chemical substance that is used for its effects on bodily processes.

Drug interaction—the modification of the action of one drug by the concurrent or prior administration of another drug.

Drug misuse—the use of any drug (legal or illegal) for a medical or recreational purpose when other alternatives are available, practical, or warranted, or when drug use endangers either the user or others with whom he or she may interact.

Drug receptor—the specific molecular substance in the body with which a given drug interacts to produce its effect.

Drug tolerance—a state of progressively decreased responsiveness to a drug.

ECT—electroconvulsive therapy.

Endorphin—a term that refers to a naturally occurring protein that causes endogenous morphine-like activity.

Enkephalin—a naturally occurring protein that causes morphine-like activity.

Enzyme—a large organic molecule that mediates a specific biochemical reaction in the body.

Enzyme induction—the increased production of drug-metabolizing enzymes in the liver, stimulated by certain drugs, such that use of these drugs increases the rate at which the body can metabolize them. It is one mechanism by which pharmacological tolerance is produced.

Epilepsy—a neurological disorder that is characterized by an occasional, sudden, and uncontrolled discharge of neurons.

Estrogen—a body hormone that is secreted primarily from the ovaries of females in response to stimulation by follicle-stimulating hormone (FSH) from the pituitary gland.

Fentanyl—a potent narcotic analgesic drug.

Fetal alcohol syndrome—a symptom complex of congenital anomalies that is seen in newborns of women who ingested high doses of alcohol during critical periods of pregnancy.

Gamma-aminobutyric acid (GABA)—an inhibitory amino acid neurotransmitter in the brain.

Generic name—the name that identifies a specific chemical entity (without specifically describing the chemical). Often marketed by multiple manufacturers.

Hallucinogen—a psychedelic drug that produces profound distortions in perception.

Haloperidol (Haldol)—an antipsychotic drug that is classified chemically as a butyrophenone.

Harmine—a psychedelic agent that is obtained from the seeds of *Peganum harmala*.

Hashish—an extract of the hemp plant *(Cannabis sativa)* that has a higher concentration of THC than does marijuana.

Heroin—a semisynthetic opiate that is produced by a chemical modification of morphine.

Hypothalamus—a structure that is located at the base of the brain, above the pituitary gland.

Ibotinic acid—a psychedelic agent that is found in *Amanita muscaria*.

Ibuprofen (Advil, Motrin)—a nonnarcotic, nonsalicylate analgesic and anti-inflammatory drug.

Ketamine (Ketalar)—a psychedelic surgical anesthetic.

Levodopa—a precursor substance to the transmitter dopamine; it is useful in ameliorating the symptoms of Parkinson's disease.

Limbic system—a group of brain structures that are involved in emotional responses and emotional expression.

β-Lipotropin—a 91–amino-acid protein that contains amino acid sequences that have morphine-like activity.

Lithium—an alkali metal that is effective in the treatment of mania and depression.

Local anesthetic—a drug that reversibly blocks nerve conduction.

Lysergic acid diethylamide (LSD)—a semisynthetic psychedelic drug.

Major tranquilizer (antipsychotic tranquilizer)—a drug that is used in the treatment of psychotic states.

Mania—a mental disorder that is characterized by an expansive emotional state, elation, hyperirritability, excessive talkativeness, flight of ideas, and increased behavioral activity.

MAO inhibitor (MAOI)—a drug that inhibits the activity of the enzyme monoamine oxidase.

Marijuana—a mixture of the crushed leaves, flowers, and small branches of both the male and female hemp plant *(Cannabis sativa)*.

MDA—a synthetically produced derivation of amphetamine.

MDMA—methylene-dioxy methamphetamine; a psychedelic drug that is related to MDA.

Meperidine (Demerol)—a synthetically produced opiate narcotic.

Meprobamate (Equanil)—a sedative-hypnotic agent that is frequently used as an antianxiety drug.

Mescaline—a psychedelic drug that is extracted from the peyote cactus *(Lophophora williamsii)*.

Methadone (Dolophine)—a synthetically produced opiate narcotic.

Methaqualone (Quaalude)—a sedative-hypnotic compound that has relatively low potency.

Methylphenidate (Ritalin)—a CNS stimulant that is chemically and pharmacologically related to amphetamine.

Minor tranquilizer—any sedative-hypnotic drug that is promoted primarily for use in the treatment of anxiety.

Mixed agonist–antagonist—a drug that attaches to a receptor, producing weak agonist effects but displacing more potent agonists, precipitating withdrawal in drug—dependent persons.

Monoamine oxidase (MAO)—an enzyme that is capable of metabolizing norepinephrine, dopamine, and serotonin to inactive products.

Monoamine oxidase inhibitor (MAOI)—*see* **MAO inhibitor.**

Morphine—the major sedative and pain-relieving drug that is found in opium, comprising approximately 10 percent of the crude opium exudate.

Muscarine—a drug extracted from the mushroom *Amanita muscaria* that directly stimulates acetylcholine receptors.

Myristin—a psychedelic agent that is obtained from nutmeg and mace.

Naloxone (Narcan)—a pure narcotic antagonist.

Naltrexone (Trexan)—a long-acting narcotic antagonist.

Neurotransmitter—an endogenous chemical that is released by one neuron and alters the electrical activity of another neuron.

Nicotine—a behavioral stimulant that is found in tobacco and is responsible for its psychedelic effects and for tobacco dependence.

Norepinephrine (NE)—a synaptic transmitter in both the central and peripheral nervous systems.

Ololiuqui—a psychedelic drug that is obtained from the seeds of the morning glory plant.

Opiate—any natural or synthetic drug that exerts actions on the body that are similar to those induced by morphine, the major pain-relieving agent obtained from the opium poppy *(Papaver somniferum).*

Opiate narcotic—a drug that has both sedative and analgesic actions.

Opium—a crude resinous exudate from the opium poppy.

Parkinson's disease—a disorder of the motor system that is characterized by involuntary movements, tremor, and weakness.

Pentylenetetrazol (Metrazol)—a convulsant drug.

Peptide—a chemical that is composed of a chain-link sequence of amino acids.

Pergonal—a preparation of follicle-stimulating hormone that is extracted from the urine of postmenopausal females.

Peyote—a cactus that contains mescaline.

Pharmacodynamics—a study of the interactions of a drug with the receptors that are responsible for the action of the drug in the body.

Pharmacokinetics—a study of the factors that influence the absorption, distribution, metabolism, and excretion of a drug.

Pharmacology—the branch of science that deals with the study of drugs and their actions on living systems.

Phencyclidine (Sernyl)—a psychedelic surgical anesthetic.

Phenothiazine—a class of chemically related compounds that are useful in the treatment of psychosis.

Phenytoin (Dilantin)—an antiepileptic drug.

Physical dependence—a state in which the presence of a drug is required for a person to function normally. Such a state is revealed by withdrawing the drug and noting the occurrence of withdrawal symptoms (abstinence syndrome). Characteristically, withdrawal symptoms can be terminated by readministration of the drug.

Physostigmine—an acetylcholine esterase (AChE) inhibitor.

Placebo—a pharmacologically inert substance that may elicit a significant reaction largely because of the mental "set" of the patient or the physical setting in which the drug is taken.

Potency—a measure of drug activity that is expressed in terms of the amount required to produce an effect of given intensity. Potency varies inversely with the amount of drug that is required to produce this effect—that is, the more potent the drug, the lower the amount required to produce the effect.

Progesterone—a hormone that is secreted from the ovaries in response to stimulation by luteinizing hormone (LH) from the pituitary gland.

Progestins—a group of synthetically produced progesterones, most frequently found in oral contraceptive tablets.

Psilocybin—a psychedelic drug that is obtained from the Mexican mushroom *Psilocybe mexicana.*

Psychedelic drug—any drug that has the ability to alter sensory perception.

Psychoactive drug—any chemical substance that alters mood or behavior as a result of alterations in the functioning of the brain.

Psychological dependence—a compulsion to use a drug for its pleasurable effects. Such dependence may lead to a compulsion to misuse a drug.

Receptor—a location at which a neurotransmitter or drug binds to exert its characteristic effect.

Reserpine (Serpasil)—an antipsychotic drug.

Reye's syndrome—a rare CNS disorder that occurs in children; it is associated with aspirin ingestion.

Risk-to-benefit ratio—an arbitrary assessment of the risks and benefits that may accrue from administration of a drug.

Scopolamine—an anticholinergic drug that crosses the blood-brain barrier to produce sedation and amnesia.

Sedative-hypnotic drug—any chemical substance that exerts a nonselective general depressant action on the nervous system.

Serotonin (5-hydroxytryptamine, 5-HT)—a synaptic transmitter that is both in the brain and in the peripheral nervous system.

Side effect—any drug-induced effect that accompanies the primary effect for which the drug was administered.

Spasticity—a state of abnormal increases in muscle tension, resulting in increased resistance of the muscle to stretching.

Tardive dyskinesia—a movement disorder that appears after months or years of treatment with neuroleptic (antipsychotic) drugs. It usually worsens with drug discontinuation. Symptoms are often masked by the drugs that cause the disorder.

Teratogen—any chemical substance that may induce abnormalities of fetal development.

Testosterone—a hormone secreted from the testes that is responsible for the distinguishing characteristics of the male.

Tetrahydrocannabinol (THC)—a major psychoactive agent that is found in marijuana, hashish, and other preparations of hemp *(Cannabis sativa).*

THC—tetrahydrocannabinol.

Tolerance, drug—a state of progressively decreasing responsiveness to a drug.

Toxic effect—any drug-induced effect that is either temporarily or permanently deleterious to any organ or system of an animal or patient to which the drug is administered. Drug toxicity includes both the relatively minor side effects that invariably accompany drug administration and the more serious and unexpected manifestations that occur in only a small percentage of persons who take a drug.

Withdrawal syndrome—the symptoms that occur when one ceases to ingest a drug. Also called drug **abstinence syndrome.**

Bibliography: A Basic Pharmacology Bookshelf

American Medical Association. *Drug Evaluations Annual 1991*. Milwaukee, Wis.: American Medical Association, 1990.

Bevan, J. A., and J. H. Thompson. *Essentials of Pharmacology: An Introduction to the Principles of Drug Action*, 3d ed. Philadelphia: Lippincott, 1983.

Cooper, J. R., F. E. Bloom, and R. H. Roth. *The Biochemical Basis of Neuropharmacology*, 5th ed. New York: Oxford, 1986.

Craig, C. R. and R. E. Stitzel, eds. *Modern Pharmacology*, 3d ed. Boston: Little, Brown, 1990.

DiPalma, J. R., and G. J. DiGregorio. *Basic Pharmacology in Medicine*, 3d ed. New York: McGraw-Hill, 1990.

Gilman, A. G., T. W. Rall, A. S. Nies, and P. Taylor, eds. *Goodman and Gilman's The Pharmacological Basis of Therapeutics*, 8th ed. New York: Pergamon, 1990.

Goth, A. *Medical Pharmacology*, 12th ed. St. Louis: Mosby, 1988.

Hollister, L. E. *Clinical Pharmacology of Psychotherapeutic Drugs*, 2d ed. New York: Churchill Livingstone, 1983.

Julien, R. M. *Drugs and the Body*. New York: W. H. Freeman, 1988.

Levine, R. R. *Pharmacology: Drug Actions and Reactions*, 3d ed. Boston: Little, Brown, 1983.

Liska, K. *Drugs and the Human Body: With Implications for Society*, 3d ed. New York: Macmillan, 1990.

Meltzer, H. Y., ed. *Psychopharmacology: The Third Generation of Progress*. New York: Raven Press, 1987.

Rang, H. P., and M. M. Dale. *Pharmacology*. Edinburgh: Churchill Livingstone, 1987.

I N D E X

Catecholamine-like Psychedelic drugs, 247–251
  classification, 241–242
  structures, 242–243
Catechol-o-methyl transferase (COMT), 401–402
Cell membranes:
  effect on drug distribution, 13–14
  fluidization, 67, 75
  structure, 12
Central nervous system (CNS), 365–375
Cerebral cortex:
  and acetylcholine neurons, 399–400
  anatomy of, 371–375
  and caffeine, 133
  and cocaine, 117
  and nicotine, 141
Charas, 269
"China white," 203, 417
Chloral hydrate, 48, 52, 54, 66
Chlorazepate (Tranxene), 100, 101
Chlordiazepoxide (Librium), 48, 55, 93, 99–101
Chloroprocaine (Nesacaine), 311
Chlorphenesin (Maolate), 305
Chlorpromazine (Thorazine), 40, 227, 228, 341
  classification, 49
  history, 219–220
  structures, 220
  (See also Phenothiazines)
Chlorprothixene (Taractan), 228
Chlorzaxone (Paraflex), 305
Chromosome damage:
  and caffeine, 138
  and LSD, 259
Cigarettes, 346–350
  and alcohol, additive effects in cancer, 80–81
  and birth control pills, 325–327
  (See also Nicotine)
Cimoxatone, 164, 175
Citalopram, 171, 417
Claviceps purpurea, 252
Clomiphene (Clomid), 331, 417
Clomipramine, 171
Clonazepam (Clonopin), 99, 100, 293, 296
Clonidine (Catapres), 188, 191, 211–212
Clozapine (Clozaril), 221, 223–226, 236
  structure, 235
Clorazepate (Tranxene), 293, 296
Cocaine, 110–120
  classification, 48, 111
  extent of use, 272
  reinforcing properties, 340, 405
  sites and mechanism of action, 116–117, 402
Codeine, 173, 202, 418
  absorption, 5
  classification, 49, 193
Cognitive-behavioral therapy, 191

Cohoba, 259
Contraceptives:
  male, 333–335
  oral, 316–327
Contragestin, 330
Cough:
  and opioids, 194, 198, 202
"Crack," 113, 114, 115, 202
"Crack Babies," 119–120
Crime:
  and alcohol, 78
  and marijuana, 284–285
  and opioid analgesics, 207–208
Cross tolerance and cross dependence:
  of LSD, 264
  of opioid analgesics, 199
  of sedative-hypnotic drugs, 199
"Crystal," 124, 262
Cyclobenaprine (Flexaril), 305

Dantrolene (Dantrium), 304, 418
  structure, 303
Datura stramonium, 246
Delirium tremens, 84, 418
Dementia, 56–57, 101, 103
Demulen, 321
Dependence, drug, 28–29
Dendrites, 376–384
Depo-Medrol, 324
Depo-Provera, 327–329, 418
Depression:
  definition of, 157–161
  effect of drugs on, 103, 161–186
  and electroconvulsive therapy, 176–177
  and oral contraceptives, 324
  and reserpine, 159
"Designer drugs," 203–204, 256
Desipramine (Norpramin), 162, 164
Dextroamphetamine (Dexedrine), 48, 120, 122, 128
Dezocine (Dalgan), 193, 194, 204, 205
Diarrhea:
  opioid analgesics for, 185–186, 198, 202
  during opioid withdrawal, 200
Diazepam (Valium), 31, 85, 106, 293, 297, 304, 305, 408
  classification, 48
  pharmacokinetics, 28, 98, 101–102
  structure, 99, 303
  uses, 100, 304
Diencephalon, 367–369
Diethylpropion (Tenuate, Tepanil), 127
Diethylstilbestrol, 329
Dimethyltryptamine (DMT), 222, 259–260, 418
  classification, 49, 241, 244–246
  structure, 244
Dissociative anesthetics, 262–265

and cocaine, 118
and caffeine, 134
and opioid analgesics, 197
Smoking and lung cancer, 5, 143–150
Smoking and oral contraceptives, 325–327
"Soldier's disease," 186
Soma (cell body), 384
Spasms, muscle, 302–305
Spasticity, drugs for, 302–305
"Speed" (*see* Methamphetamine)
"Speedball," 124
Sperm production and drugs, 282, 333–335
Spinal cord, 365–368
and caffeine, 133–134
and opioid receptors, 187–191, 410–411
Stimulants, behavioral, 110–129
classification, 48, 111
STP (*see* DOM)
Substance P, 187–191, 196, 211–212, 367, 408, 410
Sufentanyl (Sufenta), 203
Synanon Foundation, 210
Synaptic transmission, 377–380, 390–414

Tardive dyskinesia, 230–231, 423
Temazepam (Restoril), 99, 100
Teonanacatl, 260
Teratogenesis, 17, 41
and caffeine, 138
and LSD, 259
Testosterone:
and alcohol, 283
and male fertility, 333–335
and marijuana, 282–283
Tetracaine (Pontocaine), 311
Tetrahydrazoline (Tyzine), 129
Tetrahydrocannabinol (THC) (*see* Marijuana)
Thalamus, 367, 369
Theophylline, 134
Therapeutic index, 36
Thiopental (Pentothal):
classification, 48
distribution, 38, 59–60
as general anesthetic, 67
Thioridazine (Mellaril), 228
Thiothixene (Navane), 228
TMA, 247, 249–250
classification, 49, 241
structure, 243
Tobacco (*see* Nicotine)
Tolerance, 28–29
Toxic paranoid psychosis, 118, 119, 122, 247
Toxicity of drugs, 37, 39–41
(*See also* individual agents)
Tranquilizers, 103, 217
Tranylcypromine (Parnate), 164, 172–176

classification, 111, 164
Trazodone (Desyrel), 162, 164, 169–170
Triazolam (Halcion), 100
Tricyclic antidepressants, 161–168
and analgesia, 191
classification, 48
sites and mechanisms of actions, 116·117,
159–161, 163, 402, 408
Trifluoperazine (Stelazine), 228
Triflupromazine (Vesprin), 228
Trihexyphenidyl (Artane), 300
Tri-Levlin, 321
Trimethadione (Tridione), 293, 297
structure, 295
Trimipramine (Surmontil), 162, 164
Tri-Norinyl, 321
Tripelennamine, 205
Triphasil, 321
Tyramine, 175
Tryptophan, 234
Tyrosine hydroxylase, 400–401

Urine testing:
and amphetamines, 122
and barbiturates, 60
and benzodiazepines, 101
and cocaine, 116
and LSD, 255
and opioids, 195–196
and phencyclidine, 263
and THC (marijuana), 274–275

Valium (*see* Diazepam)
Valproic acid (Depakene), 180, 293, 294, 297
structure, 295
Variability, drug, 35–38
Vasectomy, 335

Withdrawal syndrome:
alcohol, 79, 84–88
amphetamines, 126
barbiturates, 63–64
benzodiazepines, 104–105
cocaine, 119
opioid analgesics, 199–200
and physical dependence, 28
Women and smoking, 347–348
Work ethos, and marijuana, 281–282

Yopo, 259

Xylometazoline (Otrivin), 129